Interventional Pulmonology

Editor

ALI I. MUSANI

CLINICS IN
CHEST MEDICINE

www.chestmed.theclinics.com

September 2013 • Volume 34 • Number 3

ELSEVIER

1600 John F. Kennedy Boulevard • Suite 1800 • Philadelphia, Pennsylvania, 19103-2899

http://www.theclinics.com

CLINICS IN CHEST MEDICINE Volume 34, Number 3
September 2013 ISSN 0272-5231, ISBN-13: 978-0-323-18848-7

Editor: Patrick Manley
Developmental Editor: Donald E. Mumford

Clinics in Chest Medicine (ISSN 0272-5231) is published quarterly by Elsevier Inc., 360 Park Avenue South, New York, NY 10010-1710. Months of issue are March, June, September, and December. Periodicals postage paid at New York, NY and additional mailing offices. Subscription prices are $329.00 per year (domestic individuals), $526.00 per year (domestic institutions), $157.00 per year (domestic students/residents), $361.00 per year (Canadian individuals), $645.00 per year (Canadian institutions), $448.00 per year (international individuals), $645.00 per year (international institutions), and $219.00 per year (international and Canadian students/residents). International air speed delivery is included in all Clinics subscription prices. All prices are subject to change without notice. **POSTMASTER:** Send address changes to Clinics in Chest Medicine, Elsevier Health Sciences Division, Subscription Customer Service, 3251 Riverport Lane, Maryland Heights, MO 63043. **Customer Service: Telephone: 1-800-654-2452** (U.S. and Canada); **1-314-447-8871** (outside U.S. and Canada). **Fax: 1-314-447-8029. E-mail: journalscustomerservice-usa@elsevier.com** (for print support); **journalsonlinesupport-usa@elsevier.com** (for online support).

Reprints. For copies of 100 or more of articles in this publication, please contact the Commercial Reprints Department, Elsevier Inc., 360 Park Avenue South, New York, NY 10010-1710. Tel.: 212-633-3812; Fax: 212-462-1935; E-mail: reprints@elsevier.com.

Clinics in Chest Medicine is covered in *MEDLINE/PubMed (Index Medicus), Current Contents/Clinical Medicine, EMBASE/ Excerpta Medica, Science Citation Index,* and *ISI/BIOMED.*

Printed and bound by CPI Group (UK) Ltd, Croydon, CR0 4YY

Transferred to digital print 2013

Contributors

EDITOR

ALI I. MUSANI, MD, FCCP
Associate Professor of Medicine and
Pediatrics, Director, Interventional
Pulmonology, Division of Pulmonary, Sleep,
Allergy and Immunology, Department of
Medicine, National Jewish Health, Denver,
Colorado

AUTHORS

CLEMENT AMMOUCHE, MD
Pediatric Intensivist, Hôpital Hautepierre,
Medico-surgical Pediatric Department,
University Hospital Strasbourg, Strasbourg,
France

RABIH I. BECHARA, MD
Division Director, Pulmonary and Critical Care
Medicine, Cancer Treatment Centers of
America/Southeastern, Atlanta; Clinical
Professor of Medicine, Georgia Regents
University, Augusta, Georgia

RAHUL BHATNAGAR, MB ChB, MRCP
Pleural Clinical Research Fellow, Academic
Respiratory Unit, University of Bristol,
Southmead Hospital, Bristol, United Kingdom

DAVID P. BREEN, MB, BA, BCh
Department of Respiratory Medicine, Galway
University Hospitals, Galway, Ireland

ROBERTO F. CASAL, MD
Interventional Pulmonology, Michael E.
DeBakey VA Medical Center, Baylor College of
Medicine, Houston, Texas

MARIO CASTRO, MD, FCCP
Professor of Medicine and Director of Asthma
and Airway Translational Research Unit,
Division of Pulmonary and Critical Care
Medicine, Department of Internal Medicine,
Washington University at St. Louis School of
Medicine, St Louis, Missouri

ALEXANDER CHEN, MD, FCCP
Assistant Professor of Medicine and Director of
Interventional Pulmonology, Division of
Pulmonary and Critical Care Medicine,
Department of Internal Medicine, Washington
University at St. Louis School of Medicine,
St Louis, Missouri

JONATHAN HERO CHUNG, MD
Assistant Professor, Department of Radiology,
National Jewish Health, Denver, Colorado

HENRI COLT, MD, FCCP
Professor Emeritus, Department of Medicine,
University of California Irvine, Orange,
California

JAVIER I. DIAZ-MENDOZA, MD
Interventional Pulmonology, Division of
Pulmonary and Critical Care Medicine, Henry
Ford Hospital, Detroit, Michigan

LEONARDO L. DONATO, MD
Pediatric Pulmonologist, Hôpital Hautepierre,
Medico-surgical Pediatric Department,
University Hospital Strasbourg, Strasbourg,
France

HERVÉ DUTAU, MD
Department of Thoracic Oncology, Pleural
Diseases and Interventional Pulmonology,
North University Hospital, Marseille, France

GEORGE A. EAPEN, MD
Department of Pulmonary Medicine,
The University of Texas MD Anderson
Cancer Center, Houston, Texas

CHRISTOPHER T. ERB, MD, PhD
Postdoctoral Fellow, Pulmonary, Critical Care
and Sleep Medicine, Yale School of Medicine,
New Haven, Connecticut

ARMIN ERNST, MHCM, MD
Professor of Medicine, Pulmonary, Critical
Care and Sleep Medicine, Tufts School of
Medicine, Boston, Massachusetts; President
and CEO, Reliant Medical Group, Worcester,
Massachusetts

DAVID I. FIELDING, FRACP, MD
Department of Thoracic Medicine, Royal
Brisbane and Women's Hospital, Herston,
Queensland, Australia

JAMES H. FINIGAN, MD
Divisions of Oncology, and Pulmonary and
Critical Care Medicine, Department of
Medicine, National Jewish Health, Denver;
Division of Pulmonary Sciences and Critical
Care Medicine, Department of Medicine,
University of Colorado, Aurora, Colorado

STEFANO GASPARINI, MD, FCCP
Director Pulmonary Diseases Unit, Azienda
Ospedaliero-Universitaria "Ospedali Riuniti",
Università Politecnica delle Marche, Ancona,
Italy

UZAIR K. GHORI, MD
Department of Medicine, Military Hospital
Rawalpindi, Rawalpindi, Pakistan

ANDREW R. HAAS, MD, PhD
Assistant Professor of Medicine, Section of
Interventional Pulmonology and Thoracic
Oncology, Division of Pulmonary, Allergy, and
Critical Care, Department of Medicine,
University of Pennsylvania Medical Center,
Philadelphia, Pennsylvania

DAVID W. HSIA, MD
Assistant Professor of Medicine, Department
of Medicine, Harbor-UCLA Medical Center,
Torrance, California

HAMZA JAWAD, MBBS
Transitional Year Resident, Grand Rapids
Medical Education Partners, Grand Rapids,
Michigan

JEFFREY A. KERN, MD
Divisions of Oncology, and Pulmonary and
Critical Care Medicine, Department of
Medicine, National Jewish Health, Denver;
Division of Pulmonary Sciences and Critical
Care Medicine, Department of Medicine,
University of Colorado, Aurora, Colorado

AHMED Y. KHAN, MD
Fellow, Pulmonary and Critical Care Medicine,
Emory University School of Medicine, Atlanta,
Georgia

SETH J. KOENIG, MD
Associate Professor, Department of Medicine,
Long Island Jewish Medical Center,
Hofstra-North Shore Long Island Jewish Health
System, New Hyde Park, New York

NORIAKI KURIMOTO, MD
Department of Surgery, Santa Marianna
Hospital, Kawasaki City, Kanagawa Prefecture,
Japan

KENNETH E. LYN-KEW, MD
Assistant Professor, Department of Medicine,
National Jewish Health, Denver, Colorado

MICHAEL S. MACHUZAK, MD
Medical Director, Center for Major Airway
Diseases; Staff, Respiratory Institute,
Cleveland Clinic; Professor of Medicine,
Lerner College of Medicine, Cleveland, Ohio

NICK A. MASKELL, DM, FRCP
Reader in Respiratory Medicine, Academic
Respiratory Unit, University of Bristol,
Southmead Hospital, Bristol, United Kingdom

ATUL C. MEHTA, MBBS, FACP, FCCP
Staff, Respiratory Institute, Cleveland Clinic;
Professor of Medicine, Lerner College of
Medicine, Cleveland, Ohio

GAËTANE C. MICHAUD, MS, MD, FRCP(C)
Assistant Professor of Medicine, Pulmonary,
Critical Care and Sleep Medicine, Yale School
of Medicine, New Haven, Connecticut

SEPTIMIU MURGU, MD, FCCP
Assistant Professor, Department of Medicine, University of Chicago Pritzker School of Medicine, Chicago, Illinois

ALI I. MUSANI, MD, FCCP
Associate Professor of Medicine and Pediatrics, Director, Interventional Pulmonology, Division of Pulmonary, Sleep, Allergy and Immunology, Department of Medicine, National Jewish Health, Denver, Colorado

TAKAHIRO NAKAJIMA, MD, PhD, FCCP
Division of Thoracic Surgery, Toronto General Hospital, University Health Network, University of Toronto, Toronto, Ontario, Canada

TATHAGAT NARULA, MD
Fellow, Respiratory Institute, Cleveland Clinic, Cleveland, Ohio

DAVID E. OST, MD
Department of Pulmonary Medicine, The University of Texas MD Anderson Cancer Center, Houston, Texas

NICHOLAS J. PASTIS, MD, FCCP
Assistant Professor of Medicine, Division of Pulmonary, Critical Care, Allergy, and Sleep Medicine; Division of Pulmonary and Critical Care Medicine, Medical University of South Carolina, Charleston, South Carolina; Division of Pulmonary Disease and Critical Care Medicine, Richmond, Virginia

JONATHAN PUCHALSKI, MD, MEd
Assistant Professor of Medicine, Director, Thoracic Interventional Program, Division of Pulmonary, Critical Care and Sleep Medicine, Yale University School of Medicine, New Haven, Connecticut

JOSEPH C. SEAMAN, MD
Clinical Assistant Professor, Department of Clinical Sciences, Florida State University College of Medicine, Lung Associates of Sarasota, Sarasota, Florida

RAY WESLEY SHEPHERD, MD, FCCP
Division of Pulmonary, Critical Care, Allergy, and Sleep Medicine, Medical University of South Carolina, Charleston, South Carolina;

Associate Professor of Medicine, Director of Interventional Pulmonology, Division of Pulmonary Disease and Critical Care Medicine, Virginia Commonwealth University Medical Center, Richmond, Virginia

AJAY SHESHADRI, MD
Fellow, Division of Pulmonary and Critical Care Medicine, Department of Internal Medicine, Washington University at St. Louis School of Medicine, St Louis, Missouri

GERARD A. SILVESTRI, MD, FCCP
Professor of Medicine, Division of Pulmonary, Critical Care, Allergy, and Sleep Medicine; Division of Pulmonary and Critical Care Medicine, Medical University of South Carolina, Charleston, South Carolina; Division of Pulmonary Disease and Critical Care Medicine, Richmond, Virginia

MICHAEL J. SIMOFF, MD
Director, Bronchoscopy and Interventional Pulmonology, Division of Pulmonary and Critical Care Medicine, Henry Ford Hospital; Associate Professor of Medicine, Wayne State University School of Medicine, Detroit, Michigan

ARLENE SIRAJUDDIN, MD
Assistant Professor of Radiology, Department of Radiology, Northwestern University Feinberg School of Medicine, Chicago, Illinois

DANIEL H. STERMAN, MD
Associate Professor of Medicine, Chief, Section of Interventional Pulmonology and Thoracic Oncology, Division of Pulmonary, Allergy, and Critical Care, Department of Medicine, University of Pennsylvania Medical Center, Philadelphia, Pennsylvania

JUSTIN M. THOMAS, MD
Interventional Pulmonary Fellow, Clinical Instructor, Division of Pulmonary and Critical Care, Department of Medicine, National Jewish Health, Denver, Colorado

THI MAI HONG TRAN, MD
Pediatric Pulmonologist, Pulmonary Department, Hanoi National Hospital of Pediatrics, Hanoi, Vietnam

THOMAS VANDEMOORTELE, MD, FRCPC, FCCP
Department of Pulmonology, Hôpital Notre-Dame, Centre Hospitalier de l'Université de Montréal (CHUM), Montreal, Quebec, Canada

KAZUHIRO YASUFUKU, MD, PhD, FCCP
Director, Interventional Thoracic Surgery Program, Division of Thoracic Surgery, Toronto General Hospital, University Health Network; Assistant Professor, University of Toronto, Toronto, Ontario, Canada

Contents

are the more recently developed endocytoscopy system and confocal fluorescence microendoscopy, currently used only for research purposes.

CLINICS IN CHEST MEDICINE

DOWNLOAD
Free App!

Review Articles
THE CLINICS

NOW AVAILABLE FOR YOUR iPhone and iPad

Preface

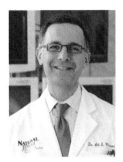

Ali I. Musani, MD, FCCP
Editor

Technological advances spurred by the untamable passion of interventional pulmonologists for providing better-than-ever diagnostic and therapeutic options to patients with chest diseases have lead to unfathomable progress in the last few decades.

Interventional pulmonology's (IP's) rapidly expanding role in common lung diseases, such as emphysema and asthma, is already starting to show promise. There are now several options for treating severe emphysema bronchoscopically in patients who are poor candidates for surgical lung volume reduction or lung transplantation, or who are awaiting lung transplantation. Modalities such as endobronchial valves, biological glue, and coils are already approved in several European countries and are undergoing studies in the United States. Similarly, bronchial thermoplasty for the treatment of poorly controlled asthma is now FDA approved and gaining momentum around the world.

In the area of lung cancer diagnosis and therapeutics, IP has successfully shifted the paradigm of mediastinal staging toward a less invasive and more comprehensive approach with endobronchial ultrasound. Navigation bronchoscopy and radial ultrasound are established and powerful tools in the evaluation of pulmonary nodules. They are safer, minimally invasive, and provide a higher diagnostic yield than a traditional bronchoscopic lung biopsy.

Currently, studies are underway that combine navigation technologies with radial ultrasound to biopsy lung lesions, diagnose them with on-site cytology, and then, using the same navigation-guided pathway, treat the lesion with ablative modalities, such as photodynamic therapy or radiofrequency ablation. Imagine a patient walking into your office with a suspicious pulmonary nodule and leaving with their lung cancer diagnosed and treated in a single outpatient procedure. That's the potential and promise of IP.

I am immensely grateful to all the esteemed authors who generously volunteered their time and shared their priceless experience and knowledge. I was fortunate to recruit many of the world's authorities in IP to contribute to this edition. Their articles will certainly enhance the practice of pulmonary medicine.

In order to give this edition the feel of a comprehensive review book on IP, I have tried to cover each major modality or group of technologies in a single article. I have also included articles on some topics that you might not have seen before in the IP literature, including pediatric IP and radiology for interventional pulmonologists. I hope you will find the entire edition informative and useful in your practice.

Finally, I am extremely thankful to my wonderful and supportive wife, Lubna and our beautiful children, Sara and Sef for their understanding and support during the preparation of this edition and in my demanding work schedule in general.

Ali I. Musani, MD, FCCP
Associate Professor of Medicine and Pediatrics
Director, Interventional Pulmonology
Division of Pulmonary, Sleep, Allergy and Immunology
Department of Medicine
National Jewish Health
Denver, Colorado, USA

E-mail address:
MusaniA@NJHealth.org

Clin Chest Med 34 (2013) xiii
http://dx.doi.org/10.1016/j.ccm.2013.08.001
0272-5231/13/$ – see front matter © 2013 Elsevier Inc. All rights reserved.

Flexible Bronchoscopy

Roberto F. Casal, MD[a], David E. Ost, MD[b],
George A. Eapen, MD[b],*

KEYWORDS

- Flexible bronchoscopy • Bronchoalveolar lavage • Transbronchial lung biopsy
- Transbronchial needle aspiration

KEY POINTS

- Although bronchoscopy technology continues to evolve at a fairly rapid pace, basic procedures, such as bronchoalveolar lavage (BAL), transbronchial lung biopsy (TBLB), and transbronchial needle aspiration (TBNA), continue to play a paramount role in the diagnosis of bronchopulmonary diseases.
- Pulmonologists should be trained in these basic bronchoscopic procedures.
- Bronchoscopy technology continues to evolve.
- Basic procedures such as bronchoalveolar lavage, transbronchial biopsies and transbronchial needle aspiration remain very important in patient care.
- Pulmonologists should achieve and maintain high skill levels in these procedures.

INTRODUCTION

The flexible bronchoscope is the most widely used invasive tool for diagnosis and treatment of bronchopulmonary diseases.[1] Its ability to reach distal airways and lung parenchyma with only mild to moderate sedation mostly accounts for its popularity. This article reviews the history and development of the flexible bronchoscope and its indications, contraindications, and basic diagnostic techniques, such as BAL, TBLB, and TBNA. Advanced diagnostic techniques, such as endobronchial ultrasound (EBUS) or electromagnetic navigation and therapeutic bronchoscopy, are discussed elsewhere in this issue.

HISTORY

More than a century after Dr Gustav Killian's introduction of the rigid bronchoscope, Shigeto Ikeda presented the first prototype flexible fiberoptic bronchoscope, developed by Machida, at the 9th International Congress on Diseases of the Chest in Copenhagen, Denmark, August 17–19, 1966.[2] This was the beginning of a revolution in the world of bronchoscopy, and this news was immediately published in the *New York Times* and spread throughout the world. The Machida flexible bronchoscope was first commercialized in 1968.[3,4] With Ikeda's feedback, further prototypes were developed by Machida and subsequently by Olympus. Substantial improvements in image quality, angulation, and the development of a working channel followed. Within a decade, the flexible fiberoptic bronchoscope was in use throughout the world. In the early 1980s, Ikeda started working on the development of a videobronchoscope. The replacement of the fiberoptic bundle with a miniature video camera at the tip of the bronchoscope was first achieved by Pentax in 1987. This provided improvement in image quality and the possibility of visualizing the images on

[a] Interventional Pulmonology, Michael E. DeBakey VA Medical Center, Baylor College of Medicine, Houston, TX 77030, USA; [b] Department of Pulmonary Medicine, The University of Texas MD Anderson Cancer Center, 1515 Holcombe Boulevard, Houston, TX 77030, USA
* Corresponding author. Department of Pulmonary Medicine, The University of Texas MD Anderson Cancer Center, 1515 Holcombe Boulevard, Unit 403, Houston, TX 77030.
E-mail address: geapen@mdanderson.org

Clin Chest Med 34 (2013) 341–352
http://dx.doi.org/10.1016/j.ccm.2013.03.001
0272-5231/13/$ – see front matter © 2013 Elsevier Inc. All rights reserved.

a color screen as opposed to being limited to the bronchoscope eyepiece. Its impact on bronchoscopy training was substantial, and this technology was eagerly adopted by most teaching institutions.

The advent of the flexible bronchoscope was rapidly followed by the development of a vast array of bronchoscopic diagnostic and therapeutic techniques. Reynolds introduced BAL in the mid-1970s, allowing the recovery of cellular and noncellular material from the lower respiratory tract.[5] Following the line of work of Andersen and Zavala and colleagues, TBLB was successfully adapted to flexible bronchoscopy, particularly for diffuse parenchymatous lung diseases and infections.[6–12] TBNA of mediastinal lymph nodes, initially described by the Argentinean thoracic surgeon, Eduardo Schiepatti,[13,14] in 1949, was first performed with flexible bronchoscopy by Wang and coworkers[15,16] from The Johns Hopkins Hospital in Baltimore in the late 1970s. Wang designed a novel needle to be used through the flexible bronchoscope, which, 30 years later, is still in use. Aside from the use of baskets and forceps for foreign body removal, the first therapeutic bronchoscopy tool used through the flexible bronchoscopy was the Nd:YAG laser, developed by Dumon and colleagues,[17] who published their experience in 1980. This technique was, and still is, used for the management of benign and malignant tracheobronchial stenosis.

Flexible bronchoscopy continues to evolve at a rapid pace, and newer techniques—both diagnostic and therapeutic—are now readily available (autofluorescence bronchoscopy, narrow band imaging, confocal microscopy, optical coherence tomography, EBUS, electromagnetic navigation, argon plasma coagulation, photodynamic therapy, bronchoscopic lung volume reduction, bronchial thermoplasty, and so forth). Although these techniques are reviewed elsewhere in this journal, we cannot fail to mention the advent of the convex probe EBUS (CP-EBUS), which was introduced in the early 2000s and has had an enormous impact in the world of bronchoscopy. CP-EBUS has an ultrasound transducer mounted at the tip of the bronchoscope, which allows for real-time visualization and sampling of mediastinal and hilar lymph nodes. Its favorable safety profile and high diagnostic yield—comparable to that of mediastinoscopy—have made it the procedure of choice in centers where technology and expertise are available.[18–21] Initially performed by interventional pulmonologists and thoracic surgeons, it is now widely accepted by general pulmonologists, and it is slowly replacing standard TBNA in most centers, in particular academic ones.

INDICATIONS AND CONTRAINDICATIONS

Indications for flexible bronchoscopy can be broadly divided into diagnostic and therapeutic categories (summarized in **Boxes 1** and **2**).[22] In several instances, a planned diagnostic bronchoscopy becomes a therapeutic one, particularly when bronchoscopic findings are unexpected or not clearly evident in preprocedure radiographic images. In a retrospective chart review of 4273 flexible bronchoscopies performed between 1988 and 1993 in an academic center, 86% were diagnostic, 10% were therapeutic, and 4% were performed in healthy volunteers for research purposes.[23]

Flexible bronchoscopy is in general a safe procedure with low rate of complications. Major complications, such as respiratory distress, arrhythmia, cardiopulmonary arrest, major bleeding, and pneumothorax, occur in less than 1% of cases. The reported mortality is low, with a death rate of 0% to 0.04% in more than 68,000 procedures.[24] Contraindications to flexible bronchoscopy are mostly relative rather than absolute.[24,25] Absolute contraindications include hemodynamic instability, life-threatening arrhythmias, severe refractory hypoxemia, absence of informed consent, inadequate facility, and inexperienced operator.[25,26] There are several other situations in which the risks of bronchoscopy are increased, and the risk/benefit ratio should be carefully analyzed in all patients. Patients with underlying coronary artery disease should be managed with extra care. Flexible bronchoscopy with moderate sedation is associated with increase in heart rate that may induce ischemia in a small number of patients.[27] Although considered safe in patients with underlying coronary artery disease, most investigators postpone elective bronchoscopy for 6 weeks post–acute coronary syndrome or decompensated heart failure. Severe hypoxemia is also a relative contraindication for a nonemergent flexible bronchoscopy. If bronchoscopy is absolutely necessary, endotracheal intubation and general anesthesia might provide a safer scenario. Uncooperative patients also increase the risk of complications, and general anesthesia is a valuable alternative for these patients as well. The relevance of bleeding diathesis depends on the bronchoscopic procedure to be performed. Airway examination and BAL can be performed without substantial risk of bleeding, but the oral route for bronchoscope insertion might be a safer alternative than the nasal route in cases of severe uncorrected coagulopathy. Coagulopathy becomes relevant when brushing, biopsies, or needle aspirations are planned. Blind biopsies (ie, TBLBs vs endobronchial biopsies) carry the highest risk.[25] Also,

---

Box 1
Indications for diagnostic flexible bronchoscopy

Signs and symptoms
- Hemoptysis
- Stridor
- Unilateral wheezing
- Hoarseness
- Unexplained chronic cough

Infections
- Pneumonia in immunocompromised host
- Nonresolving pneumonia
- Cavitary lesion

Diffuse lung disease
- Interstitial lung disease
- Diffuse alveolar damage and hemorrhage
- Drug-induced lung disease

Malignancy
- Lung nodule or mass
- Endobronchial tumor
- Suspected airway invasion by adjacent malignancies (ie, esophagus or thyroid)
- Early detection (positive sputum cytology/negative CT scan)
- Mediastinal or hilar lymphadenopathy or mass
- Mediastinal staging or restaging

Other airway disorders
- Mucus plugging
- Foreign body aspiration
- Benign airway stricture (ie, idiopathic, Wegener's granulomatosis, sarcoidosis, or tuberculosis)

Intensive care
- Bronchoscopy-guided intubation (difficult airway)
- Endotracheal tube position

Miscellaneous
- Lung transplant
- Bronchopleural fistula
- Aerodigestive fistula
- Chest trauma
- Chemical/thermal injury of airways
- Preoperative and postoperative for lung resection surgery

Box 2
Indications for therapeutic flexible bronchoscopy

Malignant central airway obstruction
- Tumor destruction (laser, argon plasma coagulation, cryotherapy, brachytherapy, or photodynamic therapy)
- Stenting (self-expandable stents)

Benign central airway obstruction
- Radial cuts
- Balloon dilation
- Stenting

Aerodigestive fistulas
- Stenting
- Laser-induced closure

Foreign body removal

Tracheobronchial toilet

Hemoptysis
- Hemostasis of centrally located bleeding lesions (laser or argon plasma coagulation)
- Airway blockers for massive bleeding

Bronchopleural fistulas closure
- Airway spigots
- Endobronchial valves
- Sealants

Miscellaneous
- Aspiration of cyst
- Abscess drainage
- Bronchial thermoplasty
- Endoscopic lung volume reduction

---

visible endobronchial bleeding locations may be easier to control with different therapeutic techniques. Platelet counts less than 50,000/mm^3, uremia with platelet dysfunction, international normalized ratio greater than 1.5, and elevated partial thromboplastin time are relative contraindications for the biopsies. These thresholds are mainly based on personal experience and expert opinions, because data on bronchoscopy-related bleeding complications are scant. Papin and colleagues[28] performed 25 TBLBs in 24 patients with a mean platelet count of 30,000/mm^3 (range 7000–60,000/mm^3). Three patients developed self-limited bleeding and 1 (platelet count 23,000/mm^3) had fatal bleeding. Low-molecular-weight heparin should be held for 12 hours and antiplatelet agents for 5 days. This is particularly important with clopidogrel. Ernst and colleagues[29] reviewed 604 cases of flexible bronchoscopy with transbronchial lung biopsies. They found that the risk of bleeding was substantially higher among those patients receiving aspirin and clopidogrel combined (100%) and clopidogrel alone (89%) in comparison with control patients (3.4%). Herth and coworkers found no increased risk of bleeding with aspirin.[30] Hence, the risk seems agent-specific.

In patients with poor respiratory function, the presence of large bullas or extensive emphysema in the proximity of the target area becomes a relative contraindication for TBLB due to higher risk of symptomatic pneumothorax. The incidence of pneumothorax is influenced by several factors: bronchoscopists, forceps type, number of biopsies performed, and imaging guidance. Although the rate varies among institutions, it is generally low, and death is even rarer.[31] Although an invaluable tool to direct TBLB in the absence of diffuse lung disease, the ability of fluoroscopy to prevent pneumothorax is somewhat controversial. Puar and coworkers[32] performed at least 3 TBLBs in 68 patients with tactile sensation technique (no fluoroscopy) and found only 1 pneumothorax. A mail survey, however, of 231 bronchoscopists in the United Kingdom reported a pneumothorax rate of 1.8% with fluoroscopy versus 2.9% without it, after TBLB.[33] Overall, flexible bronchoscopy is a safe procedure, and the likelihood of complications can be minimized by careful patient selection, strict evaluation of risk/benefit ratio in high-risk patients, and adherence to patient safety protocols.

BASIC DIAGNOSTIC PROCEDURES

During the planning phase of bronchoscopy, the most appropriate procedure or procedures are chosen. This decision is based on data from clinical presentation, radiographic images, location and extent of disease, and suspected etiology. In general terms, a combination of procedures (BAL, bronchial washings, TBLBs, and brushing) tends to increase yield. Cytology samples can be obtained from BAL, bronchial washings, cytology brushing, TBNA, and touch preparation of forceps biopsies (endobronchial biopsies and TBLB). Histology samples require forceps biopsy (endobronchial biopsy and TBLB) or needle core biopsy. Microbiological information can be obtained from any sample, but it is typically performed on BAL, washing, and protected-specimen brush.

Bronchoalveolar Lavage

Unlike bronchial washings that provide samples from the large airways, BAL obtains material from the lower respiratory tract and alveolar spaces. Its technique varies from one center to another, despite the presence of published consensus statements.[34] Essentially, after carefully examining the airway, the bronchoscope is wedged in the target bronchi, mostly at the 4th or 5th generation branches. The bronchoscope's working channel is kept in the lumen (away from the airway wall) to facilitate fluid recovery. Aliquots of 30 mL to 60 mL of sterile saline are typically instilled and subsequently aspirated either with the bronchoscope's suction (into a trap container) or with the same syringes used for instilling the saline. Although most institutions instill a total of 100 mL to 300 mL, there are no data indicating an ideal volume. Small amounts are thought to lavage small bronchi and scant alveoli; at the same time, larger amounts are associated with greater complications, such as transient hypoxia and fever. Kelly and colleagues[35] analyzed the distribution of BAL by digital subtraction radiography. They found that 60 mL of fluid only sample the proximal airways, whereas 120 mL perfuse an entire segment, and its aspiration retrieves fluid from the entire segment. Typically, 40% to 60% of instilled saline is recovered, with cell viability above 80%.[25,36,37] The following factors are associated with decreased return: obstructive lung disease, cigarette smoking, and advanced age. The loss of elastic recoil allowing the airways to collapse with suction seems to be the reason for the diminished return.

The normal cellular composition of BAL fluid is influenced by several factors, such as age, gender, and smoking status. A BAL of a healthy nonsmoker adult yields 80% to 95% macrophages, 5% to 15% lymphocytes (CD4/CD8 ratio of 1.5–1.8), less than 3% neutrophils, and less than 1% eosinophils and mast cells.[25,36,38] When looking to analyze cell count with differential, it is important to perform BAL prior to any other procedure (brush or TBLB), which can contaminate the sample, particularly with blood elements.

BAL has a prominent role in multiple scenarios: infections, inflammatory processes, and malignancies. Nevertheless, correlation with clinical and radiographic features is imperative. The findings of BAL in noninfectious diffuse pulmonary disorders are summarized in **Table 1**. Leaving aside a few exceptions in which BAL can be diagnostic (alveolar proteinosis, Langerhans cell granulomatosis, and eosinophilic pneumonia), BAL findings mostly support a suspected diagnosis or help rule out infectious etiologies that may mimic noninfectious inflammatory disorders. With the advances in radiology (specifically with high-resolution CT), the need for BAL has

Table 1
BAL findings in diffuse lung disease

Diffuse Lung Disease	Typical BAL Cellular Pattern	T Lymphocyte CD4/CD8 Ratio	Other Relevant BAL Findings
Sarcoidosis	↑Total cell count ↑Lymphocytes	↑	—
Hypersensitivity pneumonitis	↑Total cell count ↑Lymphocytes	↓	Neutrophils can be ↑ with recent exposure to antigen
Chronic beryllium disease	↑Total cell count ↑Lymphocytes	↑	BAL lymphocytes proliferation with beryllium salts
Asbestosis	↑Neutrophils	↑	Ferruginous bodies
Idiopathic pulmonary fibrosis	↑Neutrophils ↓ Lymphocytes	—	—
Cryptogenic organizing pneumonia	↑Total cell count ↑Lymphocytes	↓	Foamy macrophages
Pulmonary alveolar proteinosis	Variable	—	Milky fluid and foamy macrophages with PAS-positive material
Drug-induced lung disease	Variable	↓	Foamy macrophages with amiodarone exposure
Pulmonary Langerhans cell histiocytosis	↑Total cell count Variable differential	—	CD1$^+$ Langerhans cells
Eosinophilic pneumonia	↑↑ Eosinophils	—	Eosinophils counts greater in acute than in chronic pneumonia

diminished in several conditions: usual interstitial pneumonitis, interstitial lung disease associated with collagen-vascular disease, and pulmonary lymphangioleiomyomatosis.[39,40]

Bronchopulmonary infections are common indications for BAL, particularly in immunocompromised hosts and in cases of nonresolving pneumonias. The yield of BAL for bacterial pneumonias ranges from 30% to 75%, and it is slightly higher in ventilator-associated pneumonias.[22] The superiority of BAL, however, with respect to blinded tracheal aspirates in ventilator-associated pneumonias remains controversial.[41–43] BAL plays an important role in the diagnosis of tuberculous and nontuberculous mycobacterial infections. The average yield of BAL is approximately 70%, and it varies according to the clinical-radiographic presentation—lower in miliary cases of additional TBLB typically required to increase bronchoscopy yield.[44,45] The use of bronchoscopy in immunocompromised subjects with suspected pulmonary infections is widely accepted.[46–50] These patients typically represent a diagnostic challenge due to the wide array of potential causes of lung infiltrates (both infectious and noninfectious). Additionally, many patients are already receiving broad-spectrum antimicrobials before

bronchoscopy. BAL has a role even in patients who are already receiving broad-spectrum antibiotics and antifungals, with isolation of resistant organisms or organisms that were not targeted in up to 40% of the cases.[48] The yield of BAL in immunocompromised patients is far from perfect, but it can be increased from approximately 40% to approximately 70% when combined with TBLB.[51] Because many of these patients are also thrombocytopenic—and at high risk of bleeding with biopsies—BAL continues to be the most used technique for this population.

Transbronchial Lung Biopsy

The term, transbronchial lung biopsy, is typically used for biopsies of lung parenchyma and for biopsy of localized lesions—such as tumors. It is generally used in combination with BAL for the diagnosis of diffuse lung disease of both infectious and noninfectious origin. A survey of 1800 pulmonologists in the United States showed that 70% of bronchoscopists routinely used this technique for diffuse lung disease.[52] With advances in radiology, however, particularly with the advent of high-resolution CT, its use seems to be declining in most institutions. The yield of TBLB for diagnosis of pulmonary nodules has been largely increased with new technologies, such as radial-probe EBUS, virtual bronchoscopy, and electromagnetic navigation, which are discussed elsewhere in this issue.

Most TBLBs are performed under moderate sedation, unless patients are allergic to the commonly used sedatives, they develop excessive cough, or they cannot cooperate with the operator. The role of fluoroscopy for TBLB is discussed previously, and the authors support its use. TBLB should be performed after routine airway examination and any additional desired procedures (BAL or brushing). The bronchoscope is gently wedged in the target bronchus and the bronchoscopy forceps passed through the working channel. The advantages of keeping the bronchoscope wedged are both to isolate and tamponade potential bleeding and to minimize procedure time by taking several biopsies without withdrawing and advancing the scope each time. When the tip of the forceps is felt outside of the bronchoscope, the fluoroscope is turned on. The biopsy forceps (closed) are then advanced toward the target area. With the forceps approximately 0.5 cm to 1 cm proximal to the target, the forceps are then opened. While avoiding taking the biopsy during a cough episode, the forceps are then advanced and closed in the desired area or when hitting resistance. Some bronchoscopists instruct their patients to indicate (eg, with a hand gesture) if they experience pain when the forceps are closed in order to abort the biopsy and minimize the risk of pneumothorax[25]; however, this is not supported by scientific evidence. If patients do not manifest pain, the forceps are then slowly retracted (in its closed position) and special attention should be paid to the visceral pleural line on fluoroscopy, looking for potential tenting, in which case the forceps should be opened. If there is no pleural tenting, the forceps are entirely removed from the bronchoscope, and the sample is extracted from the forceps. A touch preparation can be prepared if on-site cytology examination is desired, and the biopsy can be placed in formalin for final pathology and in normal saline for culture when indicated. The number of biopsies taken correlates with the diagnostic yield. A study from Descombes and coworkers[53] in 530 consecutive patients with diffuse lung disease showed a yield of 38% with 1 to 3 specimens and 69% with 6 to 10 specimens ($P<.01$). Yield also varies based on the underlying disease. Unfortunately, an increase in the number of biopsies is also associated with an increase in complications, in particular pneumothorax. Although there are no strict criteria regarding the number of biopsies to take, the authors think that an average of 5 to 7 biopsies

should reach a respectable yield without compromising the risk/benefit ratio. This should also be tailored to patient needs and suspected pathology. Generally more tissue is needed for noninfectious diffuse lung disease and less tissue to culture for infectious etiologies. Regarding the biopsy forceps, there is apparently no difference in yield between toothed and cup forceps. Although larger forceps provide more tissue, it is debatable whether this increases the yield.[54,55]

As discussed previously, diffuse interstitial lung disease is one of the most common indications for TBLB. TBLB is only necessary, however, when clinical, laboratory, and radiographic information cannot reach a clear-cut diagnosis. TBLB should be pursued in younger patients, rapidly progressive disease, atypical high-resolution CT pattern, and suspected therapy responsive disorders (hypersensitivity pneumonitis and sarcoidosis) and to rule out infections before prescribing immunosuppressive agents. The overall yield of TBLBs for diffuse lung diseases is approximately 70%.[56,57] TBLB yield is higher for diseases with centrilobular distribution, such as sarcoidosis, hypersensitivity pneumonitis, eosinophilic pneumonias, and lymphangitic carcinomatosis.[56,58] The yield is lower, however, for diseases that require more tissue, especially idiopathic interstitial pneumonias (30%). Most consensus guidelines on idiopathic interstitial pneumonias recommend TBLB primarily to rule out sarcoidosis and infections.[59] Lung transplant recipients frequently undergo TBLB for surveillance and when clinically indicated. Its diagnostic yield is high in cases of acute rejection or infections and low for obliterative bronchiolitis.[60,61] TBLB and BAL are highly complementary in the diagnosis of pulmonary infections in immunocompromised subjects, with a combined yield of approximately 70%.[51] The yield is affected by the type of immunosuppression (post-transplant or HIV) and the infectious cause. A study by Ikedo and coworkers found the yield of TBLB lower than that of BAL or bronchial washings for *Mycobacterium avium* intracellulare infection.[62] Unless contraindicated, TBLB should be performed early (in addition to BAL) in most immunosuppressed patients with active pulmonary infections.

Although a relatively safe procedure, TBLB increases risk of complications of bronchoscopy, in particular the risk of pneumothorax and bleeding.[33] The risk of pneumothorax varies according to the number of biopsies, patient population, use of fluoroscopy, and bronchoscopist experience, and it usually ranges between 1% and 4%.[10,55,63,64] The risk of pneumothorax is also higher in mechanically ventilated patients, where it ranges between 7% and 14%.[65,66] Nevertheless, mechanical ventilation is not a contraindication for TBLB because it has been proved to change management in approximately 40% to 50% of patients, with a favorable risk/benefit ratio.[65,66] The incidence of significant bleeding (greater than 50 mL) is approximately 1%.[64] As discussed previously, bleeding is increased in the context of coagulopathy, uremia, and the use of antiplatelets, especially clopidogrel.[28,29] The risk of bleeding is also increased in patients with pulmonary hypertension. Three human studies, however, have shown that the risk of significant bleeding in mild to moderate pulmonary hypertension is not increased, and this should not be an absolute contraindication for TBLB.[67–69]

Transbronchial Needle Aspiration

TBNA is a well-established technique for sampling of mediastinal and hilar lymph nodes or masses and peripheral lung nodules.[15,16,70–73] Nevertheless, US and UK surveys have shown low rates of adoption of this most useful technique.[1,52,74] Responders to these surveys experienced a poor diagnostic yield, a potential reason for it being underused. The advances in bronchoscopy in the past decade, in particular the advent of CP-EBUS, has also had a negative impact on the use of standard TBNA for sampling of mediastinal and hilar nodes or masses, especially for staging of lung cancer.[19–21] This article uses the term TBNA for the standard or blind procedure. EBUS-TBNA is discussed elsewhere in this issue.

The indications for TBNA are summarized in **Box 3**. TBNA's most common indication, sampling of hilar and mediastinal lymph nodes or tumors, is in rapid decline in centers where EBUS has become available. New technologies, however, such as radial-probe EBUS, virtual bronchoscopy, and electromagnetic navigation, are boosting the use of TBNA for peripheral lung nodules and masses, both for diagnostic purposes and for insertion of fiducial markers for stereotactic body radiation therapy.[75] Despite the high yield of forceps biopsy for endobronchial lesions, in cases where tumors are covered with necrotic material, TBNA allows reaching the core of the tumor and obtain diagnosis. Also, in cases of friable tumors with high bleeding tendency, a needle aspiration is generally less traumatic than forceps biopsy.

Needle sizes range from 22G (for cytology) to 19G (for histologic sampling).[76,77] Needle length typically ranges from 10 mm to 15 mm. Longer and stiffer needles are generally used to sample mediastinal/hilar structures penetrating the tracheal/bronchial wall, whereas shorter and

---

Box 3
Indications for TBNA

Mediastinal or hilar
- Lymphadenopathies
- Tumors or masses

Mediastinal cysts
- Diagnosis
- Drainage

Mediastinal abscess
- Diagnosis
- Drainage

Peripheral nodules or masses

Insertion of fiducial markers for stereotactic body radiation therapy

Necrotic or friable endobronchial tumors

Submucosal injection (ie, cyanoacrilate glue and cidofovir)

---

more flexible needles are preferable for peripheral lung nodules or masses. In cases of endobronchial or submucosal lesions, a 22G needle is preferable because it is less traumatic. A trocar and cannula design of 21G and 19G beveled needles is used when histologic analyses are needed. All needles should be retractable to prevent bronchoscope damage. After routine airway examination and determination of target area for puncture (specific intercartilaginous space), the needle (inside the metal hub) is passed through the working channel. This should be done with the scope in neutral position to prevent damage of working channel. Once the metal hub is visible (within a few millimeters from the tip of the scope), with the bronchoscope centered in the airway lumen to avoid mucosal injury, the catheter is withdrawn, leaving the needle visible. With the needle in view, the bronchoscope is directed toward the target area, and, with an angle greater than 45°, the needle is anchored on the wall. Several techniques have been described to penetrate the tracheal/bronchial wall with the needle.[2] In the jabbing method, the bronchoscope is held still, and the needle is jabbed against the wall. In the piggyback method, the needle catheter is held firmly at the entrance to the working channel, and both the bronchoscope and needle are advanced forward as a unit. For the hub against the wall method, the metal hub is kept in contact with the target area on the wall and then the needle is pushed out of the catheter. The cough method entails keeping the needle out and against the wall and asking patients for a strong cough to allow the needle to penetrate the wall. Once the wall is penetrated, suction is applied at the proximal end of the needle. If blood is aspirated, a new site should be selected because this is a blind technique and a large vessel might be punctured. If blood is not aspirated, the needle is moved back and forth to shear cells into it. After releasing suction, the needle is brought back into the catheter and, once only the metal hub (and no needle) is visible, withdrawn through the bronchoscope. For peripheral lung nodules or masses, with the needle hub in the bronchoscopic view, the bronchoscope is positioned in the bronchial segment that leads to the lesion. Under fluoroscopic guidance (plus any additional technique, such as radial-probe EBUS or electromagnetic navigation), the needle (within the catheter) is slowly advanced until it reaches its target (keeping in mind that the needle extends another 10–15 mm when pushed out). Once the needle is out, suction is applied and the catheter moved back and forth, followed by release of suction, retraction of the needle, and complete removal of the needle apparatus form the bronchoscope. The processing of the obtained samples is a crucial step but outside the scope of this review.[78]

The yield of TBNA to detect malignant mediastinal involvement ranges from 40% to 80%.[79–83] Several factors, such as operator experience, lymph node location, lymph node size, and needle size, have been shown to influence the yield.[79,84,85] Although no randomized controlled studies have been performed comparing TBNA with CP-EBUS–TBNA for staging of lung cancer, the superiority of EBUS has been largely reported, and it is the preferred bronchoscopic technique.[18,19,21] Unlike TBNA, EBUS-TBNA also allows for biopsy of lymph nodes as small as 5 mm in short axis while preserving high yield. The availability of a 19G needle and the consequent potential for histologic sampling have suggested a major role for TBNA in the diagnosis of sarcoidosis.[86,87] Nevertheless, a recent randomized controlled study of TBNA (19G) versus EBUS-TBNA by Tremblay and coworkers[88] showed superiority of EBUS-TBNA for diagnosis of stages I and II sarcoidosis. The yield of TBNA for diagnosis of mycobacterial and fungal infections in smears or cultures from lymph node aspirates is low (40%–50%), but the finding of necrotizing granulomas along with clinical, radiographic, and serologic findings may be of great help.[89–91] The use of TBNA for peripheral lung nodules has become more popular with the advent of supplementary guidance tools, such as radial-probe EBUS and electromagnetic navigation, which have increased its yield.[92,93] These new tools are discussed elsewhere in this issue. Several investigators argue that the yield of TBNA is greater than that of forceps biopsy or cytology brush for malignancies, particularly due to its ability to penetrate through the bronchial wall.[94] Factors that influence the yield of TBNA for peripheral lung nodules include, among others, lesion location, lesion size, and relation to bronchus. Baaklini and coworkers[95] found a yield of 64% for lesions located in the inner third of the lung versus 35% for lesions located in the outer two-thirds of the lungs, with a lower yield also for smaller lesions (<2 cm). Tsuboi and coworkers[96] described 4 types of pulmonary nodules according to the tumor-bronchus relationship: type 1 (bronchus patent up to the tumor), type 2 (bronchus contained in tumor), type 3 (bronchus with intact mucosa but compressed by tumor), and type 4 (bronchus extrinsically compressed by peribronchial lymph node or submucosal infiltration). TBNA is thought especially useful for diagnosis of types 3 and 4 lesions in comparison with other bronchoscopic techniques.[2]

Overall, the use of TBNA is safe. The most common complication of TBNA is damage to a bronchoscope's working channel.[2,25] Careful manipulation of the needle (always kept inside the catheter when passing through a scope) and use of neutral position of the bronchoscope when passing a needle through the distal part of it, can minimize this risk. Significant bleeding is rare, even in the context of bleeding diathesis.[97] Kelly and coworkers[98] found no significant bleeding in 15 patients with superior vena cava syndrome. Fever and bacteremia are also infrequent.[99] Purulent pericarditis, hemomediastinum, and pneumomediastinum also are reported.[100–102]

SUMMARY

Although bronchoscopy technology continues to evolve at a rapid pace, basic procedures, such as BAL, TBLB, and TBNA, continue to play a paramount role in the diagnosis of bronchopulmonary diseases. The advent of newer and more sophisticated techniques should not prevent appropriately training pulmonologists on these basic bronchoscopic procedures.

REFERENCES

1. Colt HG, Prakash U, Offord KP. Bronchoscopy in North America: survey by the American Association of Bronchology. J Bronchol 2000;7:8–25.
2. Bolliger CT, Mathur PN, editors. Interventional bronchoscopy. Basel (Switzerland): Karger; 2000.

3. Ikeda S, Yanai N, Ishikawa S. Flexible bronchofiberscope. Keio J Med 1968;17(1):1–16.

4. Becker HD. Bronchoscopy: the past, the present, and the future. Clin Chest Med 2010;31(1):1–18. Table of Contents.

5. Reynolds HY, Newball HH. Analysis of proteins and respiratory cells obtained from human lungs by bronchial lavage. J Lab Clin Med 1974;84(4):559–73.

6. Andersen HA, Fontana RS. Transbronchoscopic lung biopsy for diffuse pulmonary diseases: technique and results in 450 cases. Chest 1972;62(2):125–8.

7. Andersen HA, Fontana RS, Harrison EG Jr. Transbronchoscopic Lung biopsy in diffuse pulmonary disease. Dis Chest 1965;48:187–92.

8. Andersen HA, Miller WE, Bernatz PE. Lung biopsy: transbronchoscopic, percutaneous, open. Surg Clin North Am 1973;53(4):785–93.

9. Zavala DC, Bedell GN. Percutaneous lung biopsy with a cutting needle. An analysis of 40 cases and comparison with other biopsy techniques. Am Rev Respir Dis 1972;106(2):186–93.

10. Hanson RR, Zavala DC, Rhodes ML, et al. Transbronchial biopsy via flexible fiberoptic bronchoscope; results in 164 patients. Am Rev Respir Dis 1976;114(1):67–72.

11. Levin DC, Wicks AB, Ellis JH Jr. Transbronchial lung biopsy via the fiberoptic bronchoscope. Am Rev Respir Dis 1974;110(1):4–12.

12. Scheinhorn DJ, Joyner LR, Whitcomb ME. Transbronchial forceps lung biopsy through the fiberoptic bronchoscope in Pneumocystis carinii pneumonia. Chest 1974;66(3):294–5.

13. Schiepatti E. La puncion mediastinal a traves del espolon traqueal. Rev Asoc Med Argent 1949;63(663–664):497–9.

14. Schiepatti E. Mediastinal lymph node puncture through tracheal carina. Surg Gynecol Obstet 1958;107:243–6.

15. Wang KP, Haponik EF, Gupta PK, et al. Flexible transbronchial needle aspiration. Technical considerations. Ann Otol Rhinol Laryngol 1984;93(3 Pt 1):233–6.

16. Wang KP, Terry P, Marsh B. Bronchoscopic needle aspiration biopsy of paratracheal tumors. Am Rev Respir Dis 1978;118(1):17–21.

17. Dumon JF, Reboud E, Garbe L, et al. Treatment of tracheobronchial lesions by laser photoresection. Chest 1982;81(3):278–84.

18. Ernst A, Anantham D, Eberhardt R, et al. Diagnosis of mediastinal adenopathy-real-time endobronchial ultrasound guided needle aspiration versus mediastinoscopy. J Thorac Oncol 2008;3(6):577–82.

19. Herth FJ, Eberhardt R, Vilmann P, et al. Real-time endobronchial ultrasound guided transbronchial needle aspiration for sampling mediastinal lymph nodes. Thorax 2006;61(9):795–8.

20. Yasufuku K, Chiyo M, Sekine Y, et al. Real-time endobronchial ultrasound-guided transbronchial needle aspiration of mediastinal and hilar lymph nodes. Chest 2004;126(1):122–8.

21. Yasufuku K, Pierre A, Darling G, et al. A prospective controlled trial of endobronchial ultrasound-guided transbronchial needle aspiration compared with mediastinoscopy for mediastinal lymph node staging of lung cancer. J Thorac Cardiovasc Surg 2011;142(6):1393–400.e1.

22. Mason RJ, Broaddus VC, Murray JF, et al, editors. Textbook of respiratory medicine. Philadelphia: Elsevier-Saunders; 2005.

23. Pue CA, Pacht ER. Complications of fiberoptic bronchoscopy at a university hospital. Chest 1995;107(2):430–2.

24. Ernst A, Silvestri GA, Johnstone D. Interventional pulmonary procedures: guidelines from the American College of Chest Physicians. Chest 2003;123(5):1693–717.

25. Wang KP, Mehta AC, Turner JF, editors. Flexible bronchoscopy. Hoboken, NJ: Wiley-Blackwell; 2012.

26. Burgher LW, Jones FL, Patterson JR, et al. Guidelines for fiberoptic bronchoscopy in adults. Am Rev Respir Dis 1987;136:1066.

27. Matot I, Kramer MR, Glantz L, et al. Myocardial ischemia in sedated patients undergoing fiberoptic bronchoscopy. Chest 1997;112(6):1454–8.

28. Papin TA, Lynch JP 3rd, Weg JG. Transbronchial biopsy in the thrombocytopenic patient. Chest 1985;88(4):549–52.

29. Ernst A, Eberhardt R, Wahidi M, et al. Effect of routine clopidogrel use on bleeding complications after transbronchial biopsy in humans. Chest 2006;129(3):734–7.

30. Herth FJ, Becker HD, Ernst A. Aspirin does not increase bleeding complications after transbronchial biopsy. Chest 2002;122(4):1461–4.

31. Sun SW, Zabaneh RN, Carrey Z. Incidence of pneumothorax after fiberoptic bronchoscopy (FOB) in community-based hospital; are routine post-procedure chest roentgenograms necessary? Chest 2003;124:145.

32. Puar HS, Young RC Jr, Armstrong EM. Bronchial and transbronchial lung biopsy without fluoroscopy in sarcoidosis. Chest 1985;87(3):303–6.

33. Simpson FG, Arnold AG, Purvis A, et al. Postal survey of bronchoscopic practice by physicians in the United Kingdom. Thorax 1986;41(4):311–7.

34. Haslam PL, Baughman RP. Report of ERS Task Force: guidelines for measurement of acellular components and standardization of BAL. Eur Respir J 1999;14(2):245–8.

35. Kelly CA, Kotre CJ, Ward C, et al. Anatomical distribution of bronchoalveolar lavage fluid as

assessed by digital subtraction radiography. Thorax 1987;42(8):624–8.

36. Hunninghake GW, Gadek JE, Kawanami O, et al. Inflammatory and immune processes in the human lung in health and disease: evaluation by bronchoalveolar lavage. Am J Pathol 1979;97(1): 149–206.

37. Pingleton SK, Harrison GF, Stechschulte DJ, et al. Effect of location, pH, and temperature of instillate in bronchoalveolar lavage in normal volunteers. Am Rev Respir Dis 1983;128(6):1035–7.

38. BAL Cooperative Group Steering Committee. Bronchoalveolar lavage constituents in healthy individuals, idiopathic pulmonary fibrosis, and selected comparison groups. Am Rev Respir Dis 1990; 141:S169–202.

39. Collard HR, King TE Jr. Demystifying idiopathic interstitial pneumonia. Arch Intern Med 2003; 163(1):17–29.

40. Raghu G, Mageto YN, Lockhart D, et al. The accuracy of the clinical diagnosis of new-onset idiopathic pulmonary fibrosis and other interstitial lung disease: a prospective study. Chest 1999; 116(5):1168–74.

41. Fagon JY, Chastre J, Wolff M, et al. Invasive and noninvasive strategies for management of suspected ventilator-associated pneumonia. A randomized trial. Ann Intern Med 2000;132(8):621–30.

42. Group CCCT. A randomized trial of diagnostic techniques for ventilator-associated pneumonia. N Engl J Med 2006;355:2619–30.

43. Ruiz M, Torres A, Ewig S, et al. Noninvasive versus invasive microbial investigation in ventilator-associated pneumonia: evaluation of outcome. Am J Respir Crit Care Med 2000;162(1):119–25.

44. Funahashi A, Lohaus GH, Politis J, et al. Role of fibreoptic bronchoscopy in the diagnosis of mycobacterial diseases. Thorax 1983;38(4):267–70.

45. Jett JR, Cortese DA, Dines DE. The value of bronchoscopy in the diagnosis of mycobacterial disease. A five-year experience. Chest 1981;80(5): 575–8.

46. Baughman RP. Use of bronchoscopy in the diagnosis of infection in the immunocompromised host. Thorax 1994;49(1):3–7.

47. Hilbert G, Gruson D, Vargas F, et al. Bronchoscopy with bronchoalveolar lavage via the laryngeal mask airway in high-risk hypoxemic immunosuppressed patients. Crit Care Med 2001;29(2):249–55.

48. Hohenadel IA, Kiworr M, Genitsariotis R, et al. Role of bronchoalveolar lavage in immunocompromised patients with pneumonia treated with a broad spectrum antibiotic and antifungal regimen. Thorax 2001;56(2):115–20.

49. Pisani RJ, Wright AJ. Clinical utility of bronchoalveolar lavage in immunocompromised hosts. Mayo Clin Proc 1992;67(3):221–7.

50. Wallace RH, Kolbe J. Fibreoptic bronchoscopy and bronchoalveolar lavage in the investigation of the immunocompromised lung. N Z Med J 1992; 105(935):215–7.

51. Jain P, Sandur S, Meli Y, et al. Role of flexible bronchoscopy in immunocompromised patients with lung infiltrates. Chest 2004;125(2):712–22.

52. Prakash UB, Stubbs SE. The bronchoscopy survey. Some reflections. Chest 1991;100(6): 1660–7.

53. Descombes E, Gardiol D, Leuenberger P. Transbronchial lung biopsy: an analysis of 530 cases with reference to the number of samples. Monaldi Arch Chest Dis 1997;52(4):324–9.

54. Loube DI, Johnson JE, Wiener D, et al. The effect of forceps size on the adequacy of specimens obtained by transbronchial biopsy. Am Rev Respir Dis 1993;148(5):1411–3.

55. Smith LS, Seaquist M, Schillaci RF. Comparison of forceps used for transbronchial lung biopsy. Bigger may not be better. Chest 1985;87(5): 574–6.

56. Ensminger SA, Prakash UB. Is bronchoscopic lung biopsy helpful in the management of patients with diffuse lung disease? Eur Respir J 2006;28(6): 1081–4.

57. Vansteenkiste J, Verbeken E, Thomeer M, et al. Medical thoracoscopic lung biopsy in interstitial lung disease: a prospective study of biopsy quality. Eur Respir J 1999;14(3):585–90.

58. Bradley B, Branley HM, Egan JJ, et al. Interstitial lung disease guideline: the British Thoracic Society in collaboration with the Thoracic Society of Australia and New Zealand and the Irish Thoracic Society. Thorax 2008;63(Suppl 5):v1–58.

59. American Thoracic Society, European Respiratory Society. American Thoracic Society/European Respiratory Society International Multidisciplinary Consensus Classification of the Idiopathic Interstitial Pneumonias. This joint statement of the American Thoracic Society (ATS), and the European Respiratory Society (ERS) was adopted by the ATS board of directors, June 2001 and by the ERS Executive Committee, June 2001. Am J Respir Crit Care Med 2002;165(2):277–304.

60. Aboyoun CL, Tamm M, Chhajed PN, et al. Diagnostic value of follow-up transbronchial lung biopsy after lung rejection. Am J Respir Crit Care Med 2001;164(3):460–3.

61. Hopkins PM, Aboyoun CL, Chhajed PN, et al. Prospective analysis of 1,235 transbronchial lung biopsies in lung transplant recipients. J Heart Lung Transplant 2002;21(10):1062–7.

62. Ikedo Y. The significance of bronchoscopy for the diagnosis of Mycobacterium avium complex (MAC) pulmonary disease. Kurume Med J 2001; 48(1):15–9.

63. Hernandez Blasco L, Sanchez Hernandez IM, Villena Garrido V, et al. Safety of the transbronchial biopsy in outpatients. Chest 1991;99(3):562–5.

64. Herf SM, Suratt PM, Arora NS. Deaths and complications associated with transbronchial lung biopsy. Am Rev Respir Dis 1977;115(4):708–11.

65. O'Brien JD, Ettinger NA, Shevlin D, et al. Safety and yield of transbronchial biopsy in mechanically ventilated patients. Crit Care Med 1997; 25(3):440–6.

66. Papin TA, Grum CM, Weg JG. Transbronchial biopsy during mechanical ventilation. Chest 1986; 89(2):168–70.

67. Diaz-Guzman E, Vadi S, Minai OA, et al. Safety of diagnostic bronchoscopy in patients with pulmonary hypertension. Respiration 2009;77(3):292–7.

68. Morris MJ, Peacock PM, Mego DM. The risk of hemorrhage from bronchoscopic lung biopsy due to pulmonary hypertension in interstitial lung disease. J Bronchol 1998;5:115–21.

69. Schulman LL, Smith CR, Drusin R, et al. Utility of airway endoscopy in the diagnosis of respiratory complications of cardiac transplantation. Chest 1988;93(5):960–7.

70. Gasparini G, Barbareschi M, Boracchi P, et al. Tumor angiogenesis predicts clinical outcome of node-positive breast cancer patients treated with adjuvant hormone therapy or chemotherapy. Cancer J Sci Am 1995;1(2):131–41.

71. Gasparini S, Ferretti M, Secchi EB, et al. Integration of transbronchial and percutaneous approach in the diagnosis of peripheral pulmonary nodules or masses. Experience with 1,027 consecutive cases. Chest 1995;108(1):131–7.

72. Katis K, Inglesos E, Zachariadis E, et al. The role of transbronchial needle aspiration in the diagnosis of peripheral lung masses or nodules. Eur Respir J 1995;8(6):963–6.

73. Wang KP. Staging of bronchogenic carcinoma by bronchoscopy. Chest 1994;106(2):588–93.

74. Smyth CM, Stead RJ. Survey of flexible fibreoptic bronchoscopy in the United Kingdom. Eur Respir J 2002;19(3):458–63.

75. Anantham D, Feller-Kopman D, Shanmugham LN, et al. Electromagnetic navigation bronchoscopy-guided fiducial placement for robotic stereotactic radiosurgery of lung tumors: a feasibility study. Chest 2007;132(3):930–5.

76. Dasgupta A, Mehta AC, Wang KP. Transbronchial needle aspiration. Semin Respir Crit Care Med 1997;18:571.

77. Wang KP. Transbronchial needle aspiration to obtain histology specimen. J Bronchol 1994;1:116.

78. Ndukwu I, Wang KP, Davis D, et al. Direct smear for cytology examination of transbronchial needle aspiration specimens [abstract]. Chest 1991; 1(100):888.

79. Schenk DA, Bower JH, Bryan CL, et al. Transbronchial needle aspiration staging of bronchogenic carcinoma. Am Rev Respir Dis 1986;134(1):146–8.

80. Shure D, Fedullo PF. The role of transcarinal needle aspiration in the staging of bronchogenic carcinoma. Chest 1984;86(5):693–6.

81. Shure D, Fedullo PF. Transbronchial needle aspiration in the diagnosis of submucosal and peribronchial bronchogenic carcinoma. Chest 1985;88(1): 49–51.

82. Utz JP, Patel AM, Edell ES. The role of transcarinal needle aspiration in the staging of bronchogenic carcinoma. Chest 1993;104(4):1012–6.

83. Wang KP, Brower R, Haponik EF, et al. Flexible transbronchial needle aspiration for staging of bronchogenic carcinoma. Chest 1983;84(5):571–6.

84. Haponik EF, Cappellari JO, Chin R, et al. Education and experience improve transbronchial needle aspiration performance. Am J Respir Crit Care Med 1995;151(6):1998–2002.

85. Hsu LH, Liu CC, Ko JS. Education and experience improve the performance of transbronchial needle aspiration: a learning curve at a cancer center. Chest 2004;125(2):532–40.

86. Morales CF, Patefield AJ, Strollo PJ Jr, et al. Flexible transbronchial needle aspiration in the diagnosis of sarcoidosis. Chest 1994;106(3):709–11.

87. Pauli G, Pelletier A, Bohner C, et al. Transbronchial needle aspiration in the diagnosis of sarcoidosis. Chest 1984;85(4):482–4.

88. Tremblay A, Stather DR, Maceachern P, et al. A randomized controlled trial of standard vs endobronchial ultrasonography-guided transbronchial needle aspiration in patients with suspected sarcoidosis. Chest 2009;136(2):340–6.

89. Baran R, Tor M, Tahaoglu K, et al. Intrathoracic tuberculous lymphadenopathy: clinical and bronchoscopic features in 17 adults without parenchymal lesions. Thorax 1996;51(1):87–9.

90. Baron KM, Aranda CP. Diagnosis of mediastinal mycobacterial lymphadenopathy by transbronchial needle aspiration. Chest 1991;100(6):1723–4.

91. Harkin TJ, Ciotoli C, Addrizzo-Harris DJ, et al. Transbronchial needle aspiration (TBNA) in patients infected with HIV. Am J Respir Crit Care Med 1998;157(6 Pt 1):1913–8.

92. Chao TY, Chien MT, Lie CH, et al. Endobronchial ultrasonography-guided transbronchial needle aspiration increases the diagnostic yield of peripheral pulmonary lesions: a randomized trial. Chest 2009;136(1):229–36.

93. Schwarz Y, Greif J, Becker HD, et al. Real-time electromagnetic navigation bronchoscopy to peripheral lung lesions using overlaid CT images: the first human study. Chest 2006;129(4):988–94.

94. Reichenberger F, Weber J, Tamm M, et al. The value of transbronchial needle aspiration in the

diagnosis of peripheral pulmonary lesions. Chest 1999;116(3):704–8.

95. Baaklini WA, Reinoso MA, Gorin AB, et al. Diagnostic yield of fiberoptic bronchoscopy in evaluating solitary pulmonary nodules. Chest 2000; 117(4):1049–54.

96. Tsuboi E, Ikeda S, Tajima M, et al. Transbronchial biopsy smear for diagnosis of peripheral pulmonary carcinomas. Cancer 1967;20(5):687–98.

97. Harrow EM, Oldenburg FA Jr, Lingenfelter MS, et al. Transbronchial needle aspiration in clinical practice. A five-year experience. Chest 1989;96(6):1268–72.

98. Kelly PT, Chin R, Adair NE, et al. Bronchosocopic needle aspration in patients with superior vena cava disease. J Bronchol 1997;4:290–3.

99. Witte MC, Opal SM, Gilbert JG, et al. Incidence of fever and bacteremia following transbronchial needle aspiration. Chest 1986;89(1):85–7.

100. Epstein SK, Winslow CJ, Brecher SM, et al. Polymicrobial bacterial pericarditis after transbronchial needle aspiration. Case report with an investigation on the risk of bacterial contamination during fiberoptic bronchoscopy. Am Rev Respir Dis 1992;146(2): 523–5.

101. Kucera RF, Wolfe GK, Perry ME. Hemomediastinum after transbronchial needle aspiration. Chest 1986; 90(3):466.

102. Wang KP, Marsh BR, Summer WR, et al. Transbronchial needle aspiration for diagnosis of lung cancer. Chest 1981;80(1):48–50.

Review of the International Association for the Study of Lung Cancer Lymph Node Classification System

Localization of Lymph Node Stations on CT Imaging

Hamza Jawad, MBBS[a], Arlene Sirajuddin, MD[b],
Jonathan Hero Chung, MD[c],*

KEYWORDS

- International Association for the Study of Lung Cancer lymph node map • Lymph node stations
- Imaging • CT

KEY POINTS

- The International Association for the Study of Lung Cancer (IASLC) map is the newest lymph node classification system. Compared with previous lymph node maps, it provides fixed, specific anatomic descriptors for all thoracic lymph node stations.
- CT imaging is one of the most important modalities used in the clinical staging of lung cancer patients.
- It is important to be familiar with the IASLC map as well as able to accurately identify the different lymph node stations on CT imaging.
- Lymph node maps have been continuously evolving in past years and may be subject to future amendments as more information becomes available from clinical trials.

INTRODUCTION

Thoracic lymphadenopathy is a common finding in patients with lung cancer and signifies metastatic nodal involvement. The location of the involved thoracic lymph node groups in relation to the primary lung tumor determines the nodal (N) designation of the tumor, node, metastasis (TNM) classification system used in the staging of lung cancer. Accurate detection and classification of the involved thoracic lymph node groups are essential for appropriate staging of lung cancer patients, also determining available treatment options and helping predict patient prognosis.

Funding Sources: Nil.
Conflict of Interest: Nil.

[a] Transitional Year Residency Program, Grand Rapids Medical Education Partners, 25 Michigan Street Northeast, Suite 2200, Grand Rapids, MI 49503, USA; [b] Department of Radiology, Northwestern University Feinberg School of Medicine, 676 North Saint Clair, Suite 800, Chicago, IL 60611, USA; [c] Department of Radiology, National Jewish Health, 1400 Jackson Street, Denver, CO 80206, USA

* Corresponding author.

E-mail address: chungj@njhealth.org

Clin Chest Med 34 (2013) 353–363
http://dx.doi.org/10.1016/j.ccm.2013.04.008
0272-5231/13/$ – see front matter © 2013 Elsevier Inc. All rights reserved.

Multiple lymph node maps have been published in the past to provide diagrammatic descriptions of thoracic lymph node groups. Although they provide an excellent visual representation of these nodal groups, they are of limited value when clinicians are faced with the challenge of identifying and classifying thoracic lymphadenopathy on CT imaging. This article reviews the most recent thoracic lymph node classification system, proposed by the IASLC in 2009.[1] It describes each of the IASLC lymph node stations with both illustrations and CT images to enable clinicians to better understand and accurately identify these lymph nodes on CT imaging. Although articles in the past have correlated CT images with the previously used Mountain-Dressler American Thoracic Society map (MD-ATS) classification,[2–4] to the authors' knowledge, this is the first attempt to depict the recently published IASLC lymph node map with representative CT images.

HISTORY OF THORACIC LYMPH NODE MAPS

Thoracic lymph node maps have been in place for the past 40 years. They were developed to provide a systematic, universal approach to gauge the degree of lymph node involvement in lung cancer patients. The general idea behind these maps was to classify the thoracic lymph nodes into numerically labeled regions with fixed anatomic boundary descriptors. The intent was to provide a universally accepted, precise lymph node classification system to guide assessment of patient treatment outcomes and planning of individual patient therapy, and to also allow for comparison of results across multiple institutions and clinical trial designs.

Because these maps directly affect patient management and treatment decisions for a disease with extremely high morbidity and mortality burden, they have been under continuous scrutiny and been revised frequently. Multiple versions of these maps arose throughout the years due to failure of consensus on a single version.

The first lymph node map was proposed by Naruke and colleagues[5] in the 1960s. This was met with widespread acceptance and used in North America, Europe, and Japan. In the 1980s/ 1990s, attempts were made to revise the anatomic descriptors proposed in the Naruke map. The first revision was the development of the American Thoracic Society (ATS) lymph node map. Subsequently, Mountain and Dressler[4] created another lymph node map, known as the MD-ATS map (Fig. 1), in an attempt to unify the Naruke and ATS maps into a single classification system. The MD-ATS map was adopted by the American Joint Committee on Cancer (AJCC) and the Prognostic Factors TNM Committee of the International Union Against Cancer (UICC) at the 1996 annual meetings of these organizations. Although the MD-ATS map was widely used in North America, it was only sporadically used in Europe. Meanwhile, Japan continued to use the initial Naruke map, as advocated by the Japan Lung Cancer Society.

THE IASLC MAP

The IASLC commenced its first lung cancer staging project in 1998. They discovered that the node (N) descriptors of the MD-ATS and Naruke classification systems had significant discrepancies, which had direct implications on the staging of lung cancer patients. The IASLC committee members were charged with the task of developing a new lymph node classification system with the purpose of (1) reconciling the differences between the MD-ATS and Naruke maps and (2) providing anatomically distinct descriptions for the proposed lymph node stations. In 2009, the IASLC committee proposed a new lymph node map. This new map, known as the IASLC map, grouped the thoracic lymph nodes into 7 specific zones: supraclavicular, upper, aorticopulmonary, subcarinal, lower, hilar-interlobar, and peripheral (Table 1).[1] The thoracic lymph nodes are further assigned to 1 of 14 numbered stations (stations 1–14); the descriptor "R" or "L" is added to denote right-sided or left-sided nodes, respectively. The TNM Classification of Malignant Tumours, 7th edition, was also published in 2009, which incorporated the newly formulated IASLC lymph node classification system into its proposals. The IASLC lymph node map is detailed in Fig. 2.

According to the new TNM edition, patients without lymph node involvement are designated as N0. N1 disease is defined as having metastatic lymph node involvement of ipsilateral peripheral or hilar zones (stations 10–14). N2 disease is present if there is extension of tumor metastasis to ipsilateral mediastinal (upper, aortopulmonary, and lower) or subcarinal zones (stations 2–9). The N3 designation signifies metastatic lymph node involvement of the ipsilateral or contralateral supraclavicular zone lymph nodes (station 1) or any nodes in the contralateral mediastinal, hilar-interlobar, and peripheral zones.

RADIOGRAPHIC ANATOMY

The IASLC lymph node classification provides precise anatomic descriptors for lymph node station boundaries. Like previous maps, however, it may

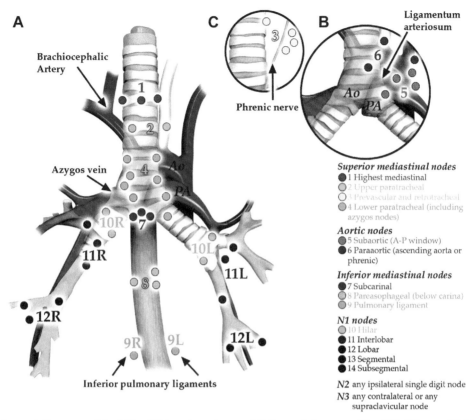

Fig. 1. Coronal diagrams of the MD—ATS lymph node map. (*A*) Coronal diagram of the MD-ATS map. (*B*) Diagram view of sub-aortic (station 5) and para-aortic (station 6) lymph nodes. (*C*) Lateral view, demonstrating prevascular and retrotracheal lymph nodes (station 3). Ao, aortic arch; L, left; PA, pulmonary artery; R, right.

be subject to modifications in the future. Already, a few areas of uncertainty within the IASLC lymph node map have been pointed out by various investigators.

The supraclavicular zone lymph nodes (station 1) were previously termed, *highest mediastinal nodes*, by the MD-ATS classification system and were defined as lymph nodes lying above a horizontal line at the upper rim of the left innominate vein where it ascends to the left, crossing in front of the trachea at its midline. The IASLC map classifies the supraclavicular zone as station 1 and further subcategorizes it into 3 separate lymph node groups—supraclavicular, lower cervical, and sternal notch nodes (**Fig. 3**, see **Table 1**). The latter 2 lymph node groups are a new addition to station 1 and were previously not included by the MD-ATS map. In a recent article, Pitson and colleagues[6] pointed out that the definition provided for the lateral aspect of the lower border of the station 1 nodes (clavicles) is unclear in terms of whether the upper or lower border of the clavicles should be used. According to the IASLC map, the

lateral borders for the superior margins for both stations 2 and 3 are the lung apex and pleura. Because clavicles can vary in position and can extend inferior to the lung apex, this leads to a region inferior to the lung apex but superior to the clavicles where stations 1, 2, and 3 can all be potentially present. This carries importance because this is a distinction between N2 and N3 disease.

Station 2 lymph nodes are part of the upper zone, and include the right and left upper paratracheal lymph node groups, 2R and 2L, respectively (**Figs. 4** and **5**). They were previously defined by the MD-ATS classification as lymph nodes lying below the lower margin of the station 1 nodes but superior to an imaginary line drawn horizontally and tangentially to the upper margin of the aortic arch. According the recent IASLC classification, the upper margin of 2R and 2L is the superior border of the manubrium medially and the lung apex and pleural space laterally. The lower margins of 2R and 2L have been differentiated, however. The inferior border of 2L is now formed by

Table 1
IASLC lymph node classification

Nodal Zone	Lymph Node Group	IASLC Station	Anatomic Boundaries		
			Superior Border	Inferior Border	Other Important Anatomic Descriptors
Supraclavicular	Lower cervical; supraclavicular; sternal notch nodes	1R and 1L (see Fig. 3)	Lower margin of cricoid cartilage	Laterally: both clavicles Medially: upper border of manubrium	Border between 1R and 1L nodes: midline of trachea
Upper	Upper paratracheal	2R (see Figs. 4–6 and 9)	Medially: superior border of manubrium Laterally: apex of right lung and pleural space	Intersection of caudal margin of left brachiocephalic (innominate) vein with trachea	Border between 2R and 2L: left lateral border of trachea
		2L (see Figs. 4 and 5)	Medially: superior border of manubrium Laterally: apex of right lung and pleural space	Superior border of the aortic arch	
	Prevascular (3a) and retrotracheal (3p)	3a (see Figs. 4 and 7)	Apex of chest	Carina	Anterior border: sternum Posterior border: SVC (on the right) and left carotid artery (on the left)
		3p (see Figs. 7 and 10)	Apex of chest	Carina	Anterior boundary: posterior aspect of trachea
	Lower paratracheal	4R (see Figs. 7–9)	Intersection of caudal margin of left brachiocephalic vein with trachea	Lower border of azygous vein	Demarcation between 4R and 4L: left lateral border of trachea Left-lateral limit of 4L: ligamentum arteriosum
		4L (see Figs. 7 and 9)	Superior border of the aortic arch	Superior rim of the left main pulmonary artery	

			Lower border	Upper border	
Aorticopulmonary	Subaortic	5 (see Figs. 7A, 8, 10 and 11)	Lower border of aortic arch	Upper rim of left main pulmonary artery	Lateral to ligamentum arteriosum
	Para-aortic	6 (see Fig. 7)	Horizontal line drawn tangentially to the upper border of aortic arch	Lower border of aortic arch	Located anterior and lateral to ascending aorta and aortic arch
Subcarinal	Subcarinal	7 (see Figs. 10, 12, and 13)	Carina of the trachea	Left: upper border of the left lower lobe bronchus; Right: lower border of the bronchus intermedius	
Lower	Paraesophageal	8	Left: upper border of left lower lobe bronchus; Right: lower border of bronchus intermedius	Diaphragm	Adjacent to esophageal wall; can be either side of midline
	Pulmonary ligament	9 (see Fig. 14)	Inferior pulmonary vein	Diaphragm	Lie within the pulmonary ligament (which is formed by inferior extension of mediastinal pleural reflections)
Hilar-interlobar	Hilar	10 (see Fig. 15)	Left: superior rim of main pulmonary artery; Right: caudal border of azygous vein	Interlobar regions	Includes lymph nodes adjacent to mainstem bronchi and hilar vessels
	Interlobar	11 (see Fig. 12)			Located distal to the bifurcation regions of mainstem bronchi
Peripheral	Lobar	12			Adjacent to lobar bronchi
	Segmental	13 (see Fig. 12)			Adjacent to segmental bronchi
	Subsegmental	14			Adjacent to subsegmental bronchi

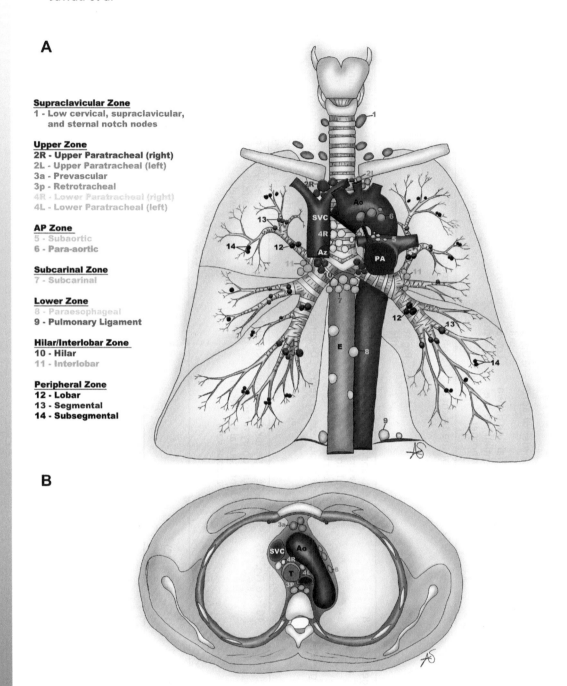

A

Supraclavicular Zone
1 - Low cervical, supraclavicular, and sternal notch nodes

Upper Zone
2R - Upper Paratracheal (right)
2L - Upper Paratracheal (left)
3a - Prevascular
3p - Retrotracheal
4R - Lower Paratracheal (right)
4L - Lower Paratracheal (left)

AP Zone
5 - Subaortic
6 - Para-aortic

Subcarinal Zone
7 - Subcarinal

Lower Zone
8 - Paraesophageal
9 - Pulmonary Ligament

Hilar/Interlobar Zone
10 - Hilar
11 - Interlobar

Peripheral Zone
12 - Lobar
13 - Segmental
14 - Subsegmental

B

Fig. 2. (*A*) Coronal and (*B*) cross-sectional diagrams of the IASLC lymph node map. Ao, aortic arch; Az, azygous vein; E, esophagus; PA, pulmonary artery; SVC, superior vena cava; T, trachea.

the superior margin of the aortic arch, whereas the inferior border of station 2R is now the caudal margin of the left innominate vein where it intersects the trachea (see **Table 1**). Recently, Ichimura and colleagues[7] pointed out that this is usually an oblique intersection and can be difficult to identify accurately on axial CT images. Those who created the IALSC map, however, have insisted that the caudal margin of the left innominate vein be followed precisely, regardless of the obliquity of the margin (**Fig. 6**).[8] Another major change from the previous classification is that the left tracheal

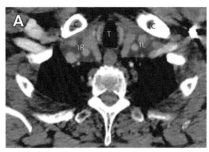
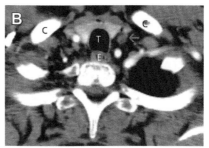

Fig. 3. Station 1. (*A*) Axial CT of the chest shows location of 1R and 1L lymph node stations (highlighted in *pink*). (*B*) Axial CT of the chest shows an enlarged 1L lymph node (*pink arrow*). C, clavicle; E, esophagus; T, trachea.

border now forms the border between stations station 2R and 2L (see **Fig. 5**). Previously, this border was set at the level of the tracheal midline, but readjusting it to the left tracheal border better conforms to the actual lymphatic drainage pattern of the paratracheal region.

Station 3 is also contained in the upper zone and consists of 2 lymph node groups—prevascular (3a) and retrotracheal (3p) (see **Fig. 4**; **Fig. 7**). Station 3a refers to the lymph nodes found anterior to the major vessels of the mediastinum. Station 3p includes the lymph nodes posterior to the trachea. The major change in station 3 from the MD-ATS classification system is that its anatomic boundaries have now been precisely defined (see **Table 1**). According to the IASLC criteria, the posterior margin of 3a is formed by the superior

vena cava on the right and the common carotid artery on the left. These 2 structures are not continuous, however, throughout the superoinferior extent of station 3a (ie, lung apex to the carina) and it may be difficult to determine the posterior margin of station 3a on some CT axial sections.

Station 4 lymph nodes are also part of the upper nodal zone, and consist of the right and left lower paratracheal nodes, 4R and 4L, respectively (see **Fig. 7**, **Table 1**). Previously, the lower border of 4R was defined as a line extending across the right main bronchus at the upper margin of the right upper lobe bronchus. The IASLC classification now sets the lower border of 4R at the lower border of the azygos vein where it meets the superior vena cava (**Fig. 8**). Previously, the lower border of 4L was defined as a line extending across the

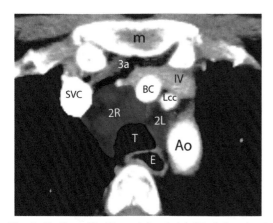

Fig. 4. Stations 2R, 2L, and 3a. Axial CT of the chest highlights the locations of 2R (*red*), 2L (*orange*), and 3a (*blue-violet*) lymph node stations. Note that the left tracheal border separates stations 2R and 2L. Also, the 3a lymph nodes lie anterior to the superior vena cava on the right and anterior to the left common carotid artery on the left. Ao, aorta; BC, right brachiocephalic artery; E, esophagus; IV, left innominate vein; Lcc, left common carotid artery; m, manubrium; SVC, superior vena cava; T, trachea.

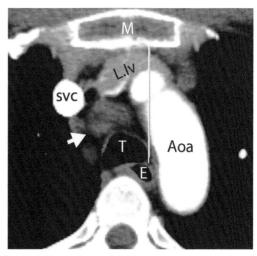

Fig. 5. Station 2R. Axial CT of chest shows an enlarged 2R lymph node (*white arrow*). Note that the left tracheal border (*green line*) forms the border between 2R and 2L lymph node stations. Aoa, aortic arch; E, esophagus; L.Iv, left innominate vein; M, manubrium; SVC, superior vena cava; T, trachea.

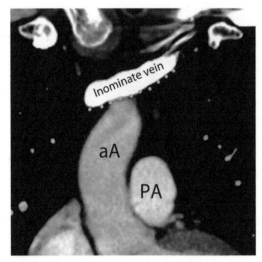

Fig. 6. Coronal CT scan of chest shows the caudal border (*blue dotted line*) of the left innominate vein which forms the inferior border of station 2R. Note that this follows an oblique course and may be hard to appreciate on axial CT images. aA, ascending aorta; PA, main pulmonary artery.

left main bronchus at the upper margin of the origin of the upper lobe bronchus. It is now at the upper rim of the left main pulmonary artery (**Fig. 9**). Similar to station 2, the border between 4R and 4L is now formed by the left tracheal border, which is more consistent with the actual lymphatic drainage patterns of the paratracheal region. Another major change from the previous MD-ATS map is that the pleural reflection, which is

generally not appreciable on CT, does not serve as a border between stations 4 and 10. The boundary descriptors of the IASLC system (see **Table 1**), which are easily recognized on CT imaging, allow for much more consistent differentiation between station 4 and station 10 lymph nodes on CT imaging.

Station 5 (subaortic) lymph nodes form a part of the aorticopulmonary zone (see **Figs. 7A and 8**; **Fig. 10**, see **Table 1**). Their superoinferior extent is from the lower border of the aortic arch to the upper rim of left main pulmonary artery. The ligamentum arteriosum separates the station 5 nodes from 4L nodes, which are located more medially (**Fig. 11**).

Station 6 (para-aortic) lymph nodes are also classified as aorticopulmonary zone nodes. They are defined as lymph nodes lying anterior and lateral to the ascending aorta and aortic arch (see **Fig. 7**). Their superoinferior extent is from the upper border of the aortic arch to the lower border of the aortic arch.

Station 7 (subcarinal) nodes are defined as lymph nodes located immediately inferior to the carina (see **Fig. 10**; **Fig. 12**). The IASLC classification system extends them more inferior than the previous classification. Their lower border is now formed by the upper border of the lower lobe bronchus on the left and by the lower border of the bronchus intermedius on the right (**Fig. 13**). This has allowed the inferior border of station 7 to match the superior border of the station 8 nodes.

Station 8 (paraesophageal) nodes lie adjacent to the esophagus, either to the right or left of midline (see **Fig. 2A**). They extend from the lower border of

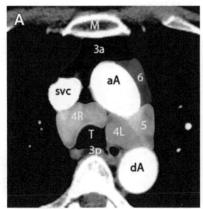
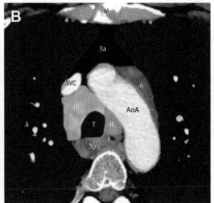

Fig. 7. Stations 3a, 3p, 4R, 4L, 5, and 6. (*A*) Axial CT of the chest at the level of aorticopulmonary window highlights the location of stations 3a (*blue-violet*), 3p (*brown*), 4R (*yellow*), 4L (*teal*), 5 (*pale pink*), and 6 (*green*). (*B*) Axial CT of chest at the level of aortic arch shows the locations of stations 3a (*blue-violet*), 3p (*brown*), 4R (*yellow*), 4L (*teal*), and 6 (*green*). aA, ascending aorta; AoA, aortic arch; dA, descending aorta; E, esophagus; M, manubrium; SVC, superior vena cava; T, trachea.

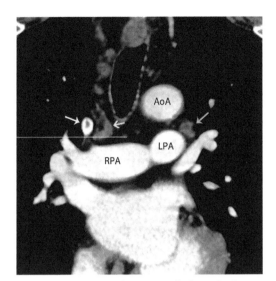

Fig. 8. Stations 4R and 5. Coronal chest CT demonstrates an enlarged station 4R lymph node (*yellow arrow*) adjacent to the azygos vein (*white arrow*). Note that lower border of the azygos vein (*yellow line*) demarcates the inferior limit of station 4R. Also shown is an enlarged station 5 lymph node (*pink arrow*). AoA, aortic arch; LPA, left main pulmonary artery; RPA, right main pulmonary artery.

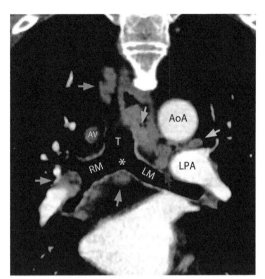

Fig. 10. Stations 3p, 4L, 5, 7, 10, and 11. Coronal CT of the chest shows multiple enlarged lymph nodes including stations 3p (*brown arrow*), 4L (*blue arrow*), 5 (*pale pink arrow*), 7 (*olive green arrow*), 10 (*magenta arrow*), and 11 (*bright green arrow*). *, carina; AoA, aortic arch; AV, azygous vein; LM, left mainstem bronchus; LPA, left main pulmonary artery; RM, right mainstem bronchus; T, trachea.

station 7 nodes superiorly to the diaphragm inferiorly. Station 9 (pulmonary ligament) nodes lie within the pulmonary ligament. They are generally situated more lateral than station 8 nodes. As

Pitson and colleagues[6] point out, it may be difficult to differentiate between station 9 nodes (**Fig. 14**) that sit inside the pulmonary ligament and station 8 nodes that sit lower, near the pulmonary ligament.[6] Rusch and Asamura, authors of the IASLC map,[8] acknowledge that this may be the case,

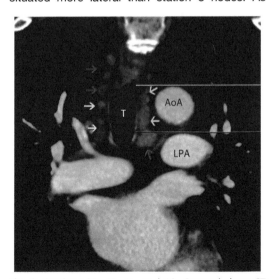

Fig. 9. Stations 2R, 4R, 4L, and 10. Coronal chest CT shows multiple enlarged lymph nodes corresponding to stations 2R (*red arrows*), 4R (*yellow arrows*), 4L (*blue arrows*), and 10 (*magenta arrow*). Superior border of the aortic arch (*yellow line*) forms the superior margin of station 4L; superior rim of left main pulmonary artery (*blue line*) forms the inferior border of station 4L. AoA, aortic arch; LPA, left main pulmonary artery; T, trachea.

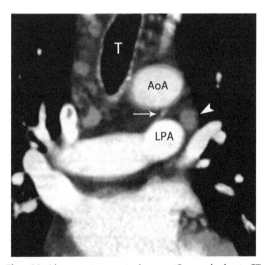

Fig. 11. Ligamentum arteriosum. Coronal chest CT demonstrates the location of ligamentum arteriosum (*white arrow*), which is partially calcified. Also shown is an enlarged station 5 lymph node (*white arrowhead*). AoA, aortic arch; LPA, left main pulmonary artery; T, trachea.

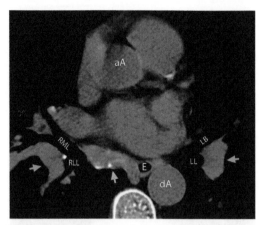

Fig. 12. Stations 7, 11, and 13. Axial CT of the chest shows multiple enlarged lymph nodes representing stations 7 (*olive green arrow*), 11 (*green arrows*), and 13 (*purple arrow*). aA, ascending aorta; dA, descending aorta; E, esophagus; LB, lingular bronchus; LL, left lower lobe bronchus; RLL, right lower lobe bronchus; RML, right middle lobe bronchus.

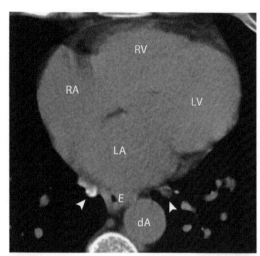

Fig. 14. Station 9. Axial CT of the chest at the level of pulmonary ligament demonstrates 2 enlarged, calcified station 9 lymph nodes (*arrowheads*). dA, descending aorta; E, esophagus; LA, left atrium; LV, left ventricle; RA, right atrium; RV, right ventricle.

although this distinction is usually straightforward at surgery.

The hilar-interlobar zone includes hilar (station 10) and interlobar (station 11) lymph node groups (see **Figs. 9** and **12**; **Fig. 15**). The peripheral zone consists of lobar (station 12), segmental (station 13), and subsegmental (station 14) lymph node groups.

Another cause of confusion, pointed out by Ichimura and colleagues,[7] are the lymph nodes that are located such that they extend across the set boundaries and theoretically can be classified into more than one lymph node station (see **Fig. 8**). This was clarified by Rusch and colleagues, who stated that such lymph nodes should be designated to stations where they predominantly reside.[8]

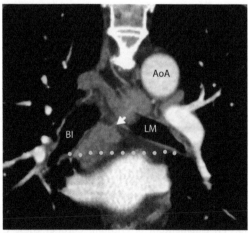

Fig. 13. Station 7. Coronal CT of the chest shows an enlarged station 7 lymph node (*white arrow*); also demonstrated is the lower border of station 7 (*dotted line*). AoA, aortic arch; BI, bronchus intermedius; LM, left mainstem bronchus.

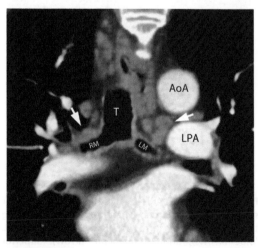

Fig. 15. Station 10. Coronal CT chest shows multiple enlarged station 10 lymph nodes (*arrows*). AoA, aortic arch; LM, left mainstem bronchus; LPA, left main pulmonary artery; RM, right mainstem bronchus; T, trachea.

SUMMARY

The IASLC map is the newest lymph node classification system. Compared with previous lymph node maps, it provides fixed, specific anatomic descriptors for all thoracic lymph node stations. CT imaging is one of the most important modalities used in the clinical staging of lung cancer patients. Therefore, it is important to be familiar with the IASLC map as well as to accurately identify the different node stations on CT imaging. It is also important to understand that lymph node maps have been continuously evolving in past years and may be subject to future amendments as more information becomes available from clinical trials.

REFERENCES

1. Rusch VW, Asamura H, Watanabe H, et al. The IASLC lung cancer staging project: a proposal for a new international lymph node map in the forthcoming seventh edition of the TNM classification for lung cancer. J Thorac Oncol 2009;4(5):568–77.

2. Ko JP, Drucker EA, Shepard JA, et al. CT depiction of regional nodal stations for lung cancer staging. AJR Am J Roentgenol 2000;174(3):775–82.

3. Suwatanapongched T, Gierada DS. CT of thoracic lymph nodes. Part I: anatomy and drainage. Br J Radiol 2006;79(947):922–8.

4. Mountain CF, Dresler CM. Regional lymph node classification for lung cancer staging. Chest 1997; 111(6):1718–23.

5. Naruke T, Suemasu K, Ishikawa S. Lymph node mapping and curability at various levels of metastasis in resected lung cancer. J Thorac Cardiovasc Surg 1978;76(6):832–9.

6. Pitson G, Lynch R, Claude L, et al. A critique of the international association for the study of lung cancer lymph node map: a radiation oncology perspective. J Thorac Oncol 2012;7(3):478–80.

7. Ichimura H, Kikuchi S, Ishikawa H. Caudal border of level 2R in the new international lymph node map for lung cancer. J Thorac Oncol 2010;5(4):579 [author reply: 579–80].

8. Rusch VW, Asamura H. Response: a critique of the international association for the study of lung cancer lymph node map. J Thorac Oncol 2012;7(3):481.

Lung Cancer Screening
Past, Present and Future

James H. Finigan, MD[a,b,c],*, Jeffrey A. Kern, MD[a,b,c]

KEYWORDS

- Lung cancer screening • National Lung Screening Trial • Low-dose computed tomography
- Chest radiograph

KEY POINTS

- The National Lung Screening Trial (NLST) proved that low-dose computed tomography (LDCT) screening for lung cancer decreases mortality.
- Most LDCT trials have investigated yearly screening.
- How more or less frequent screening would affect the sensitivity and specificity of LDCT screening is unclear.
- How long to screen individuals remains unknown.
- Almost certainly, the NLST will result in increased LDCT screening for lung cancer.

INTRODUCTION

Lung cancer is the leading cause of cancer death for men and women in the United States and worldwide.[1,2] The most effective way to decrease lung cancer morbidity and mortality would be to significantly alter current smoking patterns. Unfortunately, while smoking decreased dramatically in the 1960s and 1970s, the smoking rate more recently has plateaued. For the past 10 years, roughly 20% of the population has remained actively smoking.[3] The high mortality rate for lung cancer is heavily influenced by the fact that most cases are diagnosed at an advanced stage, when cure is no longer an option, in contrast to cancers such as breast and colon cancers, which have effective screening tests. Seventy percent of lung cancers are stage 3 or 4 at the time of diagnosis, and the 5-year mortality for lung cancer has remained relatively unchanged for the past

40 years, while survival for most other cancers has steadily improved.[2]

Outside of reducing cigarette smoking rates, arguably the most important factor that impacts lung cancer mortality has been the absence of an effective screening test to diagnose early stage, curable disease. Effective cancer screening is based on the premise that lethal malignancies can be found before they are symptomatic and when therapy can be curative. Over the past 4 decades, numerous lung cancer screening trials, primarily using serial chest radiographs or computed tomography (CT) scans, have been conducted. Despite initial negative studies, the recent publication of the National Lung Screening Trial (NLST) demonstrated improved lung cancer survival in participants screened with serial low dose CT scans; the NLST is the first trial showing screening can decrease lung cancer mortality. This trial

[a] Division of Oncology, Department of Medicine, National Jewish Health, 1400 Jackson Street, Denver, CO 80206, USA; [b] Division of Pulmonary and Critical Care Medicine, Department of Medicine, National Jewish Health, 1400 Jackson Street, Denver, CO 80206, USA; [c] Division of Pulmonary Sciences and Critical Care Medicine, Department of Medicine, University of Colorado, 12700 East 19th Avenue, Aurora, CO 80045, USA
* Corresponding author. Department of Medicine, National Jewish Health, 1400 Jackson Street, K736A, Denver, CO 80206.
E-mail address: FiniganJ@NJHealth.org

Clin Chest Med 34 (2013) 365–371
http://dx.doi.org/10.1016/j.ccm.2013.03.004

suggests that large-scale successful screening for lung cancer is possible.

LUNG CANCER SCREENING BY CHEST RADIOGRAPH

Studies of lung cancer screening began in the 1970s, with several examining the efficacy of serial chest radiographs with or without sputum cytology analysis to diagnose early stage lung cancer and decrease lung cancer mortality. The first randomized controlled trial was the Mayo Clinic trial, which randomized 9211 men, aged 45 years or older who had smoked at least 20 cigarettes a day in the past year. All patients underwent an initial prevalence screen chest radiograph and sputum cytology examination followed by a chest radiograph and sputum cytology every 4 months for the screening group versus routine recommendations of yearly chest radiograph and sputum cytology in the control arm. While the screening group had more lung cancers, and specifically more stage 1 lung cancers diagnosed and resected, there was no difference in lung cancer mortality.[4,5] Similar findings were observed in 2 other chest radiograph screening trials. The Johns Hopkins Lung Project and the Czechoslovakian experience each randomized patients to some combination of serial chest radiographs and sputum cytology versus yearly chest radiograph.[6,7] Again, both found a difference in early stage lung cancers diagnosed but no difference in mortality.

These initial screening studies highlight the importance of using mortality as an end-point in cancer screening trials and the problem of overdiagnosis bias. Overdiagnosis refers to the identification of cancers that do not progress or influence mortality. In an adequately powered, randomized controlled trial, the incidence of cancer should be equal in both the screening and control arms. If cancer occurs more frequently in the screening arm, it suggests that the difference in cancer diagnoses represents cancers that would not advance to the point of causing death. Overdiagnosis results in unneeded, often invasive tests and treatments. The Mayo Lung Project is an example of overdiagnosis. After 8.5 years of follow-up, 206 cancers were diagnosed in the screening arm compared with 160 in the control arm. After 12 years of follow-up, that difference had shrunk, but was still apparent, with 585 cancers diagnosed in the screening arm and 500 in the control arm. That there was no difference in cancer mortality further supports the likelihood that those excess cancers were the product of overdiagnosis.

The most recent trial of chest radiograph screening was the Prostate, Lung, Colorectal and Ovarian (PLCO) trial. This trial differs from previous chest radiograph screening studies in its large size (154,901 total participants) and the fact that the control arm of the study did not undergo either baseline or annual chest radiographs.[8] Importantly, PLCO was a screening trial for multiple cancers, and a requirement of a smoking history was not an inclusion criterion, making it a study of screening in a general population, not a high-risk population. Starting in 1993, men and women aged 55 to 74 years in the study group underwent annual screening for 4 years. The usual care group consisted patients given no specific recommendation regarding screening. There was high adherence to screening in the screening arm and a low rate of chest radiographs in the usual care arm. The PLCO trial demonstrated no effect of annual chest radiograph screening on diagnosing lung cancer, no difference on lung cancer stage or histology, and no difference on lung cancer mortality through 13 years of follow-up. A subanalysis of the efficacy of yearly chest radiograph screening including only patients at higher risk of lung cancer (ie, at least 30 pack-year smoking history who were either current smokers or had quit within the previous 15 years) also demonstrated no effect on lung cancer incidence or lung cancer mortality. Many of the cancers were diagnosed during the follow-up period, after active radiographic screening had ended, raising the question of whether a screening period of more than 4 years would have been more effective. An analysis limited to the period during which screening occurred, however, confirmed no increase in lung cancers diagnosed by annual chest radiograph. The PLCO trial provides a possible final confirmation that annual chest radiographs have no impact on lung cancer diagnosis or mortality when compared with no screening.

Overdiagnosis was less apparent in the PLCO trial, with a smaller difference in lung cancer rates between the screened and usual care arms (1696 cases in the chest radiograph group vs 1620 cases in the usual care arm at study end). This difference when compared with the Mayo Clinic Project might result from screening chest radiographs that were performed more frequently in the Mayo Clinic trail compared with the PLCO trial (every 4 months versus yearly). Additionally, in the Mayo Clinic trial all patients had initial chest radiographs to diagnose and exclude prevalence lung cancers at the time of study entry, following which time patients were randomized to either screening or control arms. In the PLCO trial, patients were randomized before any chest radiograph evaluation, and the usual care arm did not receive imaging as part of the protocol.

LUNG CANCER SCREENING BY CT

Chest radiographs diagnosed more early stage lung cancers; however, chest radiograph screening did not decrease the number of late-stage cancers compared with the control group, resulting in similar overall mortality rates. The emergence of CT scanning created new hope for effective lung cancer screening, as chest CTs have increased resolution compared with chest radiographs, resulting in increased sensitivity for diagnosing small cancers. This raised the possibility that chest CT scans could identify early stage lung cancers before they progressed to advanced stage disease.

The initial trials of chest CT screening for lung cancer primarily consisted of single-arm, observational studies that investigated the utility of low-dose CT (LDCT) scans to diagnose early stage cancer. LDCTs expose patients to less than 25% of the radiation than a conventional CT scan of the chest, 1.5 versus 7 mSv.[9] Two studies performed in Japan included up to 6000 people with a low lung cancer risk (minimal or no smoking history). While the prevalence of lung cancer in these studies was less than 1%, they confirmed that LDCT scans detect more cancers and benign nodules than chest radiographs.[10,11]

Investigators at the Mayo Clinic enrolled 1520 high-risk subjects, defined as at least 20 pack-year smoking history and participants could not have quit smoking more than 10 years before enrollment, in a prospective study in which participants underwent 5 annual LDCT scans (1 prevalence scan followed by 4 yearly incidence scans).[12] After these 4 years, 1118 participants (74%) had nodules of at least 4 mm detected by LDCT. Sixty-six participants (4%) were ultimately diagnosed with lung cancer. Of these, 61% were stage 1, with a lung cancer mortality rate of 2.8%. Although these numbers seem encouraging, the authors note that this was not significantly different from the mortality rates in the chest radiograph Mayo Lung Project. The authors concluded that LDCT scans could detect early stage lung cancers but had no significant effect on mortality. These findings raised the concern that, similar to chest radiographs, LDCTs might diagnose more early stage lung cancers without decreasing late-stage cancer rates, resulting in overdiagnosis with no effect on mortality. Interestingly, 26% percent of patients had nodules missed on the baseline scan (false-negative rate). Additionally, the authors noted a high rate of benign disease (false-positive rate) and warned about potential complications and expense incurred in the work-up of these benign lesions.

The Early Lung Cancer Action Program (ELCAP) screened patients aged 60 or older with at least a 10 pack-year history of cigarette smoking with LDCT.[13,14] The baseline scan (31,567 participants) detected a pulmonary nodule in 4186 (13%) participants, and the subsequent annual incidence scans (27,456 total annual screens) found a new nodule in 1460 (5%) participants. Of these, nodules found on baseline scans were confirmed as lung cancer in 405 patients or 1.2% of all baseline screening tests and 9.7% of positive baseline screens (ie, nodule identified). Of the incidence screens, 74 proved to be cancer, for a rate of 0.2% of all incidence screens and 5.1% of positive incidence screens. An additional 13 cases of lymphoma or metastasis from a distant, nonpulmonary site were diagnosed by either baseline or annual chest LDCT. Most lung cancers diagnosed (85%) were stage 1, and the estimated 10-year survival rate of this subgroup was 88%. A biopsy was performed in 535 patients, of whom 92% had cancer, with benign disease being reported in the remaining 8% of patients. These results are striking in the rate of stage 1 cancers diagnosed, the estimated low mortality associated with early diagnosis, and the arguably low rate of biopsy for benign processes. However, the absence of a control group ultimately limits this study.

The Detection and Screening of Early Lung Cancer by Novel Imaging Technology and Molecular Essays (DANTE) trial was a randomized, controlled lung cancer screening trial comparing 5 annual LDCTs to no screening.[15] The trial included 2811 men, aged 60 to 75 years with at least a 20 pack-year history of smoking, and half of the participants were randomized to the screening arm and half to the control arm. Subjects were followed for a median of 33.7 months. Similar to previous screening studies, there was a significant increase in lung cancers diagnosed with screening LDCTs (60 vs 34). However, the 2 arms had similar rates of advanced lung cancer, and screening again no effect on lung cancer-specific or all-cause mortality. The rate of invasive procedures (eg, video-assisted thoracoscopic surgery) was significantly higher in the screening arm compared with the control arm. Like prior single arm LDCT trials, DANTE indicated that lung cancer screening with LDCT scans might result in overdiagnosis and a high false-positive rate and that LDCT likely leads to unnecessary procedures that do not affect mortality. Though the DANTE trial was an advance over prior LDCT studies in that it included a control group, interpretation of its results is hampered by its small size.

THE NLST—IMPROVED SURVIVAL WITH LDCT

The NLST is the first large, randomized controlled trial of screening using LDCT in patients at high risk for lung cancer. The trial enrolled 53,454 participants (men and women) between 55 and 74 years of age with at least a 30 pack-year history of smoking. Additionally, if not currently smoking, subjects must have quit within the previous 15 years.[16] Participants were enrolled between August 2002 and April 2004, during which period the screening group (26,723 subjects) underwent an initial prevalence scan followed by 2 annual incidence scans. The control group (26,733 subjects) underwent yearly chest radiographs. The median follow-up of patients in both arms was 6.5 years, and the maximum follow-up was 7.4 years. Over 90% of participants in each arm followed the protocol during both years of screening.

Over 2 years, 24.2% of scans in the LDCT group and 6.9% of chest radiographs in the control group were classified as abnormal (ie, positive). Of these, 96.4% were ultimately found to be false positives in the LDCT arm compared with 94.5% in the chest radiograph arm. During the 2 years of screening, 649 lung cancers were diagnosed in the LDCT group compared with 279 lung cancers detected in the chest radiograph group. At the completion of follow-up, 1060 and 941 lung cancers had been diagnosed in the LDCT and chest radiograph groups, respectively. The LDCT participants were more likely to have stage 1 or 2 cancer than those who were screened with chest radiographs. The lung cancer mortality rate was 247 deaths per 100,000 person-years in the LDCT group and 309 deaths per 100,000 person-years in the chest radiograph group. The relative risk of lung cancer mortality was decreased 20.3% by LDCT screening (95% confidence interval [CI], 6.8%–26.7% $P = .004$), and the number needed to screen to prevent 1 lung cancer death with LDCT was 320. This study was the first trial to demonstrate that lung cancer screening with CT scans can decrease mortality.

POTENTIAL RISKS OF LDCT SCREENING

Although the NLST demonstrated that LDCT screening can improve survival in patients at risk for lung cancer, screening opens patients to the risk of radiation exposure as well as increased cost and physical and emotional morbidity associated with follow-up of identified nodules. Increased radiation exposure secondary to LDCT screening is a concern given the heightened risk of cancer secondary to radiation. As stated previously, the dose of radiation with an LDCT is 1.5 mSv compared with a dose of 7 mSv from a conventional chest CT.[9] However, a positive scan usually results in further imaging, including diagnostic CT or positron emission tomography

(PET) scanning, raising the cumulative radiation exposure. Even given this, it has been estimated that in high-risk patients (as defined by NLST), the benefits of LDCT screening outweigh risks of radiation-induced cancer.[17] However, in people at low risk of lung cancer, for example nonsmokers or younger individuals, the risks of radiation-induced cancer likely are greater than the risk of lung cancer.[18]

The evaluation of clinically inconsequential processes found by LDCT is an additional risk of screening. Given the increase in lung cancers detected by LDCT compared with chest radiograph during NLST, overdiagnosis of cancers that do not affect mortality is again likely. It is notable that most of the increase in lung cancers diagnosed by LDCT in the NLST consisted of bronchioalveolar carcinomas (BACs); LDCT diagnosed 119 more cancers than chest radiographs, and 75 of these were BACs. In contrast, other histologic forms of lung cancer were diagnosed at similar rates in both the LDCT and the chest radiograph arms. True BAC, newly classified as adenocarcinoma in situ (AIS), is a slowly growing process with little impact on mortality.[19,20] The evaluation and treatment of cancers that likely would not affect mortality expose patients to un-needed risk and cost. In addition, the evaluation of nodules ultimately found to be benign further raises concerns for excess morbidity and expense. In the NLST, the rate of serious complications resulting from invasive diagnostic and therapeutic procedures for patients who ultimately did not have cancer was 15%. However, the entry criteria for NLST included participants at higher risk for lung cancer when compared with other LDCT trials. Lung cancer occurs frequently in patients outside the age range of NLST and with fewer pack-years of smoking,[21] and when applied to a population defined by a broader risk profile, LDCT screening likely would detect more lung cancers but also more benign processes (false positives). The Fleischner Society, which has created guidelines for the evaluation and management of pulmonary nodules (**Table 1**), broadly categorizes patients as high risk if they have "a history of smoking or other known risk factors."[22]

Given the inherent risks of LDCT screening, there is a need to define more accurately the at-risk population that would most benefit from screening. NLST data suggest that screening is efficacious in a high-risk population, but a uniform definition of high risk does not exist. Several models have been created to help predict the risk of developing lung cancer in a given individual, using clinical risk factors such as smoking history, age, asbestos exposure, and prior history of malignancy.[23–25] Use of these models can further define

Table 1
Fleischner Society guidelines for the evaluation of noncalcified pulmonary nodules detected incidentally by nonscreening CT

Nodule Size (mm)[a]	≤4	>4–6	>6–8	>8
Low- Risk Patient[b]	No follow-up needed[c]	Repeat CT at 12 mo; if unchanged, no further follow-up[d]	Repeat CT at 6–12 mo and 18–24 mo if no change	Repeat CT at 3, 9, and 24 mo; dynamic contrast-enhanced CT, PET, and/or biopsy
High-Risk Patient[e]	Repeat CT at 12 mo; if unchanged, no further follow-up[d]	Repeat CT at 6–12 mo and 18–24 mo if no change[d]	Repeat CT at 3–6 mo and 9–12 and 24 mo if no change	Same as for low-risk patient

[a] Average of length and width.
[b] Minimal or absent history of smoking and of other known risk factors.
[c] The risk of malignancy in this category (1%) is substantially less than that in a baseline CT scan of an asymptomatic smoker.
[d] Ground-glass or partly solid nodules may require longer follow-up to exclude indolent adenocarcinoma.
[e] History of smoking or of other known risk factors.
   Data from MacMahon H, Austin JH, Gamsu G, et al. Guidelines for management of small pulmonary nodules detected on CT scans: a statement from the Fleischner Society. Radiology 2005;237(2):398.

a population at risk that might benefit from screening. Even within the inclusion criteria of the NLST, the predicted rate of lung cancer is not uniform, and increases with age, smoking history, and exposure to other lung cancer risk factors. For example, Bach and Gould have calculated that when applied to a person with a high risk of lung cancer (eg, older person with 110 pack-year history of smoking), the number needed to screen to prevent a cancer death is 82, while for a person meeting NLST study criteria but with minimal risk (eg, age 55, 30 pack-year history, recently quit smoking), the number needed to screen to prevent a single cancer death is 1236.[26] When screening is applied to a very low-risk population of 40-year-old nonsmokers, over 35,000 people would require LDCT screening to prevent 1 death.[26]

Clearly a better method to define risk of lung cancer is needed. The identification and use of biomarkers of lung cancer might refine the population of those high-risk patients who would most benefit from screening, thereby increasing specificity and decreasing the number of benign nodules identified by CT. One tool to improve specificity of CT screening for lung cancer screening is nodule volume doubling time. The Dutch-Belgian lung cancer screening trial studied the change in nodule volume over time, as measured on CT scans, as a mechanism of differentiating benign from malignant nodules. This strategy is based on the idea that cancers increase in size at a greater rate than benign processes. The authors determined that a long volume doubling

Box 1
Recommendations from the American College of Chest Physicians and the American Society of Clinical Oncology on the role of CT screening for lung cancer

Recommendation #1

Annual screening should be offered over both annual screening with chest radiograph or no screening to smokers and former smokers aged 55 to 74 years who have smoked for 30 pack-years or more and either continue to smoke or have quit within the past 15 years. Screening should only be done by centers that can deliver the evaluation and care provided to NLST participants (grade of recommendation: 2B).

Recommendation #2

No CT screening should not be performed for individuals who have accumulated fewer than 30 pack-years of smoking and are either younger than 55 years or older than 74 years, or for individuals who quit smoking more than 15 years ago, or for individuals with severe comorbidities that would preclude potentially curative treatment and limit life expectancy (grade of recommendation: 2C).

Adapted from Bach PB, Mirkin JN, Oliver TK, et al. Benefits and harms of CT screening for lung cancer: a systematic review. JAMA 2012;307(22):2427; with permission.

time (>400 days) predicted benign disease and might be used to reduce invasive follow-up diagnostic testing. Additionally, biologic markers, including changes in gene expression patterns,[27] exhaled breath analysis for volatile compounds,[28] serum measurement of proteins,[29] and tumor autoantibodies[30] have all been studied as possible diagnostic tools for early detection of lung cancer and may help define a high-risk population that might benefit from screening.

SUMMARY

The NLST proved that LDCT screening for lung cancer decreases mortality. Based on existing data, the American College of Chest Physicians and the American Society of Clinical Oncology created a clinical practice guideline for lung cancer screening using LDCT (**Box 1**).[17] However, several questions remain regarding how a screening program might be implemented. First, the optimal interval of screening is unknown. Most LDCT trials have investigated yearly screening; however, how more or less frequent screening would affect the sensitivity and specificity of LDCT screening is unclear. Additionally, how long to screen individuals remains unknown. The NLST had similar rates of lung cancer incidence in each of the 3 years of screening, as well as during the follow-up period after screening, suggesting that a longer screening period would continue to diagnose new lung cancers. Almost certainly, the NLST will result in increased LDCT screening for lung cancer. How this affects lung cancer mortality in general practice remains to be seen.

REFERENCES

1. Jemal A, Bray F, Center MM, et al. Global cancer statistics. CA Cancer J Clin 2011;61(2):69–90.
2. Siegel R, Naishadham D, Jemal A. Cancer statistics, 2012. CA Cancer J Clin 2012;62(1):10–29.
3. Centers for Disease Control and Prevention (CDC). Current cigarette smoking prevalence among working adults—United States, 2004-2010. MMWR Morb Mortal Wkly Rep 2011;60(38):1305–9.
4. Fontana RS, Sanderson DR, Woolner LB, et al. Lung cancer screening: the Mayo program. J Occup Med 1986;28(8):746–50.
5. Marcus PM, Bergstralh EJ, Fagerstrom RM, et al. Lung cancer mortality in the Mayo Lung Project: impact of extended follow-up. J Natl Cancer Inst 2000;92(16):1308–16.
6. Frost JK, Ball WC Jr, Levin ML, et al. Early lung cancer detection: results of the initial (prevalence) radiologic and cytologic screening in the Johns Hopkins study. Am Rev Respir Dis 1984;130(4):549–54.
7. Kubik A, Polak J. Lung cancer detection. Results of a randomized prospective study in Czechoslovakia. Cancer 1986;57(12):2427–37.
8. Oken MM, Hocking WG, Kvale PA, et al. Screening by chest radiograph and lung cancer mortality: the Prostate, Lung, Colorectal, and Ovarian (PLCO) randomized trial. JAMA 2011;306(17):1865–73.
9. Mettler FA Jr, Huda W, Yoshizumi TT, et al. Effective doses in radiology and diagnostic nuclear medicine: a catalog. Radiology 2008;248(1):254–63.
10. Kaneko M, Eguchi K, Ohmatsu H, et al. Peripheral lung cancer: screening and detection with low-dose spiral CT versus radiography. Radiology 1996;201(3):798–802.
11. Sone S, Takashima S, Li F, et al. Mass screening for lung cancer with mobile spiral computed tomography scanner. Lancet 1998;351(9111):1242–5.
12. Swensen SJ, Jett JR, Hartman TE, et al. CT screening for lung cancer: five-year prospective experience. Radiology 2005;235(1):259–65.
13. Henschke CI, McCauley DI, Yankelevitz DF, et al. Early lung cancer action project: overall design and findings from baseline screening. Lancet 1999;354(9173):99–105.
14. Henschke CI, Yankelevitz DF, Libby DM, et al. Survival of patients with stage I lung cancer detected on CT screening. N Engl J Med 2006;355(17):1763–71.
15. Infante M, Cavuto S, Lutman FR, et al. A randomized study of lung cancer screening with spiral computed tomography: three-year results from the DANTE trial. Am J Respir Crit Care Med 2009;180(5):445–53.
16. Aberle DR, Adams AM, Berg CD, et al. Reduced lung-cancer mortality with low-dose computed tomographic screening. N Engl J Med 2011; 365(5):395–409.
17. Bach PB, Mirkin JN, Oliver TK, et al. Benefits and harms of CT screening for lung cancer: a systematic review. JAMA 2012;307(22):2418–29.
18. Berrington de Gonzalez A, Kim KP, Berg CD. Low-dose lung computed tomography screening before age 55: estimates of the mortality reduction required to outweigh the radiation-induced cancer risk. J Med Screen 2008;15(3):153–8.
19. Travis WD, Brambilla E, Noguchi M, et al. International Association for the Study of Lung Cancer/American Thoracic Society/European Respiratory Society international multidisciplinary classification of lung adenocarcinoma. J Thorac Oncol 2011; 6(2):244–85.
20. Russell PA, Wainer Z, Wright GM, et al. Does lung adenocarcinoma subtype predict patient survival? A clinicopathologic study based on the new International Association for the Study of Lung Cancer/American Thoracic Society/European Respiratory Society international multidisciplinary lung adenocarcinoma classification. J Thorac Oncol 2011;6(9):1496–504.

21. Heuvers ME, Aerts JG, Hegmans JP, et al. History of tuberculosis as an independent prognostic factor for lung cancer survival. Lung Cancer 2012;76(3): 452–6.

22. MacMahon H, Austin JH, Gamsu G, et al. Guidelines for management of small pulmonary nodules detected on CT scans: a statement from the Fleischner Society. Radiology 2005;237(2):395–400.

23. Tammemagi CM, Pinsky PF, Caporaso NE, et al. Lung cancer risk prediction: prostate, lung, colorectal, and ovarian cancer screening trial models and validation. J Natl Cancer Inst 2011;103(13):1058–68.

24. Cassidy A, Myles JP, van Tongeren M, et al. The LLP risk model: an individual risk prediction model for lung cancer. Br J Cancer 2008;98(2):270–6.

25. Spitz MR, Etzel CJ, Dong Q, et al. An expanded risk prediction model for lung cancer. Cancer Prev Res (Phila) 2008;1(4):250–4.

26. Bach PB, Gould MK. When the average applies to no one: personalized decision making about potential benefits of lung cancer screening. Ann Intern Med 2012;157(8):571–3.

27. Spira A, Beane JE, Shah V, et al. Airway epithelial gene expression in the diagnostic evaluation of smokers with suspect lung cancer. Nat Med 2007; 13(3):361–6.

28. Mazzone PJ. Analysis of volatile organic compounds in the exhaled breath for the diagnosis of lung cancer. J Thorac Oncol 2008;3(7):774–80.

29. Ostroff RM, Bigbee WL, Franklin W, et al. Unlocking biomarker discovery: large-scale application of aptamer proteomic technology for early detection of lung cancer. PLoS One 2010;5(12):e15003.

30. Boyle P, Chapman CJ, Holdenrieder S, et al. Clinical validation of an autoantibody test for lung cancer. Ann Oncol 2011;22(2):383–9.

Early Lung Cancer
Methods for Detection

Takahiro Nakajima, MD, PhD[a],
Kazuhiro Yasufuku, MD, PhD[a,b],*

KEYWORDS

- Lung cancer • Early detection • Autofluorescence bronchoscopy • Narrow-band imaging
- Endobronchial ultrasonography • Optical coherence tomography • Endocytoscopy

KEY POINTS

- Recent advances in bronchology have allowed bronchoscopists to evaluate the airway with advanced high-resolution imaging modalities.
- Centrally arising squamous cell carcinoma of the airway, especially in heavy smokers, is thought to develop through multiple stages from squamous metaplasia to dysplasia, followed by carcinoma in situ, progressing to invasive cancer.
- Early detection is the key to improved survival.
- It would be ideal to be able to detect and treat preinvasive bronchial lesions, defined as dysplasia and carcinoma in situ before progressing to invasive cancer.

INTRODUCTION

Lung cancer is the leading cause of cancer mortality worldwide.[1] Despite evolving knowledge of lung cancer, molecular genetics, and improved technology for the detection of lung cancer, the overall survival for lung cancer is still quite poor (5 year survival 17%).[2] A recent study showed a dramatic, 20% relative decrease in lung cancer–specific mortality with low-dose computed tomography (CT) screening in high-risk groups,[3] proving the concept that early detection of lung cancer that allows prompt surgical intervention offers survival benefit. However, although screening CT of the thorax detects smaller, central, and peripheral lung lesions, it is insensitive for detection of microscopic tumors arising from the airways.[4]

Microscopic tumors arising in the central airways require other techniques for early detection.

Squamous cell carcinomas, accounting for approximately 25% to 30% of all lung cancers, arise in central airways. Pathobiologically, progression from normal bronchial epithelium to squamous metaplasia followed by dysplasia, carcinoma in situ (CIS), and finally invasive carcinoma, has been well described.[5,6] Studies have shown that patients with moderate to severe dysplasia progress to develop invasive carcinoma over the course of 3 to 4 years. Approximately 11% of patients with moderate dysplasia, and 19% to as much as 50% of patients with severe dysplasia develop invasive carcinoma.[7–9] Patients with chronic obstructive pulmonary disease (COPD) or heavy smoking history were associated

Funding Sources: Kanae Foundation for the Promotion of Medical Science (T. Nakajima); None (K. Yasufuku).
Conflict of Interest: None (T. Nakajima); unrestricted grant from Olympus Medical Systems Corp for Continuing Medical Education (K. Yasufuku).
a Division of Thoracic Surgery, Toronto General Hospital, University Health Network, University of Toronto, 200 Elizabeth Street, 9N-957, Toronto, Ontario M5G 2C4, Canada; b Interventional Thoracic Surgery Program, Division of Thoracic Surgery, Toronto General Hospital, University Health Network, University of Toronto, 200 Elizabeth Street, 9N-957, Toronto, Ontario M5G 2C4, Canada
* Corresponding author.
E-mail address: kazuhiro.yasufuku@uhn.ca

with a higher risk of development of lung cancer or CIS from dysplasia.[10] Therefore, prompt detection through screening of high-risk patients (especially heavy smokers) could potentially offer early diagnosis of preinvasive or invasive lesions, allowing for prompt therapeutic intervention and improved survival. However, the conventional airway imaging modality, white-light bronchoscopy (WLB), has been shown to be relatively insensitive in inspection of the bronchial mucosa, with only 30% sensitivity in detecting early-stage carcinoma in the central airways.[11]

New bronchoscopic modalities with higher spatial resolution are able to take advantage of intrinsic properties of healthy and abnormal tissues to change their appearance when illuminated with different wavelengths of light. These methods have been developed to serve the purpose of more advanced central airway imaging for the purpose of abnormal airway diagnosis. Currently available clinical practice modalities include autofluorescence bronchoscopy (AFB), high-magnification bronchovideoscopy (HMB), and narrow-band imaging (NBI). More precise airway inspection can be obtained with radial probe endobronchial ultrasonography (EBUS) and optical coherence tomography (OCT).[4] Recently, the endocytoscopy bronchoscopy system has allowed in vivo microscopic imaging of the bronchial mucosa and has enabled the differential diagnosis of normal bronchial epithelial cells, bronchial squamous dysplastic cells, and malignant squamous cells.[12] Confocal fluorescence microendoscopy is another useful technique, allowing in vivo microscopic assessment of the airway basement membrane and alveolar components.[13] However, the endocytoscopy system and confocal fluorescence microendoscopy are currently only used in an experimental research setting.

AUTOFLUORESCENCE BRONCHOSCOPY

AFB improves the sensitivity for detection of preinvasive lesions in the central airway.[11] AFB increases the diagnostic accuracy for squamous dysplasia, CIS, and early lung carcinoma when used simultaneously with conventional WLB.[11] It is a technique of advanced mucosal airway examination, taking advantage of the property of the normal, preneoplastic, and neoplastic tissues to change appearance when illuminated with different wavelengths of light depending on differential epithelial thickness, tissue blood flow, and fluorophore concentration. Preinvasive and neoplastic tissues express diminished red and subsequently green autofluorescence in comparison with normal tissues when illuminated with

blue light (440–480 nm wavelength).[14] Natural tissue chromophores (elastin, collagen, flavins, nicotinamide adenine dinucleotide, nicotinamide adenine dinucleotide hydrogen [NADH]) emit light when their electrons return to ground level after being excited with light of a specific wavelength. The low level of tissue autofluorescence cannot be picked up with WLB, given the "noise" from the high degree of background reflected and backscattered light. However, AFB selectively picks up the subtle changes in natural tissue autofluorescence patterns. Tissue metaplasia, dysplasia, and neoplasia reduce natural concentrations of airway chromophores (diminished expression of riboflavin, flavin, and NADH owing to increased anaerobic metabolism and lactic acid production).[15] Higher neoplastic tissue blood flow increases light absorption by the hemoglobin. Malignant tissue proliferation, even if only microscopic at first, results in a higher degree of light scattering by tissue hyperplasia. These changes result in an overall diminished green autofluorescence in tissue, with the abnormal tissue assuming a red-brown color.[16] These initially subtle mucosal changes are identifiable by WLB in less than 30% of cases, even by experienced bronchoscopists. AFB is highly sensitive for the detection of preinvasive and invasive lesions, but lacks specificity for detection of preinvasive lesions. It often cannot differentiate between the areas of high blood flow and metabolism occurring in chronic inflammatory states such as bronchitis.

Different AFB imaging systems have been developed with slightly different sensitivity for the detection of the mucosal abnormalities. Continuous improvement of AFB devices allows for increased specificity. LIFE (Xillix Technologies, Vancouver, Canada) uses a helium-cadmium laser light source, with 2 image-intensifier charge-coupled device (CCD) cameras and a color video monitor for imaging. In the SAFE-1000 system (Pentax; Asahi Optical, Tokyo, Japan), a conventional Xenon light equipped with a special filter was used as an excitation light source instead of laser light. The SAFE-3000 system (Pentax; HOYA Corp, Tokyo, Japan) incorporated single-action image switching and simultaneous display. Storz D-light (Storz, Tuttlingen, Germany) and Onco-LIFE systems (Xillix Technologies) combine autofluorescence and reflected light, resulting in slightly different sensitivities in comparison with WLB for the detection of premalignant and malignant mucosal abnormalities. Autofluorescence imaging (AFI) (Olympus Medical System Corp, Tokyo, Japan) is a new AFB system. AFI demonstrated improvement over the LIFE AFB system for specificity (83% vs 36.6%), but had slightly lower sensitivity (80% vs 96.7%) in the detection of preinvasive and invasive bronchial lesions.[17] The improved discriminatory nature of the AFI system results from its ability to integrate 3 signals: an autofluorescence signal with reflected green and red light signals.[18] The composite image displayed depicts normal epithelium as light green; areas of abundant blood flow, seen not only in malignant epithelium but also in areas of chronic benign inflammation, as dark green; and malignant tissue as a magenta color (**Fig. 1**).[17]

Multiple studies demonstrated that AFB improves detection of preinvasive central airway lesions and, when combined with WLB, also of squamous dysplasia, CIS, and early lung carcinoma.[11,14–29] A recent meta-analysis of 21 studies comparing WLB used with AFB versus WLB alone in the diagnosis of intraepithelial neoplasia and invasive lung cancer involving 3266 patients reported a pooled relative sensitivity of 2.04 (95% confidence interval [CI] 1.72–2.42) on a per-lesion basis in favor of a combined AFB and WLB approach.[18] However, as documented in previous individual studies, the sensitivity for detection of CIS and early invasive carcinomas was not superior to WLB alone (relative risk of 1.15 at 95% CI 1.05–1.26).[18] This finding suggests that while screening invasive cancer, WLB may be sufficient and more cost effective.

Use of the Raman spectrophotometry system in addition to AFB and WLB may offer improved specificity (91%) in the detection of preinvasive lesions, with only minor compromise in sensitivity (96%) as documented by a recent pilot study.[30] Laser Raman spectroscopy (LRS), currently used only in an experimental setting, involves exposing the tissue to low-power laser light and collecting the scattered light for spectroscopic analyses.[31] This technology collects spectra nondestructively, and light scattered from tissues with different molecular composition can be easily differentiated. Using this technology can potentially reduce the number of false-positive biopsies in the detection of preneoplastic lesions. Use of Raman spectra with AFB and WLB can offer a more objective airway mucosal assessment and detect more preneoplastic lesions. Also, Raman may be able to identify biomolecular changes in histologically preneoplastic and non-preneoplastic lesions that could be markers for development of late-stage malignancy. More studies are needed to assess the addition of this technology to the armamentarium of tools for the detection of endobronchial neoplasia.

AFB has also been shown to increase detection sensitivity of recurrent or new intraepithelial neoplasias and invasive carcinomas when added to WLB (from 25% for WLB alone to 75% when AFB is used in conjunction with WLB) in postoperative surveillance of patients who underwent curative resection for non–small cell lung cancer.[32] AFB combined with CT of the thorax in patients with radiographically suspicious and occult lung cancer has shown to be an effective staging and tumor extension assessment modality for lung cancer, with some impact on choice of therapeutic strategy.[33,34]

AFB can become a useful tool in the screening detection of endobronchial premalignant and malignant lesions, especially in high-risk groups (patients with head and neck cancers and COPD, and smokers), given that the incidence of synchronous lesions ranges from 0.7% to 15% and that metachronous lesions might occur in as many as 5% of high-risk patients annually.[35,36] However, more studies are needed to determine how the

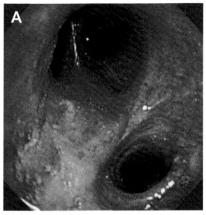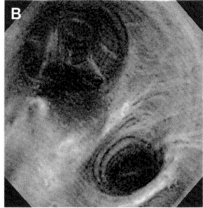

Fig. 1. Autofluorescence bronchoscopy images of representative cases of carcinoma in situ. White-light bronchoscopy (*A*) and corresponding autofluorescence bronchoscopy image (*B*). (*Courtesy of* Olympus Medical Systems Corp, Tokyo, Japan; with permission.)

AFB can best be incorporated into clinical practice in an economically efficient way and with reasonable reduction in mortality from lung cancer.

The molecular mechanism of the development of squamous cell carcinoma through multiple stages from squamous metaplasia to dysplasia, followed by CIS, and progressing to invasive cancer, has been revealed by research using biopsy samples during AFB. Increased telomerase activity and elevated hTERT (human telomerase reverse transcriptase) mRNA expression is reported to be associated with early as well as later stages of carcinogenesis.[37] Recently, biomarkers that can predict the risk of lung cancer in AFB-detected squamous metaplastic lesions were analyzed, and the presence of specific DNA copy-number alterations predicted cancer development with 97% accuracy.[38]

NARROW-BAND IMAGING

Focusing on the visualization of the vascular network in the bronchial mucosa, a new imaging technology termed narrow-band imaging was developed after the high-magnification broncho-videoscope.[39,40] NBI is a new optical imaging technology classified as an image-enhancement endoscopy using special blue and green light wavelengths, allowing for enhanced visualization of microvascular structures in the mucosal and submucosal layers.[41–44] NBI is an optical image technology that enhances vessels in the surface mucosa by using the light absorption characteristics of hemoglobin at a specific wavelength. NBI uses wavelengths at 415 nm (blue light) and 540 nm (green light). Narrow bandwidths reduce the mucosal light scattering and enable enhanced visualization of endobronchial microvasculature structures. The 415-nm blue light is absorbed by the superficial capillary vessels, whereas the 540-nm wavelength is absorbed by the

hemoglobin in the deeper, submucosal vessels. Blood vessels near the surface of the mucosa appear brown, and vessels deeper in the mucosa appear as cyan (**Fig. 2**).

In addition to molecular changes allowing autonomous progression of cell cycle that imparts metastatic potential, cancer cells must develop extended angiogenic capabilities allowing for rapid growth and invasion. A multistep angiogenesis process has been described in epithelial tumors.[45,46] To fulfill the high metabolic demands of a rapidly dividing tumor, neoplastic cells have to develop enhanced angiogenic capabilities. Animal and human invasive neoplasia pathogenesis studies suggest that a so-called angiogenic switch occurs in preinvasive lesions before the formation of invasive tumor.[47,48] Because squamous cell cancer is thought to progress through its developmental stage from squamous cell metaplasia to dysplasia and CIS, detection of each of these stages could have a significant impact on therapeutic interventions and prognosis.

NBI shows higher sensitivity than AFB in the detection of metaplastic and moderately dysplastic bronchial mucosal squamous lesions. It has equivalent sensitivity to AFB in the detection of early preinvasive malignant lesions (CIS) and invasive cancer (ranging between 90% and 100% for NBI and 83% and 89.2% for AFB). However, NBI has a higher specificity than AFB for the detection of early lung cancer.[49]

Combining AFB and NBI increases both sensitivity (93.7%) and specificity (86.9%) of the detection of early lung cancer, but the improvement is small in comparison with each technique alone. Therefore, combining the 2 technologies in the detection of cancerous and precancerous lesion does not have a significant impact on diagnostic accuracy, and may result in unnecessary cost without significant clinical benefit. Judging by the results of the studies, NBI can be used as an

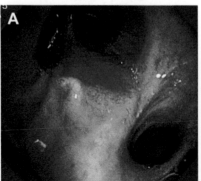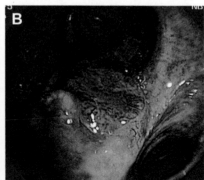

Fig. 2. Narrow-band imaging. White-light bronchoscopy (*A*) and narrow-band (*B*) images of carcinoma in situ. Dotted vessel and tortuous vessels are identified on narrow-band imaging.

alternative to AFB in the screening of cancerous and precancerous lesion of the endobronchial epithelium, without compromising sensitivity and with significant improvement in specificity.[50]

Before NBI and AFB can be incorporated into screening for lung cancer, certain issues need to be addressed. First, the natural history of the squamous cell carcinoma and bronchial dysplasia must be better characterized. Squamous cell carcinoma represents a third of all lung cancers diagnosed in the United States.[1] It is thought that pathologically, invasive cancer results from a stepwise process that begins with metaplasia, then dysplasia, followed by CIS and, finally, invasive cancer. Previous studies showed development of invasive carcinoma in 40% to 83% of patients with severely dysplastic lesions.[7,51] However, animal models and human studies show spontaneous regression of some of the lesions.[52,53] Breuer and colleagues[53] documented a 9% to 32% rate of malignant transformation for all dysplastic lesions in 52 patients followed over an 8-year period. Fifty-four percent of spontaneous regressions of all preinvasive lesions, as well as non-stepwise transformation with development of invasive carcinoma at sites previously characterized as normal in appearance, have also been described. These findings suggest that development of squamous cell carcinoma may not always follow a classic stepwise transformation pattern. In addition, the population of patients at risk must be clearly identified and those with the highest risk lesions (most likely to progress to invasive cancer) should be screened. Finally, appropriate therapeutic options and a follow-up surveillance schedule must be developed, based on evidence, to decrease overall cancer mortality and recurrence.[54] Until all these issues have been addressed, AFB and NBI will be used predominantly in a research setting.

HIGH-MAGNIFICATION BRONCHOVIDEOSCOPY

HMB is a system that was developed to enhance detailed white-light observation of bronchial dysplasia. Increased thickening of the bronchial epithelium and increased vessel growth are thought to be related to the appearance of areas of abnormal fluorescence, suggesting roles for neovascularization or increased mucosal microvascular growth in bronchial dysplasia.[25,26] However, the only abnormality seen on WLB in dysplasia is swelling and redness at the bronchial bifurcations. HMB is a direct-view WLB system that has an outer diameter of 6 mm and can easily be inserted into the tracheobronchial tree. HMB combines 2 systems: a video observation system for high-magnification observation and a fiberoptic observation system for orientation of the bronchoscope tip. By combining 2 technologies in 1 bronchoscope, the 6-mm diameter bronchovideoscope allows bronchoscopists to use this for observation with a magnification 4-fold higher than that of the regular bronchovideoscope with a depth of 1 to 3 mm. The bronchial mucosa is observed minutely on a 14-inch TV monitor at a high magnification of $110\times$ at the nearest point.[55]

HMB has enabled observation of vascular networks within the bronchial mucosa in patients with respiratory disease such as asthma, chronic bronchitis, sarcoidosis, and lung cancer. Areas of increased vessel growth and complex networks of tortuous vessels in the bronchial mucosa that are detected using HMB at sites of abnormal fluorescence may allow clinicians to differentiate between bronchitis and dysplasia. In areas of abnormal fluorescence on AFB, HMB can detect dysplasia more accurately than AFB alone, with sensitivity of 70% and specificity of 90%.[55] HMB observation in patients with asthma showed that the vessel-area density and vessel-length density are significantly increased in comparison with control subjects.[56]

By using NBI and HMB, previous studies have shown angiogenesis and alteration in microvascular structure of bronchial dysplastic lesions at sites detected as abnormal autofluorescence.[57] Using NBI combined with HMB, Shibuya and colleagues[46] showed a statistically significant increase in capillary blood vessel diameter occurring as a tissue progresses from angiogenic squamous dysplasia (ASD) to CIS, microinvasive cancer, and invasive squamous cell carcinoma. Architectural organization of the vessels also differed between the premalignant and malignant lesions. A classification system was proposed based on the vascular appearance of endobronchial lesions of varying invasiveness, which showed a high correlation with the lesions' histopathologic features.[46,58] However, more studies using the classification are needed for further validation (**Fig. 3**).

The endocytoscopy system (ECS; Olympus Medical System Corp) is a recently introduced, emerging endoscopic imaging technique enabling real-time in vivo diagnosis of cellular patterns at extremely high magnification.[59] The tip of the instrument contains an optical magnifying lens system and CCD. This endoscope can be inserted through the 4.2-mm biopsy channel and Olympus mother bronchoscope to become an "endocytoscope". The ECS has a 570-fold magnification and provides an observation field of 300×300 μm, an observation depth of 0 to 30 μm, and spatial

	Squamous dysplasia	Angiogenic squamous dysplasia	Carcinoma in situ	Micro invasive	Invasive
Tortuous vessel networks	+	+	−	−	−
Dotted vessels	−	+	+	+ +	+ + +
Spiral and screw type vessels	−	−	+	+ +	+ + +

Fig. 3. Classification of narrow-band imaging. Classification of vessel morphology based on narrow-band imaging during pathogenesis of lung cancer. (*From* Shibuya K, Nakajima T, Fujiwara T, et al. Narrow band imaging with high-resolution bronchovideoscopy: a new approach for visualizing angiogenesis in squamous cell carcinoma of the lung. Lung Cancer 2010;69:201; with permission.)

resolution of 4.2 μm for bronchial imaging.[12] Shibuya and colleagues[12] reported that ECS was useful to discriminate between normal bronchial epithelial cells, dysplastic cells, and malignant cells during ongoing bronchoscopy (Fig. 4). Another group used ECS in 4 patients for the immediate in vivo diagnosis of small cell lung cancer during ongoing bronchoscopy. ECS was able to reliably identify numerous small blue cells with hyperchromatic nuclei, which were confirmed in an in vivo diagnosis of small cell lung cancer by corresponding histopathologic diagnosis.[60]

The confocal laser endomicroscopy system is another in vivo microscopic imaging device allowing the endoscopist to obtain real-time in vivo optical biopsies during ongoing endoscopy. The probe-based endomicroscopy system (Cellvizio; Mauna Kea Technologies, Paris, France), which is capable of passage through the accessory channel of a standard endoscope, is available.[61] Thiberville and colleagues[61] observed 27

preinvasive lesions (metaplasia and dysplasia) and 2 invasive lesions, and reported some specific basement membrane alterations within preinvasive lesions. Methylene blue is a potent fluorophore, and its application to the target makes it possible to reproducibly image the epithelial layer of the main bronchi as well as cellular patterns of peripheral solid lung nodules.[62] However, whether confocal laser endomicroscopy can discriminate among diseases requires additional studies.[13]

ENDOBRONCHIAL ULTRASONOGRAPHY AND OPTICAL COHERENCE TOMOGRAPHY

Two types of EBUS are currently available for clinical use. Radial-probe EBUS, first described in 1992, is used for the evaluation of bronchial-wall structure, visualization of detailed images of the surrounding structures for assisting transbronchial needle aspiration (TBNA), as well as detection of peripheral intrapulmonary nodules.[63] On the other

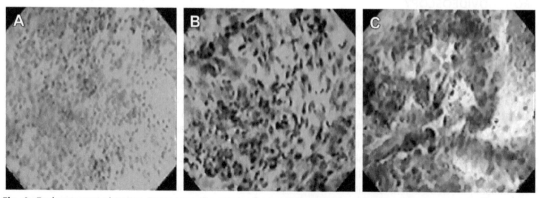

Fig. 4. Endocytoscopy images. Representative cases of normal bronchial epithelium (*A*), squamous cell carcinoma (*B*), and adenocarcinoma (*C*).

hand, the convex-probe EBUS first described in 2004 has a built-in ultrasound probe on a flexible bronchoscope, which enables bronchoscopists to perform real-time TBNA of mediastinal and hilar lesions.[63]

Premalignant lesions or small intrabronchial radiologically invisible tumors are being detected more frequently as a result of new advanced mucosal imaging technologies. The decision to use endoscopic therapeutic intervention depends on the extent of tumor within the different layers of the bronchial wall. Conventional radiologic imaging alone is not capable of distinguishing the tumor extent. Radial-probe EBUS is a sensitive method for the detection of alterations in the multilayer structure of the bronchial wall, even in small tumors. A comparison between the ultrasonographic and histologic findings in 24 cases of lung cancer revealed that the depth diagnosis was the same in 23 lesions (95.8%).[64] In another

study of a series of 15 patients, EBUS showed a high diagnostic yield of 93% for predicting tumor invasion into the tracheobronchial wall.[65] EBUS also improves the specificity (from 50% to 90%) for predicting malignancy in small AFB-positive lesions that were negative on WLB.[66]

Photodynamic therapy (PDT) is an alternative treatment for selected patients with central type early-stage lung cancer. EBUS was performed to evaluate tumor extent in 18 biopsy-proven early-stage squamous cell carcinomas (including 3 CIS).[67] Nine lesions were diagnosed as intracartilaginous by EBUS, and PDT was subsequently performed. The other 9 patients had extracartilaginous tumors unsuspected by CT and were considered candidates for other therapies such as surgical resection, chemotherapy, and radiotherapy. Using EBUS, a remission rate of 100% was achieved in the endoluminal-treated group (**Fig. 5**).

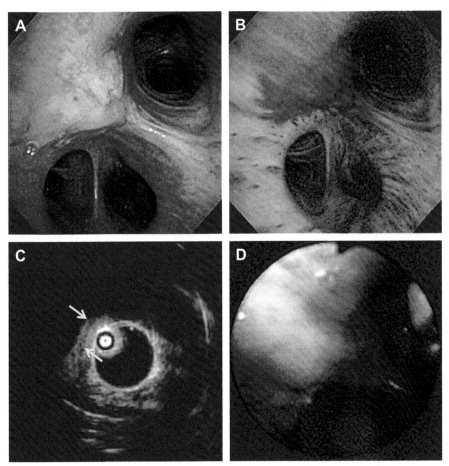

Fig. 5. Representative case of carcinoma in situ treated with photodynamic therapy. (*A*) Irregularity of mucosa was observed by white-light bronchoscopy (bifurcation of left upper and lower lobe bronchus). (*B*) Autofluorescence imaging showed magenta color for malignant tissue. (*C*) The lesion was diagnosed as intracartilaginous by radial-probe endobronchial ultrasonography. (*D*) Photodynamic therapy was subsequently performed. Arrows represent cartilaginous layer.

OCT is an optical imaging method that uses properties of light waves instead of sound waves.[68] OCT can generate high-resolution cross-sectional images of complex, living tissues in real time. Lam and colleagues[69] investigated the ability of OCT to discern the pathology of lung lesions identified by AFB in a group of high-risk smokers, and reported that normal or hyperplastic mucosa is characterized by 1 or 2 cell layers above a highly scattering basement membrane and upper submucosa. As the epithelium changes from normal/hyperplasia to metaplasia, various grades of dysplasia, and CIS, the thickness of the epithelial layer increases.[69] The basement membrane was still intact in CIS but became discontinuous or no longer visible with invasive cancer.[69] Michel and colleagues[70] examined 5 patients with endobronchial masses on chest imaging with OCT. OCT images showed differences between neoplasms and normal bronchial mucosa, and neoplastic lesions displayed irregular, ragged, dark lines between 2 light areas, which had the appearance of a fracture in the subepithelium.[70]

LRS is a novel technology that uses the Raman effect. Raman spectra can capture a fingerprint of specific molecular species and can therefore be potentially used to provide biochemical information about a given tissue or disease state.[68] Recently, results of a pilot study showed that LRS analysis in addition to autofluorescence bronchoscopic examination reduced the false-positive rate and achieved high sensitivity and specificity.[30]

SUMMARY

Recent advances in bronchology have allowed bronchoscopists to evaluate the airway with advanced high-resolution imaging modalities discussed herein. Centrally arising squamous cell carcinoma of the airway, especially in heavy smokers, is thought to develop through multiple stages from squamous metaplasia to dysplasia, followed by CIS, progressing to invasive cancer. Early detection is key to improved survival. It would be ideal to be able to detect and treat preinvasive bronchial lesions, defined as dysplasia and CIS before progressing to invasive cancer. Bronchoscopic imaging techniques capable of detecting preinvasive lesions currently available in clinical practice, including AFB, NBI, HMB, and EBUS, are discussed in this article. In addition, emerging techniques such as ECS, confocal laser endomicroscopy, OCT, and LRS are also introduced. These technologies are currently only available in a research setting, but may have a potential impact on the role of early detection of lung cancer.

AFB increases the diagnostic accuracy for squamous dysplasia, CIS, and early lung carcinoma when used simultaneously with conventional WLB. However, the specificity of AFB for detecting preinvasive lesions is moderate. AFB displays areas of epithelial thickness and hypervascularity as abnormal fluorescence, which suggests a role for neovascularization or increased mucosal microvascular growth in bronchial dysplasia. HMB enables visualization of these vascular networks. HMB can detect increased vessel growth and complex networks of tortuous vessels of various sizes in the bronchial mucosa. To further evaluate the vascular network in the bronchial mucosa, a new imaging technology, NBI, was developed and is now commercially available.

AFB and NBI are complementary for the evaluation of preinvasive bronchial lesions. The strength of AFB is its high sensitivity, acting as a monitor to pick up potentially neoplastic lesions. However, its potential limitation is moderate specificity. NBI, on the other hand, enhances the mucosal and vascular patterns, which is best suited for detailed inspection of the mucosa. A combination of autofluorescence and NBI into a single bronchovideoscope system would decrease the time for the procedure as well as unnecessary biopsies. For a bronchoscopist, AFB, NBI, and HMB are the same as performing a routine WLB without any necessary complicated procedures. Interpretation of the results seems to be fairly straightforward. Radial-probe EBUS is an excellent tool for the evaluation of the airway structure, which is useful for the determination of the depth of tumor invasion. Minimally invasive treatment may be suitable for selected patients with central type early-stage lung cancer.

REFERENCES

1. Siegel R, Ward E, Brawley O, et al. Cancer statistics, 2011: the impact of eliminating socioeconomic and racial disparities on premature cancer deaths. CA Cancer J Clin 2011;61:212–36.
2. Siegel R, Desantis C, Virgo K, et al. Cancer treatment and survivorship statistics, 2012. CA Cancer J Clin 2012;62:220–41.
3. The National Lung Screening Trial Research Team. Reduced lung cancer mortality with low-dose computed tomographic screening. N Engl J Med 2011;365:395–409.
4. Yasufuku K. Early diagnosis of lung cancer. In: Mehta A, editor. Clinics in chest medicine. Interventional Pulmonology. 2010:31(1);40–7.
5. Niklinski J, Niklinski W, Chyczewskis L, et al. Molecular genetic abnormalities in premalignant lung

lesions: biological and clinical implications. Eur J Cancer Prev 2001;10:213–26.

6. Thiberville L, Payne P, Vielkinds J, et al. Evidence of cumulative gene losses with progression of the premalignant epithelial lesions to carcinoma of the bronchus. Cancer Res 1995;155:5133–9.

7. Band PR, Feldstein M, Saccomanno G. Reversibility of bronchial marked atypia: implication for chemoprevention. Cancer Detect Prev 1986;9:157–60.

8. Venmans BJ, van Boxem TJ, Smith EF, et al. Outcome of bronchial carcinoma in situ. Chest 2000;117:1572–6.

9. Ikeda N, Hayashi A, Iwasaki K, et al. Comprehensive diagnostic bronchoscopy of central type early stage lung cancer. Lung Cancer 2007;56:295–302.

10. Alaa M, Shibuya K, Fujiwara T, et al. Risk of lung cancer in patients with preinvasive bronchial lesions followed by autofluorescence bronchoscopy and chest computed tomography. Lung Cancer 2011;72:303–8.

11. Lam S, Kennedy T, Unger M, et al. Localization of bronchial intraepithelial neoplastic lesions by fluorescence bronchoscopy. Chest 1998;113:696–702.

12. Shibuya K, Fujiwara T, Yasufuku K, et al. In vivo microscopic imaging of the bronchial mucosa using an endo-cytoscopy system. Lung Cancer 2011;72:184–90.

13. Filner JJ, Bonura EJ, Lau ST, et al. Bronchoscopic fibered confocal fluorescence microscopy image characteristics and pathologic correlations. J Bronchology Interv Pulmonol 2011;18:23–30.

14. Keith RL, Miller YE, Gemmill RM, et al. Angiogenic squamous dysplasia in bronchi of individuals at high risk for lung cancer. Clin Cancer Res 2000;6:1616–25.

15. Interventional bronchoscopy. In: Bolliger, editor. Progress in respiratory research, vol. 30. Cape Town, Mathur PN, Indianapolis, Switzerland: Springer Karger; 2000. p. 243.

16. Colt H, Murgu S. Interventional bronchoscopy form bench to bedside: new techniques for early lung cancer detection. In: Mehta A, editor. Clinics in chest medicine. Interventional pulmonology. 2010:31(1);29–37.

17. Chiyo M, Shibuya K, Hoshino H, et al. Effective detection of bronchial preinvasive lesions by a new autofluorescence imaging bronchovideoscope system. Lung Cancer 2005;48:307–13.

18. Sun J, Garfield D, Lam B. The role of autofluorescence bronchoscopy combined with white light bronchoscopy compared with white light alone in diagnosis of intraepithelial neoplasia and invasive lung cancer. J Thorac Oncol 2011;6:1336–44.

19. Van Rens M, Schramel F, Elbers J, et al. The clinical value of lung imaging autofluorescence endoscope for detecting synchronous lung cancer. Lung Cancer 2001;32:13–8.

20. Kusunoki Y, Imamura F, Uda H, et al. Early detection of lung cancer with laser-induced fluorescence endoscopy and spectrofluorometry. Chest 2000;118:1776–82.

21. Sato M, Sakurada A, Sagawa M, et al. Diagnostic results before and after induction of autofluorescence bronchoscopy in patients suspected of having lung cancer detected by sputum cytology in lung cancer mass screening. Lung Cancer 2001;32:247–53.

22. Pierard P, Martin B, Verdebout J, et al. Fluorescence bronchoscopy in high-risk patients—a comparison of LIFE and Pentax systems. J Bronchol 2001;8:254–9.

23. Chhajed PN, Shibuya K, Hoshino H, et al. A comparison of video and autofluorescence bronchoscopy in patients at high risk of lung cancer. Eur Respir J 2005;25:951–5.

24. Weigel TL, Kosco PJ, Dacic S, et al. Postoperative fluorescence bronchoscopic surveillance in non-small cell lung cancer patients. Ann Thorac Surg 2001;71:967–70.

25. Shibuya K, Fujisawa T, Hoshino H, et al. Fluorescence bronchoscopy in detection of preinvasive bronchial lesions in patients with sputum cytology suspicious or positive for malignancy. Lung Cancer 2001;32:19–25.

26. Haussinger K, Becker H, Stanzel F, et al. Autofluorescence bronchoscopy compared with white light bronchoscopy alone for the detection of precancerous lesions: a European randomised controlled multicentre trial. Thorax 2005;60:496–503.

27. Hirsch FR, Prindiville SA, Miller YE, et al. Fluorescence versus white light bronchoscopy for detection of preneoplastic lesions: a randomised study. J Natl Cancer Inst 2001;93:1385–91.

28. Ernst A, Simoff MJ, Mathur PN, et al. D-light autofluorescence in the detection of premalignant airway changes: a multicenter trial. J Bronchol 2005;12:133–8.

29. Edell E, Iam S, Pass H, et al. Detection and localization of intraepithelial neoplasia and invasive carcinoma using fluorescence-reflectance bronchoscopy—an international multicenter clinical trial. J Thorac Oncol 2009;4:49–54.

30. Short MA, Lam S, McWilliams AM, et al. Using laser Raman spectroscopy to reduce false positive of autofluorescence bronchoscopies. A pilot study. J Thorac Oncol 2011;6:1206–14.

31. Tu AT. Raman spectroscopy in biology: principles and applications. New York: Wiley; 1982.

32. Weigel TL, Yousem S, Dacic S, et al. Fluorescence bronchoscopic surveillance after curative surgical resection for non-small-cell lung cancer. Ann Surg Oncol 2000;7:176–80.

33. Sutedja TG, Codrington H, Risse EK, et al. Autofluorescence bronchoscopy improves staging of

radiographically occult lung cancer and has an impact on therapeutic strategy. Chest 2001;120: 1327–32.

34. Zaric B, Becker HD, Perin B, et al. Autofluorescence imaging videobronchoscopy improves assessment of tumor margins and affects therapeutic strategy in central lung cancer. Jpn J Clin Oncol 2010;40:139–45.

35. Furukawa K, Ikeda N, Miura T, et al. Is autofluorescence bronchoscopy needed to diagnose early bronchogenic carcinoma? Pro: autofluorescence bronchoscopy. J Bronchol 2003;10:64–9.

36. Pierard P, Vermylen P, Bosschaerts T, et al. Synchronous roentgenographically occult lung carcinoma in patients with resectable primary lung cancer. Chest 2000;7:176–80.

37. Shibuya K, Fujisawa T, Hoshino H, et al. Increased telomerase activity and elevated hTERT mRNA expression during multistage carcinogenesis of squamous cell carcinoma of the lung. Cancer 2001;92:849–55.

38. van Boerdonk RA, Sutedja TG, Snijders PJ, et al. DNA copy number alterations in endobronchial squamous metaplastic lesions predict lung cancer. Am J Respir Crit Care Med 2011;184:948–56.

39. Yamada G, Shijubo N, Kitada J, et al. Decreased subepithelial microvasculature observed by high magnification bronchovideoscope in the large airways of smokers. Intern Med 2008;47(18):1579–83.

40. Shibuya K, Hoshino H, Chiyo M, et al. High magnification bronchovideoscopy combined with narrow band imaging could detect capillary loops of angiogenic squamous dysplasia in heavy smokers at high risk for lung cancer. Thorax 2003;58:989–95.

41. Gono K, Obi T, Yamaguchi M, et al. Appearance of enhanced tissue features in narrow-band endoscopic imaging. J Biomed Opt 2004;9:568–77.

42. Gono K, Igarashi M, Obi T, et al. Multiple-discriminant analysis for white light-scattering spectroscopy and imaging of two layered tissue phantoms. Opt Lett 2004;29:971–3.

43. Tajiri H, Niwa H. Proposal for a consensus terminology in endoscopy: how should different endoscopic imaging techniques be grouped and defined? Endoscopy 2008;40:775–8.

44. Kaltenbach T, Sano Y, Friedland S, et al. American Gastroenterological Association (AGA) institute technology assessment on image-enhanced endoscopy. Gastroenterology 2008;134(3):27–40.

45. Hirsch FR, Franklin WA, Gazdar AF, et al. Early detection of lung cancer: clinical perspectives of recent advances in biology and radiology. Clin Cancer Res 2001;7:5–22.

46. Shibuya K, Nakajima T, Fujiwara T, et al. Narrow band imaging with high-resolution bronchovideoscopy: a new approach for visualizing angiogenesis in squamous cell carcinoma of the lung. Lung Cancer 2010;69:194–202.

47. Hanahan D, Folkman J. Patterns and emerging mechanisms of the angiogenic switch during tumorigenesis. Cell 1996;86:353–64.

48. Hanahan D, Inoue H, Nagai K, et al. The hallmarks of cancer. Cell 2000;100:57–70.

49. Herth FJ, Eberhardt R, Anantham D, et al. Narrow-band imaging bronchoscopy increases the specificity of bronchoscopic early lung cancer detection. J Thorac Oncol 2009;4:1060–5.

50. Zaric B, Perlin B, Becker H, et al. Combination of narrow band imaging (NBI) and autofluorescence imaging (AFI) videobronchoscopy in endoscopic assessment of lung cancer extension. Med Oncol 2012;29:1638–42.

51. Risse EK, Vooijs GP, van't Hoff MA. Diagnostic significance of 'severe dysplasia' in sputum cytology. Acta Cytol 1988;32:629–34.

52. Sawyer RW, Hammond WG, Teplitz RL, et al. Regression of bronchial epithelial cancer in hamsters. Ann Thorac Surg 1993;56:74–8.

53. Breuer RH, Pasic A, Smith EF, et al. The natural course of preneoplastic lesions in bronchial epithelium. Clin Cancer Res 2005;11:537–43.

54. Vincent B, Fraig M, Silvestri G. A pilot study of narrow-band imaging compared to white light bronchoscopy for evaluation of normal airways and premalignant and malignant airways disease. Chest 2007;131:1794–9.

55. Shibuya K, Hoshino H, Chiyo M, et al. Subepithelial vascular patterns in bronchial dysplasias using a high magnification bronchovideoscope. Thorax 2002;57:902–7.

56. Tanaka H, Yamada G, Sakai T, et al. Increased airway vascularity in newly diagnosed asthma using a high-magnification bronchovideoscope. Am J Respir Crit Care Med 2003;168:1495–9.

57. Kumaji Y, Inoue H, Nagai H, et al. Magnifying endoscopy, stereoscopic microscopy, and the microvascular architecture of superficial esophageal carcinoma. Endoscopy 2002;34:369–75.

58. Shibuya K, Nakajima T, Yasufuku K, et al. Narrow band imaging with high resolution bronchovideoscopy: a new approach to visualize angiogenesis in squamous cell carcinoma of the lung. Eur Respir J 2006;28(Suppl 50):601s.

59. Neumann H, Fuchs FS, Vieth M, et al. Review article: in vivo imaging by endocytoscopy. Aliment Pharmacol Ther 2011;33:1183–93.

60. Neumann H, Vieth M, Neurath MF, et al. In vivo diagnosis of small-cell lung cancer by endocytoscopy. J Clin Oncol 2011;29:e131–2.

61. Thiberville L, Moreno-Swirc S, Vercauteren T, et al. In vivo imaging of the bronchial wall microstructure

using fibered confocal fluorescence microscopy. Am J Respir Crit Care Med 2007;175:22–31.

62. Thiberville L, Salaün M, Lachkar S, et al. Confocal fluorescence endomicroscopy of the human airways. Proc Am Thorac Soc 2009;6:444–9.

63. Yasufuku K. Current clinical applications of endobronchial ultrasound. Expert Rev Respir Med 2010;4:491–8.

64. Kurimoto N, Murayama M, Yoshioka S, et al. Assessment of usefulness of endobronchial ultrasonography in determination of depth of tracheobronchial tumor invasion. Chest 1999;115:1500–6.

65. Tanaka F, Muro K, Yamasaki S, et al. Evaluation of tracheo-bronchial wall invasion using transbronchial ultrasonography (TBUS). Eur J Cardiothorac Surg 2000;17:570–4.

66. Herth FJ, Becker HD. EBUS for early lung cancer detection. J Bronchol 2003;10:249.

67. Miyazu Y, Miyazawa T, Kurimoto N, et al. Endobronchial ultrasonography in the assessment of centrally located early-stage lung cancer before photodynamic therapy. Am J Respir Crit Care Med 2002;165:832–7.

68. Ohtani K, Lee AM, Lam S. Frontiers in bronchoscopic imaging. Respirology 2012;17:261–9.

69. Lam S, Standish B, Baldwin C, et al. In vivo optical coherence tomography imaging of preinvasive bronchial lesions. Clin Cancer Res 2008;14:2006–11.

70. Michel RG, Kinasewitz GT, Fung KM, et al. Optical coherence tomography as an adjunct to flexible bronchoscopy in the diagnosis of lung cancer: a pilot study. Chest 2010;138:984–8.

EBUS-TBNA/Staging of Lung Cancer

David I. Fielding, FRACP, MD[a],*, Noriaki Kurimoto, MD[b]

KEYWORDS

- Endobronchial ultrasound • Transbronchial needle aspiration • Positron emission tomography/computed tomography • Lung cancer

KEY POINTS

- In the staging of mediastinal lymph nodes before lung cancer surgery, endobronchial ultrasound transbronchial needle aspirations (EBUS-TBNA) has proven to be highly sensitive and specific as well as safe.
- Although positron emission tomography/computed tomography (PET/CT) has been a major development in the preoperative workup of patients with lung cancer, EBUS-TBNA has superior test performance and PET/CT cannot be regarded as a substitute for tissue sampling with EBUS-TBNA.
- In general, EBUS-TBNA staging is needed for any patient with CT nodes greater than 1 cm in short axis, or PET-positive mediastinal nodes.
- Large studies of EUS staging have confirmed the place of sampling mediastinal nodes via the esophagus, giving complementary access to posterior and inferior lymph node stations.
- EBUS-TBNA can detect micrometastatic disease in CT-negative and PET-negative mediastinal nodes.

RADIOLOGY INVESTIGATIONS AND STAGING—COMPUTED TOMOGRAPHY, POSITRON EMISSION TOMOGRAPHY, POSITRON EMISSION TOMOGRAPHY/COMPUTED TOMOGRAPHY

By convention, computed tomography (CT) of mediastinal lymph nodes regarded nodes greater than 1 cm in the short axis to be abnormal.[1–4] It is widely known that this criterion lacks both sensitivity and specificity. Reported predictive ability of CT for mediastinal lymph node metastasis shows sensitivity ranges of 57% to 68% and specificity range of 76% to 82%. The advent of positron emission tomography (PET) scanning radically improved mediastinal node staging. Using the fluorine-18 fluorodeoxyglucose (FDG) tracer, positron emission tomography (PET) demonstrates abnormal metabolic uptake, which often precedes change in node size, providing a sensitivity of 79% to 85% and a specificity of 87% to 92%.[1–4]

Further studies over the last 10 years have demonstrated the additional benefits of PET/CT, which was an advantage because of the poor anatomic detail of PET.[5,6] An early study by Antoch and coworkers showed in 27 patients that PET/CT findings led to a treatment change for 4 patients (15%) when compared with PET alone.[7] Differences in the accuracy of overall tumor staging between PET/CT and PET ($P = .031$) were significant.

Another study showed that in 129 patients integrated PET-CT is a better predictor than PET for N status (78% vs 56%, $P = .008$).[8] It was more accurate for the total N2 nodes (96% vs 93%, $P = .01$) and for the total N1 nodes (90% vs 80%, $P = .001$).

[a] Department of Thoracic Medicine, Royal Brisbane and Women's Hospital, Butterfield Street, Herston, Queensland 4029, Australia; [b] Department of Surgery, Santa Marianna Hospital, Kawasaki City, Kanagawa Prefecture, Japan
* Corresponding author.
E-mail address: david_fielding@health.qld.gov.au

Clin Chest Med 34 (2013) 385–394
http://dx.doi.org/10.1016/j.ccm.2013.06.003
0272-5231/13/$ – see front matter © 2013 Elsevier Inc. All rights reserved.

Integrated PET-CT was significantly more sensitive at the 4R, 5, 7, 10L, and 11 stations and more accurate at the 7 and 11 lymph nodes stations than dedicated PET. A more recent study by Bille and colleagues[9] studied 1001 nodes in 159 patients before lung resection who were clinically N0 in the mediastinum. Of 71 nodes that were ultimately found to be positive histologically, PET/CT correctly identified 41 metastatic lymph node stations (57.7%; 19 N1, 22 N2). False negative results were obtained in 30 nodal stations (5 N1, 24 N2, 1 N3), and false positive results in 14 (5 N1, 9 N2). The most common lymph node station for occult metastatic involvement was in the subcarinal level (8 of 30 [26.6%]) followed by right upper and lower paratracheal and hilar levels (4 each of 30). Through systematic pulmonary and mediastinal lymph node dissection, 22 patients (13.8%) were falsely understaged and 9 patients (5.7%) were falsely overstaged. These authors concluded, "PET/CT was well below the threshold of 95% at which the test could replace invasive staging procedures."

A recent meta-analysis has explored the negative predictive value of PET/CT in evaluating the mediastinum in clinical T1 and T2 tumors with no enlarged mediastinal nodes on CT.[10,11] Ten studies were analyzed and all used mediastinoscopy and/or surgical staging to confirm nodal status. Negative predictive value of PET/CT ranged from 94% in T1 to 89% for T2 tumors.

MEDIASTINOSCOPY

In 2003 Toloza and colleagues[11] published a meta-analysis of mediastinoscopy for lung cancer staging in 5687 patients. Results are as shown in **Table 1**. Major morbidity was seen in 2% including recurrent laryngeal nerve paresis (0.55%), hemorrhage (0.32%), tracheal injury (0.09%), and pneumothorax (0.09%). Mortality occurred in 0.08%. Results for a large, single-center experience by Lemaire and coworkers are also shown.[12]

Table 1
Patients with lung cancer mediastinoscopy results

	N	Sensitivity	Specificity	Positive Predictive Value	Negative Predictive Value	Accuracy	Study Type
PET							
Dwamena et al,[4] 1999	514	79% (76–82)	91% (89–93)	90%	93%	92%	Meta-analysis
PET/CT							
Bille et al,[9] 2009	159	54%	92%	74%	82%	83%	1 center
Fischer et al,[5] 2009	98	64% (52–75)	100%			79% (69–86)	Randomized study
Mediastinoscopy							
Toloza et al,[3,11] 2003	5687	81%	100%	100%	93%		Meta-analysis
Lemaire et al,[12] 2006	1019	86%	100%	100%	95%		1 center
EBUS-TBNA staging							
Gu et al,[14,52]	1300	93% (91–95)					Meta-analysis
Adams et al,[13] 2009	800	88% (79–94)					Meta-analysis
Yasufuku	102	92	100	100	97	98	1 center
Yasufuku							
Herth et al,[15,21] 2008	97						1 center
EBUS plus EUS							
Sharples et al,[28] 2012		85 (74–92)			85%		4 centers

ENDOBRONCHIAL ULTRASOUND TRANSBRONCHIAL NEEDLE ASPIRATIONSSTAGING STUDIES

Two meta-analyses have been published on endobronchial ultrasound transbronchial needle aspirations (EBUS-TBNA) in the presurgical staging of operable patients with lung cancer, as shown in **Table 1**.[13,14] All of the studies reported on the convex probe bronchoscope but in the report of Adams and coworkers,[13] 2 early studies that used 2-step balloon EBUS and standard TBNA are included. **Table 1** also shows the single-center experience of Herth and colleagues.[15] They performed EBUS-TBNA in 97 patients with presumed or known non-small-cell lung cancer (NSCLC) and PET and CT-negative mediastinum. They sampled 156 nodes, with a diameter of 7.9 $\pm$ 0.7 mm, and all patients had node tissue confirmed by mediastinoscopy or node dissection. There was a prevalence of malignancy of 9 patients, 8 of which were detected by EBUS. The node that was missed was at station 10.

Studies directly comparing EBUS-TBNA staging and mediastinoscopy have shown no advantage to mediastinoscopy and excellent diagnostic performance of EBUS-TBNA.[16] Ernst and colleagues[16] studied 61 patients with known or suspected lung cancer; a final diagnosis of cancer was made in 57 patients. Comparison was made for nodes larger than 1 cm at stations 2, 4, and 7. A total of 120 nodes were sampled, with a mean diameter of 15 mm in the short axis. The diagnostic yield of EBUS-TBNA was 109/120 compared with 94/120 for mediastinoscopy (P = .007). The combination of EBUS and mediastinoscopy gave a yield of 115/120, which was not significantly better than EBUS alone. These authors therefore concluded that a normal EBUS-TBNA could allow a patient to proceed to surgery without mediastinoscopy.

A comparison to PET was important given the potential of this technique in stratifying risk of mediastinal involvement. In an important study, Yasufuku and colleagues[17] performed a direct comparison of CT, PET, and mediastinal node sampling by EBUS-TBNA. They studied 102 patients with 147 mediastinal and 53 hilar lymph nodes of whom EBUSTBNA proved malignancy in 37 lymph node stations in 24 patients. The sensitivities of CT, PET, and EBUS-TBNA for the correct diagnosis of mediastinal and hilar lymph node staging were 76.9%, 80.0%, and 92.3%, respectively; specificities were 55.3%, 70.1%, and 100%, and diagnostic accuracies were 60.8%, 72.5%, and 98.0%. All values for EBUS-TBNA were significantly better than both CT and PET.

Cerfolio and colleagues[18] reported a retrospective series of EBUS (and EUS) staging in suspicious enlarged N2 nodes. Of 234 patients, 72 patients had an EBUS. Sixteen were true positive for N2 disease; however, 12 were false negative. The median diameter of the false-negative nodes was 12 mm. Four passes of the node were performed and rapid on-site evaluation of samples was made. The authors state the series was relatively early in their EBUS experience and the results do not state whether adequate lymph node material was obtained at EBUS. As expected, they concluded that negative sampling in suspicious nodes should be followed by mediastinoscopy or surgical staging. In an article supporting the preoperative staging of the mediastinum by surgeons using EBUS and EUS, Groth and Andrade[19] also recommended that nonmalignant EBUS or EUS cytologic findings should be confirmed with mediastinoscopy or thoracoscopy if the pretest probability of malignancy is high.

In 2011 Yasufuku and coworkers[20] reported a large series of 153 patients with lung cancer undergoing surgical staging. These cases were mostly radiological N0 or N1 (64% of cases), and the short-axis diameter of nodes sampled was only 6.9 $\pm$ 3 mm. In the same anaesthetic, patients had EBUS-TBNA by 1 of 3 operators followed by mediastinoscopy. The average number of nodes sampled by EBUS was 3 and by mediastinoscopy was 4. The sensitivity, specificity, negative predictive value, and diagnostic accuracy of EBUS-TBNA were 81%, 100%, 91%, and 93%, respectively. The results for mediastinoscopy were 79%, 100%, 90%, and 93%, respectively. There were 8 false negative lymph node stations on EBUS-TBNA compared with 14 false negative lymph node stations on mediastinoscopy. Inadequate lymph node sampling was seen in 122 lymph nodes on EBUS-TBNA; these nodes were mostly less than 5 mm, and none were subsequently shown to have metastatic cancer at mediastinoscopy or thoracotomy. Conversely 10 lymph node stations were thought to have inadequate sampling on mediastinoscopy (lacking lymphoid tissue). This very detailed study demonstrates a great deal of skill on the part of the EBUS operators sampling very small nodes. However, by including these small nodes, the authors have shown the maximal capability of the technique. Others doing EBUS-TBNA for staging may not necessarily attempt such detailed staging of small nodes in CT and PET-negative cases except in a relatively select group of patients, as mentioned above.

EBUS-TBNA has also been reported in several studies as restaging after preoperative therapy for lung cancer. Herth and colleagues[21] reported a series of 124 patients restaged with EBUS-TBNA after induction chemotherapy. Of these, 66 had a partial response by CT criteria. Overall the sensitivity by EBUS-TBNA for detecting persistent disease was 76%; however, the negative predictive value was only 20%, indicating the need for surgical restaging in EBUS-TBNA-negative samples in this group of patients. The lower sensitivity was attributed to nodes being altered by necrosis and fibrosis from chemotherapy.

EUS COMBINED WITH EBUS IN STAGING

Numerous studies investigated EUS as a staging and diagnostic tool for mediastinal nodes.[22,23] In one large study by Annema and colleagues,[22] operable patients were randomized to either surgical staging or EUS plus surgical staging. Node metastases were found in 41 and 56 patients, respectively; sensitivity for surgical staging alone was 79% compared with 85% with the addition of EUS. Unnecessary thoracotomy occurred in significantly fewer patients with the addition of EUS (21 vs 9, $P = .02$).

In view of the clear complementary anatomic reach of EBUS and EUS, studies combining the 2 modalities were undertaken. Vilmann and Puri[24] demonstrated the concept in a 2005 study in 33 patients. Twenty patients had abnormal nodes and 13 had masses. EUS sampled 59 lesions, and EBUS sampled 60 lesions. With combined EUS-fine needle aspiration [FNA] plus EBUS-TBNA in 28 of the 31 patients in whom a final diagnosis was obtained in the evaluation of mediastinal cancer, 20 patients were found to have mediastinal involvement, whereas no mediastinal metastases were found in 8 patients. The accuracy of EUS-FNA and EBUS-TBNA, in combination, for the diagnosis of mediastinal cancer was 100% (95% CI, 83%–100%). With EBUS-TBNA, 11 additional cancer diagnoses were made compared with EUS, and 3 had "suspicious cells" that had not been obtained by EUS-FNA. Conversely, with EUS-FNA, 12 additional cancers were found compared with EBUS, as well as one "suspicious cells" case and 1 sarcoidosis in addition to EBUS-TBNA.

Rintoul and colleagues[25] studied EBUS and EUS-FNA for mediastinal staging in 18 patients with 26 lymph nodes. All had EBUS-TBNA. An additional EUS examination was performed in patients in whom the staging CT scan had demonstrated enlarged lymph nodes inaccessible by EBUS (ie, stations 5, 8, and 9, and posteroinferiorly placed lymph nodes in station 7). Seven patients had both procedures, and of these 5 patients had additional pathologic banormality detected

on EUS compared with EBUS (3 true positive, 2 true negative).

Ohnishi and colleagues[26] showed that in 110 patients the combination of EBUS and EUS had a combined sensitivity and negative predictive value of 72% and 89%, compared with PET/CT, which had results of 47% ($P<.0001$) and 76%.

EBUS and EUS-FNA combined have been studied in the radiologically normal mediastinum in NSCLC staging. In a study by Szlubowski and colleagues[27] of 120 patients clinically CT N0, nodes were abnormal for malignancy by FNA in 31/318 nodes (10%). Extensive mediastinal node dissection with TEMLA (transcervical extended bilateral mediastinal lymphadenectomy) was performed as confirmation in aspirate negative cases; 99 patients with negative FNA had TEMLA with 9 patients positive (8%). This low figure of false negative sampling for the combined technique in micrometastatic disease demonstrates its sensitivity. These authors had a sensitivity of 68%, which is understandable given the low prevalence of positive cases in this series. They concluded, "In the radiologically normal mediastinum, EBUS/EUS is a highly effective and safe technique in NSCLC staging and, if negative, a surgical diagnostic exploration of the mediastinum may be omitted."

In a large randomized series conducted at 4 centers, Sharples and colleagues[28] have reported results of surgical staging alone (n = 118) compared with endosonography (EBUS plus EUS) followed by surgical staging if endosonography was negative (n = 123). Sensitivity for detecting N2/N3 metastases was 79% (41/52; 95% confidence interval [CI] 66%–88%) for the surgical arm compared with 94% (62/66; 95% CI 85%–98%) for the endosonography strategy ($P = .02$). In the sonography arm it was possible to separate out sensitivity and negative predictive value for sonography alone (85% and 85%) versus surgical staging alone (79% and 86%).

The ASGE recommendations for EUS staging and combined EBUS/EUS staging are as follows[29]:

- EUS-FNA in patients with paraesophageal, posterior, and inferior mediastinal adenopathy, if the expertise if available.

- EBUS-FNA in patients with paratracheal mediastinal adenopathy if this information adds to the staging of the lung cancer.

- EUS-FNA and EBUS-FNA have been shown to be safe and potentially cost-effective compared with mediastinoscopy, although individually each has a high false negative rate that warrants surgical confirmation before proceeding with resection.

- In patients with known or suspected potentially resectable lung cancer whose imaging shows no evidence of mediastinal adenopathy, the authors suggest combined EUS-FNA/EBUS-FNA for staging.
- Combined EUS-FNA/EBUS-FNA has been shown to have a negative predictive value comparable to that of mediastinoscopy. However, expertise in both modalities is not readily available at most institutions.

EUS USING A CONVEX PROBE BRONCHOSCOPE

Pulmonologists have used an EBUS-TBNA scope in the esophagus to perform sampling that had previously only been performed by EUS endoscopes.[30,31] This method is known as either EUS-B-FNA or EBUS TENA (Trans Esophageal Needle aspiration). The potential advantages are that only one scope needs to be used per case, no additional training in using the scope is required and it builds on the experience of other specialties accessing organs through the esophagus such as trans-esophageal echo by cardiologists and anesthetists. Herth and colleagues[30] studied 139 consecutive patients, with a primary lung cancer with nodes larger than 1 cm needing evaluation with PET having been performed as clinically indicated. EBUS and EBUS-TENA were performed in all patients with a mean of 1 to 2 nodes sampled by each method. From 71 patients with malignant nodes, the numbers positive by the bronchus, esophagus, and combined were as follows: 65, 63, and 68 (96% sensitivity), which meant that by adding the esophageal examination, an additional 3 patients were found abnormal.

A contemporaneous study was performed by Hwangbo and coworkers.[31] In 150 patients with lung primary, following PET scan, staging EBUS-TBNA was performed followed by EUSB-FNA on nodes that were inaccessible or difficult. EBUS sampled 310 lesions (mostly nodes), and then EUSB-FNA was performed in 64 lesions in 54 patients. The reasons were as follows: 12 nodes were inaccessible by EBUS, 47 nodes were technically difficult by EBUS, and 5 had poor sampling by EBUS. By patient, overall there were also 3 patients where EUSB FNA was abnormal when EBUS was normal or impossible. One of the EBUS-negative and EUS-positive cases was 4L; it was accessible by EBUS but easier to sample by EUS. The overall success of sampling was high (41 of 45 nodes); 2 of the 4 negative nodes in the series were in sites unreachable by either method (stations 3 and 6).

In a 2012 study Szlubowski and coworkers compared a sampling of the esophageal route by EBUS scope with EUS scope.[32] It was a non-randomized study of 214 patients undergoing preoperative staging. EUS-FNA was performed in 110 patients (CUS), whereas 104 patients had EUS-B-FNA plus EBUS-TBNA (CUSb). In patients with normal results, an appropriate pulmonary resection with the systemic lymph node dissection (SLND) of the mediastinal nodes was performed. Overall, no significant differences were observed with sensitivity and specificity for the EUS scope being 92% and 98% and with the EBUS scope being 85% and 93%, respectively. In 55 CUS-negative (50%) and 53 (51%) CUSb-negative patients with NSCLC, the subsequent SLND revealed metastatic nodes in 5 patients (4.5%) and in 9 patients (8.7%), respectively ($P = NS$). There was "minimal N2" in 11 of these 14 patients (5 in the CUS group and 6 in the CUSb group)—with no predominance for any nodal station (except 3 patients with right upper lobe tumor, all with false negative results in station 2R/4R). In 3 patients with false negative results of CUSb, a multilevel N2 was diagnosed by means of SLND. This interesting study, although not randomized, shows promise for the use of the EBUS-TBNA bronchoscope in this way. The authors were surgeons and adept at use of both endoscope and bronchoscope, which supports such a comparison being done.

The EUS endoscope has a better radial range of imaging: 120° to 180° compared with 70° of the EBUS scope.[33] Furthermore, it is reported to be easier to orient and allows deeper penetration of both the ultrasound image and the needle, also allowing sampling of the adrenal gland in selected cases. As an editorial commenting on the EBUS/esophageal studies stated, "If only an EBUS scope is available for the detection of mediastinal nodes, a transesophageal (EUS) investigation should be performed with it as well to improve preoperative tumor staging. That said, we still believe that a dedicated EUS scope has additional benefit and should be part of a complete diagnostic unit." That is, gastroenterologists in mediastinal staging support the use of the EUS scope, although the studies suggest in practice the EBUS scope gives satisfactory sampling.

Although it is possible to use an EBUS scope in this way, authors have questioned whether it is worthwhile given the relatively few extra cases it picks up (3 extra from 150 cases).[34] Also, although EUS accesses station 5 well, if that node is enlarged, 4L usually is as well, and accessible by EBUS. Furthermore, it is very uncommon to see isolated station 8 or 9 nodes without, for example, associated station 7 nodes.

Overall, in mediastinal staging there are real but small benefits to staging by adding EUS. It could well be possible to anticipate those cases whereby EUS-FNA was needed (predominantly low and posterior lymph nodes on preprocure PET/CT), or to use rapid on-site assessment of specimens and move between modalities in difficult node stations such as 2L or 4L. Also, it seems using an EBUS scope seems to have the same benefits as a full EUS scope; however, different training expectations in different countries are likely to affect uptake of the method.

WHICH PATIENTS NEED MEDIASTINAL NODE TISSUE SAMPLING FOR STAGING?

Given the previous considerations, it is clear that where a patient is operable, a positive PET scan requires tissue confirmation of mediastinal nodes with abnormal uptake. If a PET scan is normal, there are some situations whereby node staging should be performed.[35] These situations include if the tumor is central, if positive N1 nodes on CT or PET are seen, if mediastinal nodes larger than 1 cm on CT are seen, and in the setting of low FDG uptake in the primary tumor. If a PET scan is normal, there are some situations whereby node staging should be performed. These situations include the following:

- If the primary tumor is central; in a study of the role of preoperative PET/CT, test performance of PET/CT was relatively poorer in central tumors in predicting N stage, with Cohen's kappa statistic of 0.39, only a fair correlation with tissue sampling.[36]
- If positive N1 nodes on CT or PET are seen.
- If mediastinal nodes larger than 1 cm on CT are seen, with negative PET uptake; in the study by Fischer and colleagues,[37] there was a lower negative predictive value for larger lymph nodes than those less than 1 cm (70% compared with 96% for small nodes). This lower negative predictive value could be accounted for by a higher overall prevalence of tumor cells in larger nodes; with similar sensitivity and specificity it meant there were more falsely negative nodes by PET/CT in the larger nodes. Although there is value in a negative PET/CT in normal-sized mediastinal lymph nodes, the risk of a false negative diagnosis is 30% in enlarged lymph nodes without FDG uptake.
- In the setting of low FDG uptake in the primary tumor.

PRACTICAL ASPECTS OF EBUS-TBNA STAGING AND TIPS

Before the procedure, it is important to consider which nodes would be N3 in a given patient and sample that first, preferably with onsite cytology examination. Demonstrating negative N3, the next nodes to be sampled are N2 followed last by N1 if N2 is negative. It is not sufficient to flush needles with saline between stations, as some cells from the first aspirate may contaminate subsequent samples. If no onsite assessment is possible, it may be necessary to change needles, therefore, between sampling of N3 and N2 and N1 nodes, depending on the situation.

Lymph nodes being sampled in staging procedures are often small and can be difficult to access. An understanding of the way metastatic cells occupy nodes is important to maximize the chance of obtaining true positive aspirates. Furthermore, where aspirated material is equivocal on cytology, it may be possible to use the features of the actual EBUS image to support a benign tissue diagnosis, which includes both the vascular patterns and the grayscale pattern of the nodes.

The flow of lymph into lymph nodes occurs via channels that drain predominantly into the subcapsular sinusoids and then to the parenchymal sinusoids.[38] This flow pattern is responsible for the observation that small metastases of breast cancer identified on hematoxylin & eosin sections are usually located in the subcapsular sinusoids. Viale and colleagues[39] reported that metastases were largely found in the subcapsular zone where afferent lymphatics enter lymph nodes. Cserni[40] studied the localization of metastases in the sentinel lymph nodes of patients with breast cancer. In 23 (72%) of sentinel nodes of 32 node-positive patients, metastases were more likely to be localized or more voluminous on the inflow side of the lymphatics draining from the tumor.

While puncturing the lymph node using EBUS, it is easier to puncture the center area than the marginal area (Fig. 1). Kurimoto and colleagues[41] histopathologically investigated 124 resected metastatic lymph nodes in patients with lung cancer. In 20% to 25% of lymph nodes, metastases were only detected in the marginal area of the lymph node. Therefore, if the onsite cytologic evaluation by EBUS-TBNA is negative after puncturing into the center of the lymph node, it is recommended to puncture the needle into the marginal area of the lymph node.

For obtaining sufficient specimens, the authors usually perform the "outer sheath method." This outer sheath method comprises pressing the outer sheath of the puncture needle against the

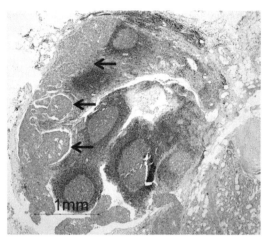

Fig. 1. A representative metastatic lymph node (squamous cell carcinoma). Metastasis (*arrow*) was largely found in the subcapsular zone.

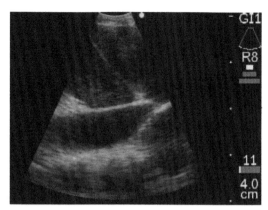

Fig. 2. The interface echo. The hyperechoic interface echo between lymph nodes means that the surface of the lymph nodes is relatively flat and the space between lymph nodes exists.

bronchial wall immediately before puncture, then moving the entire bronchoscope back up the wall and performing the puncture after the tip of the outer sheath is caught in a concavity between 2 rings of cartilage, which can be observed on the monitor, watching the top right of the image for the sheath to "drop" between 2 cartilages.

During aspiration biopsy, it is important to avoid necrotic areas in lymph nodes—this can be achieved by targeting areas of the node with maintained blood supply as demonstrated by power Doppler.[42,43] Use of power Doppler imaging to detect nodal vessels and biopsy of perivascular tissue may possibly increase the rate of diagnosis, particularly when metastasis of squamous cell carcinoma or small cell carcinoma is suspected. In the authors' experiences, vessels in metastatic lymph nodes wind irregularly, and vessels in sarcoidosis run straight inside lymph nodes. Also, in sarcoidosis, the hyperechoic interface echo between clumped lymph nodes is always found (**Fig. 2**). The surface of these nodes is relatively flat. Diagnostic accuracy of 92% is obtained using the presence of this flat interface for ruling in sarcoid (plus absence of the interface indicating malignancy).

Patterns of intranodal vessels with power Doppler are classified as (1) straight vessels from the hilum (**Fig. 3**), (2) aberrant vessels (**Fig. 4**), (3) subcapsular vessels, and (4) decreased perfusion. Three patterns (aberrant vessels, subcapsular vessels, decreased perfusion of intranodal vessels) in metastatic nodes were found in metastatic lymph nodes, diagnostic accuracy also 92%. Combining the appropriate vascular and interface echo patterns gives diagnostic accuracies of 95% and 94% for sarcoid and malignancy, respectively.

ASSESSMENT OF EBUS IMAGES USING COMPUTER ANALYSIS

There is a long history of attempting to use aspects of B-mode images to "support" a tissue diagnosis. Adibelli and colleagues[44] investigated cervical lymph node echogenicity, contour, longitudinal-to-transverse diameter ratio, and the presence of the hilus and identified only the presence of the hilus as a significant discriminator. Cole and colleagues[45] documented that, in node metastases with maximum diameter ≥15 mm, sensitivity and specificity of ultrasonography were 81.3% and 81.6%, respectively. Kebudi and colleagues[46] diagnosed axillary lymph node metastasis of breast cancer using B-mode ultrasound based on centric echogenicity, cortical thickening, length/width ratio, and lymph node diameter and reported a sensitivity of 79.1%, specificity of 77.7%, positive predictive value of 82.6%, and negative predictive value of 73.6%.

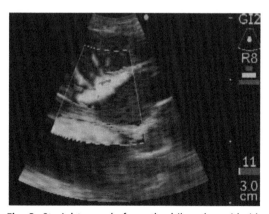

Fig. 3. Straight vessels from the hilum (sarcoidosis). Straight Intra-nodal vessels branching from hilum.

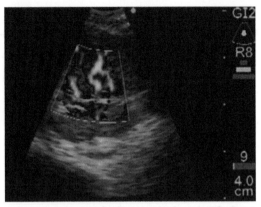

Fig. 4. Aberrant vessels (metastasis of adenocarcinoma). Intra-nodal vessels run irregularly.

Starting around 1986, research began on computer-assisted support systems known as artificial neural networks (ANN).[47] ANN has been studied as a system mimicking the biologic nervous system[48] and is currently used in pattern recognition. The diagnostic sensitivity, specificity, and accuracy of ANN using ultrasound of cervical lymph node metastasis from oral cancer have been reported at 80.6%, 94.6%, and 93.6%, respectively,[49] and these figures are comparable to CT and magnetic resonance imaging. Tagaya and colleagues[50] reported that the diagnostic accuracy of ANN for peribronchial lymph node malignancy was 91.2%, significantly higher than that for the surgeon with 5 years of experience at 78%.

Automated grayscale analysis of EBUS images has shown correct classification of benign versus malignant in 44 of 51 lymph nodes (86.3%).[51]Other new technologies in computer-aided diagnosis will appear in the near future.

MICROMETASTATIC DISEASE AND ISOLATED TUMOR CELLS

The clinical significance of occult disease in N2 nodes is relevant to this review because numerous studies now report positive aspirates in normal-sized and PET-negative nodes.[15] The term micrometastatic disease refers to lymph nodes, which have been surgically resected and undergone immunohistochemistry to detect malignant cells that were not seen on standard hematoxylin & eosin sections. Several studies have in fact documented life expectancy in cohorts of patients with such nodes compared with those with no micrometastic disease in surgically resected nodes; 3 groups found a significant survival reduction.[52–54] More relevant to the present discussion are nodes with isolated tumor cells (ITC), defined as single tumor cells or small clusters of cells, smaller than

0.2 mm in greatest diameter, whereas micrometastases are clusters of tumor cells measuring between 0.2 and 2 mm in greatest diameter.[55] Rena and colleagues[55] reported a series of 87 patients resected for T1 carcinoma, of whom 19 nodes in 14 patients had either micrometastases or ITC. Two-year and 5-year recurrence-free survival was similar for patients with either micrometstases or ITC, and these authors concluded that the significance of the detection of this remained controversial.

REFERENCES

1. Birim O, Kappetein A, Stijnen T, et al. Meta-analysis of positron emission tomographic and computed tomographic imaging in detecting mediastinal lymph node metastases in nonsmall cell lung cancer. Ann Thorac Surg 2005;79:375–82.
2. Gould M, Kuschner W, Rydzak C, et al. Test performance of positron emission tomography and computed tomography for mediastinal staging in patients with non-small-cell lung cancer: a meta-analysis. Ann Intern Med 2003;139:879–92.
3. Toloza E, Harpole L, McCrory D. Noninvasive staging of non-small cell lung cancer: a review of the current evidence. Chest 2003;123(Suppl 1): 137S–46S.
4. Dwamena B, Sonnad S, Angobaldo J, et al. Metastases from non-small cell lung cancer: mediastinal staging in the 1990s—meta-analytic comparison of PET and CT. Radiology 1999;213:530–6.
5. Fischer B, Lassen U, Mortensen J, et al. Preoperative staging of lung cancer with combined PET-CT. N Engl J Med 2009;361:32–9.
6. Hwangbo B, Kim SK, Lee HS, et al. Application of endobronchial ultrasound-guided transbronchial needle aspiration following integrated PET/CT in mediastinal staging of potentially operable non-small cell lung cancer. Chest 2009;135:1280–7.
7. Antoch G, Stattaus J, Nemat AT, et al. Non–small cell lung cancer: dual-modality PET/CT in preoperative staging. Radiology 2003;229(2):526–33.
8. Cerfolio RJ, Ojha B, Bryant AS. The accuracy of integrated PET-CT compared with dedicated PET alone for the staging of patients with nonsmall cell lung cancer. Ann Thorac Surg 2004;78:1017–23.
9. Bille A, Pelosi E, Skanjeti A. Preoperative intrathoracic lymph node staging in patients with non-small-cell lung cancer: accuracy of integrated positron emission tomography and computed tomography. Eur J Cardiothorac Surg 2009;36: 440–5.
10. Wang J, Welch K, Wang L, et al. Negative predictive value of positron emission tomography and computed tomography for stage T1-2N0 non-small-cell lung cancer: a meta-analysis. Clin Lung Cancer 2012;13:81–9.

11. Toloza EM, Harpole L, Detterbeck F, et al. Invasive staging of non-small cell lung cancer: a review of the current evidence. Chest 2003;123(Suppl 1): 157S–66S.

12. Lemaire A, Nikolic I, Petersen T, et al. Nine-year single center experience with cervical mediastinoscopy: complications and false negative rate. Ann Thorac Surg 2006;82:1185–9.

13. Adams K, Shah PL, Edmonds L, et al. Test performance of endobronchial ultrasound and transbronchial needle aspiration biopsy for mediastinal staging in patients with lung cancer: systematic review and meta-analysis. Thorax 2009;64:757–62.

14. Gu P, Zhao YZ, Jiang LY, et al. Endobronchial ultrasound-guided transbronchial needle aspiration for staging of lung cancer: a systematic review and meta-analysis. Eur J Cancer 2009;45: 1389–96.

15. Herth FJ, Eberhardt R, Krasnik M, et al. Endobronchial ultrasound-guided transbronchial needle aspiration of lymph nodes in the radiologically and positron emission tomography-normal mediastinum in patients with lung cancer. Chest 2008;133: 887–91.

16. Ernst A, Anantham D, Eberhardt R, et al. Diagnosis of mediastinal adenopathy-real-time endobronchial ultrasound guided needle aspiration versus mediastinoscopy. J Thorac Oncol 2008;3:577–82.

17. Yasufuku K, Nakajima T, Motoori K, et al. Comparison of endobronchial ultrasound, positron emission tomography, and CT for lymph node staging of lung cancer. Chest 2006;130:710–8.

18. Cerfolio RJ, Bryant AS, Eloubeidi MA, et al. The true false negative rates of esophageal and endobronchial ultrasound in the staging of mediastinal lymph nodes in patients with non-small cell lung cancer. Ann Thorac Surg 2010;90:427–34.

19. Groth SS, Andrade RS. Endobronchial and endoscopic ultrasound-guided fine-needle aspiration: a must for thoracic surgeons. Ann Thorac Surg 2010;89:S2079–83.

20. Yasufuku K, Pierre A, Darling G, et al. A prospective controlled trial of endobronchial ultrasound-guided transbronchial needle aspiration compared with mediastinoscopy for mediastinal lymph node staging of lung cancer. Thorac Cardiovasc Surg 2011;142:1393–400.

21. Herth FJ, Annema JT, Eberhardt R. Endobronchial ultrasound with transbronchial needle aspiration for restaging the mediastinum in lung cancer. J Clin Oncol 2008;26:3346–50.

22. Annema JT, van Meerbeeck JP, Rintoul RC, et al. Mediastinoscopy vs endosonography for mediastinal nodal staging of lung cancer: a randomized trial. JAMA 2010;304:2245.

23. Yasuda I, Kato T, Fumihiro Asano F, et al. Mediastinal lymph node staging in potentially resectable non-small cell lung cancer: a prospective comparison of CT and EUS/EUS-FNA. Respiration 2009;78: 423–31.

24. Vilmann P, Puri R. The complete 'medical' mediastinoscopy (EUS-FNA + EBUS-TBNA). Minerva Med 2007;98:331–8.

25. Rintoul RC, Skwarski KM, Murchison JT. Endobronchial and endoscopic ultrasound-guided real-time fine-needle aspiration for mediastinal staging. Eur Respir J 2005;25:416–21.

26. Ohnishi R, Yasuda I, Kato T. Combined endobronchial and endoscopic ultrasound-guided fine needle aspiration for mediastinal nodal staging of lung cancer. Endoscopy 2011;43:1082–9.

27. Szlubowski A, Zielinski M, Soja J, et al. A combined approach of EBUS and EUS FNA in the radiologically normal mediastinum in NSCLC. Eur J Cardiothorac Surg 2010;37:1175.

28. Sharples LD, Jackson C, Wheaton E, et al. Clinical effectiveness and cost-effectiveness of endobronchial and endoscopic ultrasound relative to surgical staging in potentially resectable lung cancer: results from the ASTER randomised controlled trial. Health Technol Assess 2012;16:1–75.

29. ASGE Standards of Practice Committee, Jue TL, Sharaf RN, et al. Role of EUS for the evaluation of mediastinal adenopathy. Semin Respir Crit Care Med 2011;32:62–8.

30. Herth FJ, Krasnik M, Kahn N, et al. Combined endoscopic-endobronchial ultrasound-guided fine-needle aspiration of mediastinal lymph nodes through a single bronchoscope in 150 patients with suspected lung cancer. Chest 2010;138: 790–4.

31. Hwangbo B, Lee GK, Lee HS, et al. Transbronchial and transesophageal fine-needle aspiration using an ultrasound bronchoscope in mediastinal staging of potentially operable lung cancer. Chest 2010;138:795–802.

32. Szlubowski A, Soja J, Kocon P, et al. A comparison of the combined ultrasound of the mediastinum by use of a single ultrasound bronchoscope versus ultrasound bronchoscope plus ultrasound gastroscope in lung cancer staging: a prospective trial. Interact Cardiovasc Thorac Surg 2012;15:442–6.

33. Annema J, Rabe KF. Endonography for lung cancer staging: one scope fits all? Chest 2010;138: 765–7.

34. Wang KP, Feller-Kopman D, Mehta A, et al. Endobronchial ultrasound and esophageal ultrasound: just because we can, does not necessarily mean we should. Chest 2011;140(1):271–2.

35. Schuhmann M, Eberhardt R, Herth FJ. Direct nodal sampling by echoendoscopy in lung cancer: the clinician's expectations: direct nodal sampling by echoendoscopy in lung cancer. Insights Imaging 2011;2:133–40.

36. Macia I, Moya J, Escobar I, et al. Quality study of a lung cancer committee: study of agreement between preoperative and pathological staging. Eur J Cardiothorac Surg 2010;37:540–5.

37. Fischer BM, Mortensen B, Hansen H. Multimodality approach to mediastinal staging in non-small cell lung cancer. Faults and benefits of PET-CT: a randomised trial. Thorax 2011;66: 294–300.

38. Kurimoto N, Murayama M, Yoshioka S, et al. Analysis of the internal structure of peripheral pulmonary lesions using endobronchial ultrasonography. Chest 2002;122:1877–94.

39. Viale G, Sonzogni A, Pruneri G, et al. Histopathological examination of axillary sentinel lymph nodes in breast carcinoma patients. J Surg Oncol 2004; 85:123–8.

40. Cserni G. Mapping metastases in sentinel lymph nodes of breast cancer. Am J Clin Pathol 2000; 113:351–4.

41. Kurimoto N, Osada H, Miyazawa T, et al. Targeting area in metastatic lymph nodes in lung cancer for endobronchial ultrasonography-guided transbronchial needle aspiration. J Bronchology 2008; 15:134–8.

42. Muller N, Colman N, Pare C, et al. Fraser and Pare's diagnosis of diseases of the chest. 4th edition. Oxford (United Kingdom): W.B. Saunders Company; 1999. p. 462.

43. Rosai J, Ackerman L. Rosai and Ackerman's surgical pathology. 9th edition. Philadelphia: Mosby, Elsevier Inc; 2004. p. 1127.

44. Adibelli ZH, Unal G, Gul E, et al. Differentiation of benign and malignant cervical lymph nodes: value of B-mode and color Doppler sonography. Eur J Radiol 1998;23(3):230–4.

45. Cole I, Chu J, Kos S, et al. Metastatic carcinoma in the neck: a clinical computerized tomography scan and ultrasound study. Aust NZ J Surg 1993;63(6): 468–74.

46. Kebudi A, Caliskan C, Yetkin G, et al. The role of pre-operative B mode ultrasound in the evaluation of the axillary lymph node metastases in the initial staging of breast carcinoma. Acta Chir Belg 2005;105(5):511–4.

47. Rumelhart DE, McClellend JL, The PDP Research Group. Parallel distributed processing. Cambridge (United Kingdom): MIT Press; 1986.

48. Yoshino S, Kobayashi A, Yahagi T, et al. Quantitative diagnose using neural networks. IEICE Trans Fundamentals 1994;E77A-11:1846–50.

49. Kawazu T, Araki K, Yoshiura K, et al. Application of neural networks to the prediction of lymph node metastasis in oral cancer. Oral Radiol 2003;19:137–42.

50. Tagaya R, Kurimoto N, Osada H, et al. Automatic objective diagnosis of lymph nodal diseases by B-mode endobronchoscopy. Chest 2008;133:137–42.

51. Nguyen P, Bashirzadeh F, Hundloe J, et al. Optical differentiation between malignant and benign lymphadenopathy by grey scale texture analysis of endobronchial ultrasound convex probe images. Chest 2012;141:709–15.

52. Gu CD, Oyama T. Detection of micrometastatic tumor cells in pN0 lymph nodes of patients with completely resected nonsmall cell lung cancer. Ann Surg 2002;235:133–9.

53. Wu J, Ohta Y, Minato H, et al. Nodal occult metastasis in patients with peripheral lung adenocarcinoma of 2.0 cm or less in diameter. Ann Thorac Surg 2001;71:1772–8.

54. Osaki T, Oyama T, Gu CD. Prognostic impact of micrometastatatic tumor cells in the lymph nodes and bone marrow of patients with completely resected stage I non-small cell lung cancer. J Clin Oncol 2002;13:2930–6.

55. Rena O, Carsanna L, Cristina L, et al. Lymph node isolated tumor cells and micrometastases in pathological stage I non-small cell lung cancer: prognostic significance. Eur J Cardiothorac Surg 2007;32:863–7.

Newer Modalities in the Work-up of Peripheral Pulmonary Nodules

Tathagat Narula, MD[a], Michael S. Machuzak, MD[b],
Atul C. Mehta, MBBS[c],*

KEYWORDS

- Peripheral pulmonary nodule • Flexible bronchoscopy • Endobronchial ultrasound
- Electromagnetic navigation • Ultrathin bronchoscopy • Virtual bronchoscopic navigation

KEY POINTS

- Major strides have been made in bronchology, and technological advancements promise a future that is likely to witness many more innovations.
- The challenge lies not just in understanding the science behind these ideas and innovations but also in incorporating these in diagnostic pathways that can be consistently applied across different landscapes.
- Although available evidence and recommendations are presented, the authors appreciate that recommendations, by their very nature, cannot encompass all possible scenarios that occur in day-to-day clinical practice.
- From the preceding discussion, it can be safely inferred that the search for an ideal modality for the diagnosis of peripheral pulmonary nodules is still going on.
- The final decision for using a modality, alone or in combination, may be based not just on what technique works best but also on expertise that is available and affordable.

INTRODUCTION

We are in an era of increasing reliance on obtaining imaging studies, including computed tomography (CT) scans of the chest, for diverse medical problems. Consequently, many pulmonary nodules are detected incidentally.[1,2] These nodules are typically small, focal, radiographic opacities that may be solitary or multiple. By definition, a single, spherical, well-circumscribed, radiographic opacity surrounded completely by aerated lung and measuring less than or equal to 3 cm in diameter is referred to as a *solitary pulmonary nodule* (SPN). *Peripheral pulmonary nodules* (PPN) are defined as lesions that are present beyond the visualized segmental bronchi. With improving resolution of the CT scan, these nodules are seldom detected in solitude. For the purpose of uniformity, the authors address these lesions as PPN.

With the findings of the recently released National Cancer Institute–sponsored National Lung Screening Trial suggesting a reduction in lung cancer–specific mortality with CT screening in at-risk people, the number of patients diagnosed with PPN could increase substantially in the near future.[3] It warrants mentioning that as many as

Conflicts of Interest: T. Narula and A.C. Mehta: None; M.S. Machuzak: Consultant for Olympus, USA.
[a] Respiratory Institute, Cleveland Clinic, 9500 Euclid Avenue, A90, Cleveland, OH 44195, USA; [b] Center for Major Airway Diseases, Respiratory Institute, Cleveland Clinic, 9500 Euclid Avenue, A90, Cleveland, OH 44195, USA; [c] Lerner College of Medicine and Respiratory Institute, Cleveland Clinic, 9500 Euclid Avenue, A90, Cleveland, OH 44195, USA
* Corresponding author.
E-mail address: mehtaa1@ccf.org

25% to 30% of newly diagnosed lung cancers present initially as a peripheral lung lesion, thus making any newly detected lung nodule a cause for potential concern.[4] In nodules larger than 2 cm, the incidence of primary lung cancer ranges from 64% to 82%.[1] Small, subcentimeter nodules, on the other hand, are much less likely to be malignant, difficult to accurately characterize radiologically, and significantly more challenging to approach bronchoscopically.[5]

Managing patients with PPN requires an organized approach that incorporates an in-depth history taking and a thorough physical examination. Emphasis must be laid on eliciting potential risk factors and clues for malignant, infectious, or inflammatory causes. This evaluation should be accompanied by defining the radiological characteristics of the nodule that may provide clues to a benign versus a malignant cause. The pattern of calcification, if present within the nodule, must be elaborated. Historically, diffuse, central, laminated and popcorn patterns of calcification suggest a benign diagnosis.[6] If one of these patterns is clearly evident, literature suggests that no additional evaluation is necessary. Comparison with old films can provide invaluable information. If a PPN is stable on imaging studies for at least 2 years, it is unlikely to be malignant and further diagnostic evaluation may not be needed. Pure ground-glass nodules that often represent slowly growing preinvasive adenocarcinoma in situ necessitate a longer duration of follow-up.[5,7]

With advances in imaging modalities, our capability to characterize PPN has improved immensely. The traditional chest radiographic image can now be supplemented with dual-energy digital subtraction radiography. CT of the chest with dynamic contrast enhancement can provide accurate descriptions of the features of a nodule. As a metabolically active tool, fluorodeoxyglucose–positron emission tomography (FDG-PET) can direct tissue biopsy by identifying lesions that are metabolically active and most likely to yield a diagnostic result on biopsy.[8] Integrated PET-CT imaging can have synergistic value in increasing the diagnostic veracity for a pulmonary nodule.[9]

Even with a thorough clinical examination and radiological evaluation, distinguishing between a benign and a malignant nodule can be challenging and sampling of the nodule is frequently required. In such situations, the value of the preliminary investment in clinicoradiological definition lies in the generation of qualitative and quantitative models for estimating the clinical pretest probability of malignancy. The American College of Chest Physician's guidelines recommend using these models to guide the need for further work-up or diagnostic testing.[5] Evidence-based widely accepted guidelines are also available to facilitate decisions regarding radiological follow-up of PPN detected on chest imaging (**Table 1**).[10]

Based on the assessment and after factoring in patient suitability and preferences, the management alternatives for a pulmonary nodule range

Table 1
Recommendations for follow-up and management of nodules smaller than 8 mm detected incidentally at nonscreening CT

Nodule Size (mm)[a]	Low-Risk Patients[b]	High-Risk Patients[c]
≤4	No follow-up needed[d]	Follow-up CT at 12 mo; if unchanged, no further follow-up[e]
>4–6	Follow-up CT at 12 mo; if unchanged, no further follow-up[e]	Initial follow-up CT at 6–12 mo, then at 18–24 mo if no change[e]
>6–8	Initial follow-up CT at 6–12 mo then at 18–24 mo if no change	Initial follow-up CT at 3–6 mo, then at 9–12 and 24 mo if no change
>8	Follow-up CT at around 3, 9, and 24 mo, dynamic contrast-enhanced CT, PET, and/or biopsy	Same as for low-risk patients

Note: Newly detected indeterminate nodule in people 35 years of age or older.
[a] Average of length and width.
[b] Minimal or absent history of smoking and of other known risk factors.
[c] History of smoking or of other known risk factors.
[d] The risk of malignancy in this category (<1%) is substantially less than that in a baseline CT scan of an asymptomatic smoker.
[e] Nonsolid (ground-glass) or partly solid nodules may require longer follow-up to exclude indolent adenocarcinoma.
Adapted from MacMahon H, Austin JH, Gamsu G, et al. Guidelines for management of small pulmonary nodules detected on CT scans: a statement from the Fleischner Society. Radiology 2005;237:395–400; with permission.

from watchful waiting with serial imaging studies to various techniques of invasive testing, including those that can potentially offer therapeutic excision. If a decision is made to proceed with sampling of a pulmonary nodule, a broad range of modalities are now available, consistent with a wide array of technological advancements. The chosen modality would vary based on clinical context and institutional expertise. In the following sections, the authors discuss the spectrum of modalities available for invasive testing, focusing primarily on the newer bronchoscopic techniques for approaching PPN.

ROLE OF SURGERY

Surgical resection is the diagnostic gold standard for a pulmonary nodule. It comes with the additional benefit of potentially being therapeutic. Depending on the clinical context, video-assisted thoracoscopic surgery, thoracotomy, and mediastinoscopy may be used alone or in combination in patients with PPN. The surgical techniques have undergone considerable refinement over the years. Localizing techniques are increasingly being used to assist resection of smaller nodules. Methods like wire localization, radiotracer guidance, electromagnetic navigation guided–dye marking, CT guidance, and ultrasound (both intrathoracic and extrathoracic) have been used successfully.[11–18] The details of these techniques are beyond the scope of this review.

For obvious reasons, surgical resection cannot be an option for every patient. A less invasive option should be pursued in nodules that have a lower pretest probability of malignancy.[5]

PERCUTANEOUS RADIOLOGICAL TECHNIQUES

During the last few decades, numerous studies have evaluated the accuracy and yield of radiologically guided transthoracic lung biopsy procedures. CT guidance is now routinely used for transthoracic needle aspiration (TTNA) of pulmonary nodules with varying characteristics.[19–21] For malignant disease, the reported mean sensitivity and specificity are 90% and 97%, respectively. A meta-analysis by Lacasse and colleagues[22] that included 48 studies and 5 other meta-analysis of CT-guided fine-needle aspiration of PPN reported a sensitivity of 86.1% and specificity of 98.8%. Even though these numbers are impressive, it is important for practitioners to recognize the right candidates for this approach. Suggested contraindications for the procedure are summarized in **Box 1**.[23–25]

Various factors can affect the diagnostic yield of TTNA for PPN.

Box 1
Contraindications to percutaneous TTNA

Bleeding diathesis

Contralateral pneumonectomy or pneumothorax

Severe emphysematous disease or large bullae in biopsy path

Intractable cough

Mechanical ventilation

Patients unable to cooperate with procedure

- Unable to hold breath consistently
- Inability to lie in required position
- Unable to give informed consent
- Unable to follow directions

FEV_1 less than 0.8 L

Abbreviation: FEV_1, forced expiratory volume in the first second of expiration.

Data from Refs.[23–25]

Effect of Size

For subcentimeter pulmonary nodules, TTNA using CT guidance has a lower diagnostic accuracy.[26] Wallace and colleagues[27] reported a sensitivity of only 50% for lesions that measure from 0.5 to 0.7 cm in diameter. In another study looking at the impact of nodule size on diagnostic accuracy of CT-guided needle aspiration, nodules more than 1.5 cm were statistically more likely to result in a diagnostic specimen (73.5%) than nodules less than or equal to 1.5 cm (51.4%).[28]

Effect of Nature of Pathology

The overall accuracy of TTNA ranges from 70% to 100% and approaches 90% to 95% for the diagnosis of thoracic malignancies. Rivera and colleagues[29] performed a meta-analysis of published series extending from 1967 to 2003 and concluded that the sensitivity of TTNA in detecting lung cancer was 90%. However, the ability of TTNA to establish a specific benign diagnosis, as in the case of a granulomatous illness like tuberculosis or fungal infection, is quite variable, ranging from 16% to 68%.[30] Multiple samplings of the lesion, the use of cutting-needle biopsy, and routine culturing of aspirated specimens have been suggested to circumvent this limitation.[31]

Effect of Distance from Pleura

Distance from the pleura also affects the diagnostic accuracy, which tends to decrease to less than 60% when the needle path exceeds 40 mm.[32]

A frequently cited limitation of CT-TTNA is the inability to provide sufficient sample volume for ancillary testing.[33] With the advent of targeted therapy for the management of patients with lung cancer, the need for ancillary testing, including molecular testing, is of critical importance, especially in patients with non–small cell lung carcinoma because it can have significant therapeutic and prognostic implications.[34]

As is the case with any invasive diagnostic procedure, poorly chosen patients run the risk of having a lower diagnostic yield coupled with a higher likelihood of procedural complications. A recent study looking at population-based estimates of TTNA reported a significant morbidity of this procedure. In 15,865 patients, they documented a pneumothorax rate of 15.0%, with 6.6% requiring chest tube placement, and a rate of hemorrhage of 1.0%, with 18.0% of those requiring blood transfusion.[35] The risk of pneumothorax increases with the depth and size of the lesion, gauge of the biopsy needle, presence and severity of emphysema, increased number of pleural passes, and the acuity of the angle of needle entry.[36–39]

In summary, percutaneous radiologically guided sampling techniques have an excellent diagnostic yield for the diagnosis of PPN that comes at the cost of a high rate of complications, especially pneumothorax. As the development of alternative safer approaches with comparative diagnostic yield continues to be pursued, small peripheral nodules in candidates at low risk of complications from TTNA should still be sampled percutaneously under radiological guidance.

BRONCHOSCOPY FOR PERIPHERAL PULMONARY NODULE

The assessment of the available literature on the yield of bronchoscopic approach to PPN is impeded by the lack of standardization across different studies. Most studies are either retrospective or prospective case series, far from the rigors of a prospective, double-blind, randomized, controlled trial. Difficulties in interpreting the available literature stems from many different factors:

- There are differences in the definition of PPN.
- There is variability in the location and size of the lesions sampled. (Of note, the location of the pulmonary nodules is not reported in some of the studies.)
- There is a lack of uniformity in patient selection across different studies.
- There is a wide spectrum of techniques used alone or in combination.

- The effect of operator ability and experience that can affect the yield is not accounted for in most studies.

Most studies use diagnostic yield (number of positive tests/number of tests performed) as a primary outcome measure. On the surface, it is easy to surmise the practical and informative nature of this approach. However, this parameter assumes the absence of false positives and makes calculations of negative predictive value impossible. It can also be significantly influenced by the characteristics of the population being studied, limiting the feasibility of making valid comparisons between different studies.[30,40,41]

CONVENTIONAL TECHNIQUES

Conventional flexible bronchoscopic approaches include the following:

- Bronchoalveolar lavage (BAL)
- Use of cytology brush
- Transbronchial biopsy (TBBx)
- Transbronchial needle aspiration (TBNA)
- Curette

For the evaluation of central airway lesions and large masses, the overall reported diagnostic sensitivity of flexible bronchoscopy is as high as 88%.[29] However, these numbers are not replicated when it comes to diagnosing PPN using conventional bronchoscopic techniques. In 1967, Tsuboi and coworkers[42] in Japan described the technique of using a specially designed curette with a high diagnostic yield for PPN. However, the independent use of a curette has been infrequent in the United States, and data on its diagnostic yield are limited.[42–44] For the other aforementioned techniques, when used independently, the diagnostic sensitivity of various conventional modalities ranges between 43% for BAL/washings and 65% for TBNA (Table 2).[44–83] However, the overall sensitivity for various modalities when combined together in the diagnosis of peripheral lesions is 78%.[29] Using fluoroscopic guidance adds to the diagnostic yield with bronchoscopy for PPN.[51,74,76,84] The presence of a visible air bronchogram extending into a nodule (the bronchus sign) has also been associated with a higher diagnostic yield.[56,85] Popovich and colleagues[86] demonstrated that diagnostic yield from PPN increases with the number of pieces of tissue sampled. In their study, the initial biopsy of a PPN had a sensitivity of 45%, which increased to 70% by the sixth sample.

The most important determinant of the yield of bronchoscopy for a PPN is the size of the nodule. An analysis of 10 studies that reported on the

Table 2
Sensitivity of conventional bronchoscopic procedures for PPN diagnosis

Author, Year	Patients	All Methods	TBLB	Brush	BAL	TBNA
van't Westeinde et al,[83] 2012	308	0.13	0.08	0.04	—	0.33
Roth et al,[82] 2008	—	0.16	0.25	0.16	0.06	0.19
Ost et al,[81] 2008	23	0.76	—	—	—	—
Sawabata et al,[80] 2006	1487	0.74	—	—	—	—
Kawaraya et al,[79] 2003	1372	0.88	0.77	0.57	—	0.35
Trkanjec et al,[78] 2003	50	0.86	0.62	0.16	0.29	—
Bandoh et al,[44] 2003	97	0.60	—	—	—	—
Baba et al,[77] 2002	87	0.75	0.53	0.44	—	0.67
Baaklini et al,[76] 2000	129	0.61	—	—	—	—
Gasparini et al,[75] 1999	480	0.76	0.50	—	—	0.70
Reichenberger et al,[74] 1999	103	—	0.39	0.36	0.28	0.47
Aristiazabal et al,[73] 1998	64	—	0.34	—	—	—
Bilaceroglu et al,[72] 1998	92	0.64	—	—	—	—
Wongsurakiat et al,[71] 1998	30	0.50	0.17	—	0.47	—
Sing et al,[70] 1997	22	—	—	0.22	—	—
Castella et al,[69] 1995	45	—	—	—	—	0.69
Debeljak et al,[68] 1994	39	—	0.77	0.59	0.36	—
de Gracia et al,[67] 1993	55	—	—	—	0.33	—
Torrington & Kern,[66] 1993	91	—	0.20	—	—	—
Utz et al,[65] 1993	—	—	—	—	—	—
Pirozynski,[64] 1992	145	—	0.33	0.30	0.65	0.58
Buccheri et al,[63] 1991	337	—	0.75	0.44	0.33	—
Popp et al,[62] 1991	87	—	0.80	0.83	—	—
Mak et al,[61] 1990	63	0.56	0.37	0.29	0.38	—
Rennard et al,[60] 1990	730	—	—	—	0.47	—
Gay & Brutinel,[59] 1989	20	—	—	—	—	0.65
Wagner et al,[58] 1989	—	—	—	—	—	—
Mori et al,[57] 1989	85	0.84	—	0.84	0.42	—
Naidich et al,[56] 1988	65	0.48	—	—	—	—
Cox et al,[55] 1984	22	0.36	0.29	0.22	0.36	—
Lam et al,[54] 1983	155	0.86	0.61	0.52	0.52	—
Pilotti et al,[53] 1982	84	—	—	0.29	—	—
Wallace & Deutsch,[52] 1982	143	—	0.19	—	—	—
McDougall & Cortese,[51] 1981	130	0.62	0.48	0.36	0.36	—
Radke et al,[50] 1979	82	0.51	—	—	—	—
Stringfield et al,[49] 1977	29	—	0.48	—	—	—
Kvale et al,[48] 1976	29	—	0.27	0.21	0.12	—
Zavala,[47] 1975	137	0.71	0.69	0.70	—	—
Hattori et al,[46] 1971	208	—	—	0.83	—	—
Oswald et al,[45] 1971	435	—	0.28	—	—	—

sensitivity of bronchoscopy for peripheral lesions by size revealed that the sensitivity was much lower for nodules that were less than 2 cm in size (34%) as compared with nodules with a diameter of more than 2 cm (63%).[29] The effect of nodule size was reinforced in a recent prospective study evaluating the role of conventional bronchoscopy in the work-up of test-positive participants in a lung cancer–screening program. The overall sensitivity of conventional bronchoscopy in this study was only

13.5%. Nodule size, once again, was demonstrated as an independent predictor of diagnostic yield.[83]

Stratification based on size and location has demonstrated a diagnostic yield of 14% for SPNs less than 2 cm in diameter that are located in the outer one-third of the lung. For lesions less than 2 cm in size located in the middle one-third of the lung, a higher yield of 31% has been reported.[87]

In summary, without a visible air bronchogram extending into the nodule, the diagnostic yield of conventional bronchoscopy for PPN, particularly those that are less than 2 cm in size, is limited. Conventional bronchoscopy is being superseded by newer bronchoscopic techniques that are elaborated further in this review. However, it is important to recognize that logistic constraints limit their availability in many parts of the world. In such settings, we recommend performing conventional bronchoscopic testing using a combination of modalities (BAL, Transbronchial lung biopsy (TBLB), brush, TBNA) to assist in diagnosing PPN, especially those that are larger than 2 cm or the ones that have an air bronchogram leading to the nodule.

NEWER MODALITIES

Bronchoscopy has evolved considerably during the past decade, and several promising procedures with new devices have been developed.

RADIAL PROBE ENDOBRONCHIAL ULTRASOUND
Basis

Radial probe endobronchial ultrasound (R-EBUS) is a technique that uses ultrasound to visualize structures within and adjacent to the airway wall. Principally, it uses a transducer to produce and transmit sound waves and then receive back the reflected sound waves. A processor integrates the sound waves (or echoes) reflected by the tissues (dependent on absorption, scatter, and reflection) and by the tissue interfaces (different acoustic impedances) to generate 2-dimensional (2D) ultrasound images.[88]

First introduced to evaluate the central airway structures, especially the mediastinal and hilar lymph nodes, advances in R-EBUS technology have permitted the visualization and performance of transbronchial biopsies of PPN without exposure to radiation.[89] To this end, a 20- or 30-MHz R-EBUS with a rotating transducer that provides 360° images of the airway wall and surrounding structures is commonly used. Depending on the diameter of the probe, a bronchoscope with a 2.0-mm or a 2.8-mm working channel can be used. A methodological limitation of R-EBUS is that the procedure does not provide real-time ultrasound guidance. The ultrasonic probe must be removed from the bronchoscope to introduce biopsy instruments after the target lesion is localized. To overcome this limitation, a technique using a guide sheath, which acts as an extended working channel beyond the reach of the bronchoscope for repeated biopsy, has been developed.[90,91] Although R-EBUS has been used extensively without the guide sheath, most recent trials focused on R-EBUS–TBBx incorporate the guide sheath (GS) method.[92–95]

Technique

Once the conventional bronchoscopy is performed, the bronchoscope tip is placed in the bronchus nearest to the nodule. The ultraminiature radial probe is placed inside the GS. Both the probe and the GS are advanced through the working channel of the bronchoscope until the nodule is visualized. Although normal air-containing lung tissue has a snowstormlike whitish image, a solid lesion appears darker. It can be distinguished from the lung tissue by a bright border (**Fig. 1**).[96] The radial probe is then removed, leaving the GS in position. The GS in effect serves as an extended working channel. Sampling instruments are inserted through the GS to obtain pathologic specimens from the nodule for analysis (**Fig. 2**).[91]

Diagnostic Yield

The overall diagnostic yield of R-EBUS ranges from 34% to 84%. Of note, even for nodules less than

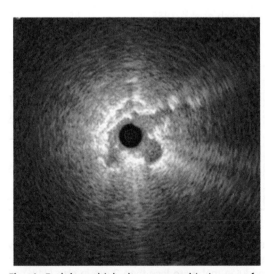

Fig. 1. Endobronchial ultrasonographic image of a single pulmonary nodule distinguished from pulmonary parenchyma by a bright border.

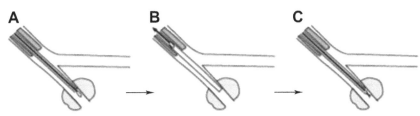

Fig. 2. R-EBUS–GS–guided biopsy. (*A*) R-EBUS is advanced to PPN via a flexible bronchoscope. (*B*) After confirmation by R-EBUS imaging, the R-EBUS probe is pulled out. (*C*) Sampling instruments are introduced through the GS. (*From* Kikuchi E, Yamazaki K, Sukoh N, et al. Endobronchial ultrasonography with guide-sheath for peripheral pulmonary lesions. Eur Respir J 2004;24:533–7; with permission.)

30 mm, the diagnostic yield of R-EBUS–TBBx approaches close to 80%.[90,93,95,97–99] Recently published retrospective data on the yield of R-EBUS for benign peripheral processes revealed a significantly higher yield compared with historical controls (58% vs 28%).[100] In fact, in a prospective randomized pragmatic trial comparing the effectiveness of R-EBUS–TBBx and the CT-guided percutaneous needle biopsy (PNB-TTNA) in the work-up of PPN, the diagnostic accuracy of R-EBUS–TBBx was shown to be no inferior to that of CT-guided PNB-TTNA and with a significantly lower complication rate.[101] Many fluoroscopically invisible lesions can also be localized with R-EBUS.[102]

A systematic review of the published literature evaluating R-EBUS accuracy comprising 16 studies with 1420 patients revealed that there was significant interstudy variation in the R-EBUS technique. Overall, R-EBUS had a pooled sensitivity of 73% for the detection of lung cancer.[94] **Table 3** summarizes the published literature for R-EBUS for PPN.

The combination of R-EBUS with other modalities has been shown to result in an improved diagnostic yield. Eberhardt and colleagues[118] studied electromagnetic navigational bronchoscopy (ENB) alone, R-EBUS alone, and ENB combined with R-EBUS. The diagnostic yield of ENB, R-EBUS, and the combination of the two was 59%, 69%, and 88%, respectively. Although R-EBUS alone was better than ENB alone, the combination increased the yield to levels comparable with TTNA, suggesting that a combination of modalities may improve the diagnostic yield.

Mizugaki and colleagues[123] studied the incremental yield of combining R-EBUS with imaging modalities, including x-ray fluoroscopy and FDG-PET. A total of 69.2% PPN were diagnosed by TBBx using R-EBUS combined with x-ray fluoroscopy. The diagnostic yield of FDG-PET independently was 78.5%. The yield with the combination of R-EBUS–TBBx and FDG-PET (90.7%) was significantly higher when compared with either procedure alone. Improved diagnostic yield with a combination of R-EBUS and fluoroscopy guidance as compared with fluoroscopy guided bronchoscopy alone (79.3 vs 33.3%) for PPN smaller than 20 mm in diameter has recently been reported.[105]

An additional advantage of R-EBUS is that it permits the visualization of the internal structure of PPN, and this information may suggest the histology of the lesion. Three classes (and 6 subclasses) of the PPN can be distinguished with R-EBUS:

Type I: a homogeneous nodule
Type II: a nodule with hyperechoic dots and linear arcs
Type III: a heterogeneous nodule

In a retrospective study, 92% of the type I lesions were benign (n = 25) and 99% of the type II and III lesions were malignant (n = 99).[124] Other characteristics of R-EBUS image patterns, including low level echoes and the halo sign, have also been recently described to help distinguish benign from malignant PPN. The presence of either of these two echo features had a diagnostic sensitivity of 94.6% for malignant lesions, and the coexistence of the two features had a specificity of 93% for a diagnosis of malignant lesions.[125]

Factors that affect the diagnostic yield of R-EBUS–TBBx have been investigated. The position of the probe relative to a peripheral lung lesion has been noted to be associated with a significant impact on the diagnostic yield of R-EBUS–guided TBLB.[99] The location of the probe directly within the lesion was 8.17 times more likely to have a successful TBBx than when the probe was adjacent to the lesion.[103] The size of the lesion has also been suggested to be a factor in determining the diagnostic yield.[91,98] Similar to conventional techniques, a retrospective study found that the diagnostic yield with R-EBUS increased from 65% to 97% with increasing number of biopsy samples, with 5 samples being the optimum number.[116]

In summary, R-EBUS is an excellent addition to the bronchoscopic tool set for the diagnosis of PPN. Although the yield still does not match up

Table 3
Diagnostic yield of R-EBUS for PPN

Study, Year	Design	Technology	Lesions	Yield (%)
Lin et al,[103] 2012	Retro	R-EBUS	39	76.9
Ishida et al,[104] 2012	Retro	R-EBUS, GS	65	64.6
Shinagawa et al,[100] 2012	Retro	R-EBUS, GS	171	58.0
Boonsarngsuk et al,[105] 2012	Retro	R-EBUS, GS	57	82.5
Oki et al,[106] 2012	Pro	R-EBUS, GS, U	203	63.5
Kuo et al,[107] 2011	Pro	R-EBUS	408	64.2
Fujita et al,[108] 2011	Retro	R-EBUS, GS	51	80.4
Ishida et al,[109] 2011	Pro	R-EBUS, GS	95	67.4
Roth et al,[110] 2011	Pro	R-EBUS, GS	124	36.0
Eckardt et al,[111] 2010	Retro	R-EBUS	95	43.0
Disayabutr et al,[112] 2010	Pro	R-EBUS	152	66.4
Oki et al,[113] 2009	Pro	R-EBUS, U	71	69.0
Eberhardt et al,[96] 2009	Pro	R-EBUS, GS	100	46.0
Huang et al,[98] 2009	Retro	R-EBUS	83	53.0
Chao et al,[92] 2009	Pro	R-EBUS	182	69.2
Fielding et al,[114] 2008	Pro	R-EBUS, GS	140	66.4
Asano et al,[115] 2008	Pro	R-EBUS, GS, VB, U	32	84.4
Yamada et al,[116] 2007	Retro	R-EBUS, GS	158	67.1
Yoshikawa et al,[117] 2007	Pro	R-EBUS, GS	123	86.2
Dooms et al,[97] 2007	Pro	R-EBUS	50	68.0
Eberhardt et al,[118] 2007	Pro	R-EBUS, GS	39	69.0
Chung et al,[119] 2007	Pro	R-EBUS	158	49.0
Herth et al,[102] 2006	Pro	R-EBUS, GS	54	70.4
Asahina et al,[120] 2005	Pro	R-EBUS, GS, VB, U	30	63.3
Paone et al,[95] 2005	Pro	R-EBUS	87	75.8
Kurimoto et al,[90] 2004	Pro	R-EBUS, GS	150	77.3
Kikuchi et al,[91] 2004	Pro	R-EBUS, GS	24	58.3
Yang et al,[121] 2004	Retro	R-EBUS	122	65.6
Shirakawa et al,[122] 2004	Pro	R-EBUS, GS	51	82.4
Herth et al,[93] 2002	Pro	R-EBUS	50	80.0

Abbreviations: Pro, prospective; Retro, retrospective; U, ultrathin bronchoscopy; VB, virtual bronchoscopy.

with radiologically guided TTNA, R-EBUS has a much better safety profile. If available, the authors suggest using R-EBUS for PPN diagnosis, especially for patients with smaller nodules and in those whereby TTNA carries a significant risk of complications.

ELECTROMAGNETIC NAVIGATION
Basis

Electromagnetic navigation (EMN) is a novel technology that facilitates approaching PPN and mediastinal lymph nodes that are difficult to sample with conventional flexible bronchoscopy (FB). The navigation system involves creating an electromagnetic (EM) field around the patient's chest and then directing endoscopic accessories using a microsensor placed on previously acquired CT images. In other words, EMN is an image-guided localization device, operating on the principles of electromagnetism that assists in placing endobronchial accessories in the target areas of the lung.[126–130] The components of the EMN include the following:

Electromagnetic location board
The electromagnetic location board (EMLB) is placed under the cephalic end of the bronchoscopy table mattress. It generates low-frequency EM waves and produces an EM field over the patient's chest (**Fig. 3**A).

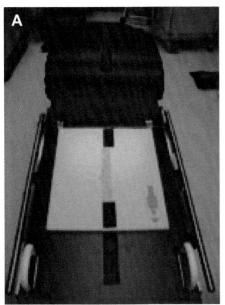
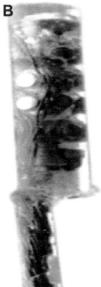
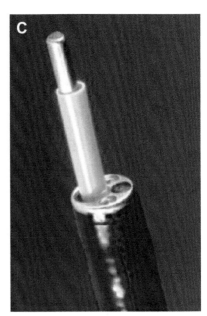

Fig. 3. (*A*) EMLB. (*B*) Microsensor. (*C*) Extended working channel (*blue*) with locatable guide in place.

Microsensor probe

A retractable microsensor probe on the tip of a flexible locatable guide (LG) is placed within the EM field (see **Fig. 3**B). Its position in the x, y, and z axes and in motion (roll, pitch, and yaw) is captured by the EMN system and displayed on the monitor in real time superimposed on previously acquired CT images.

Steerable guide

The LG also has a feature that allows its distal end to be steered in 360°, in 45° increments. The terms *steerable* and *locatable* guide are used interchangeably. The LG also provides a socket for connecting a wire, which relays the information from the sensor to the main computer.

Extended working channel

The LG is inserted into a 130-cm-long, 1.9-mm-diameter flexible catheter, serving as an extended working channel (EWC) (see **Fig. 3**C). Once the tip of the bronchoscope is wedged into the segmental bronchus of interest, the LG is advanced along with the EWC under the guidance provided by the navigation system. On reaching the desired target, the LG is withdrawn leaving the EWC in place. Endobronchial accessories are inserted through the EWC to sample the target.

CT

A high-resolution spiral CT scan of the chest is performed and reconstructed with a protocol specific to the scanner manufacturer. This recommended

reconstruction protocol optimizes CT images suitable for planning and navigational purposes.

Computer interphase

The EMN system is provided with 2 separate computers: a laptop with a dedicated program for *planning* and a main system computer used for *registration* and *navigation*.

ENB system

A new generation of the EMN bronchoscopy system was introduced in 2009. Improvements include a new software platform with a simplified planning and navigational system that improves the ease of use and enhances visualization for the physician.

Technique

EMN is performed in the following steps:

1. CT imaging

A spiral CT scan of the chest is performed. The scanner type should be a multi-slice, 4-detector or greater, with 16-detector or greater preferred. Reconstruction parameters are recommended by manufacturer type to optimize generation of a 3D map.

2. Planning module overview and workflow

Digitized information from the CT scan is downloaded into the software of the dedicated laptop. This information is used to reconstruct graphic axial, coronal, and sagittal views of the chest, a virtual bronchoscopic image (**Fig. 4**), and a 3D

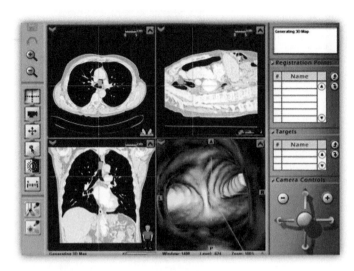

Fig. 4. CT cross sections and virtual bronchoscopy image.

representation of the patients' tracheobronchial tree and pleura. Using these views, a plan is created that will be used during the procedure.

Procedure planning comprises 4 phases:
a. Registration planning
   Registration is the process of matching the patients' CT images to the patients' body. Planning is not required for automatic registration. If a 3D map is not available, manual registration points are marked using the CT cross sections and the virtual view. These registration points are matched to actual anatomic landmarks in patients during the procedure. Five (or more) registration points are advised, specifically the main carina and 2 points in each lung, one in the upper lobe and one in the middle/lower lobe.
b. Marking target locations and dimensions
   Scrolling through the CT cross sections is performed to identify targets. Once identified, the location of the target is marked using the CT cross sections and the target dimensions are set.
c. Pathway planning
   If a 3D map is available, one or more automatic pathways to each target can be constructed to assist in navigation (**Fig. 5**). The suggested pathway can be modified, extended with waypoints, or it can be accepted for use as is.
d. Saving the plan and exiting
   When the procedure plan is complete, it is exported to a CD, a removable disk (USB), or to a network storage location for transfer to the procedure system.

3. Registration

The information gathered during the planning stage is uploaded to the systems main computer using the external memory device. FB is performed in the bronchoscopy suite where the EMN system is mapped for its surrounding metallic objects. When patients are placed on the examination table, 3 reference electrodes are fixed on the chest wall to accommodate for respiratory motion and nominal patient movement. FB is performed in a usual fashion. The LG is inserted via the working channel of the scope.

During the automatic registration process, the system records the location of the LG while the physician performs a bronchoscopic survey of

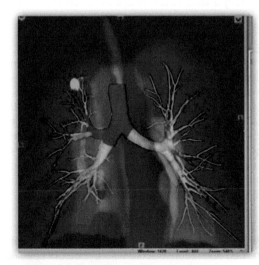

Fig. 5. Automatic pathway.

the lungs, creating a virtual cloud of navigation points that approximates the tracheobronchial tree. The system completes the registration process by matching the navigation cloud to the 3D map.

4. Real-time navigation

Following a successful registration, the scope with the LG in place is advanced toward the segmental bronchus of interest with multiple view ports available to aid navigation. In addition to pathway guidance, steering directions are provided to specific navigation objects using the tip view that represents the steering wheel on the LG handle (**Fig. 6**). This view shows the direction to rotate the steering wheel to turn the LG toward the selected navigation object. Once the LG reaches the desired target location, the EWC is fixed at the proximal end of the biopsy channel of the bronchoscope by a special locking mechanism and the LG is withdrawn. Bronchoscopic accessories are then inserted via the EWC to obtain a tissue specimen.

Yield

Several studies have been published establishing the effectiveness of the EMN in the diagnosis of PPN (**Table 4**).

After Schwarz and colleagues[127] performed the first animal trial to determine the practicality, accuracy, and safety of the real-time EMN in locating peripheral lung lesions in a swine model, Becker and colleagues[126] published results of a pilot study in humans. They obtained biopsies of PPN under the guidance of EMN in 29 patients. A definitive diagnosis was established in 20 patients

Table 4 Diagnostic yield of electromagnetic navigation for PPN				
Study, Year	Design	Lesions	Size (mm)	Yield (%)
Pearlstein et al,[131] 2012	Retro	104	28.0	85
Mahajan et al,[132] 2011	Retro	48	20.0	77
Seijo et al,[133] 2010	Pro	51	25.0	67
Eberhardt et al,[134] 2010	Pro	54	23.3	76
Bertoletti et al,[135] 2009	Pro	54	28.0	71
Lamprecht et al,[136] 2009	Retro	13	30.0	77
Wilson et al,[137] 2007	Retro	248	21.0	70
Makris et al,[138] 2007	Pro	40	23.5	63
Eberhardt et al,[118] 2007	Pro	120	26.0	59
Ebenhardt et al,[139] 2007	Pro	89	24.0	67
Schwarz et al,[128] 2006	Pro	13	33.5	69
Gildea et al,[130] 2006	Pro	60	22.8	74
Becker et al,[126] 2005	Retro	29	39.8	69

Abbreviations: Pro, prospective; Retro, retrospective.

(69%). There was one pneumothorax requiring chest tube insertion. Schwartz and colleagues[128] reported a similar diagnostic yield for PPN ranging in size from 1.5 to 5.0 cm. Hautmann and colleagues[129] performed a prospective validation study evaluation of an EMN system and concluded that EMN was safe and useful in localizing small and fluoroscopically invisible lung lesions with an acceptable level of accuracy.

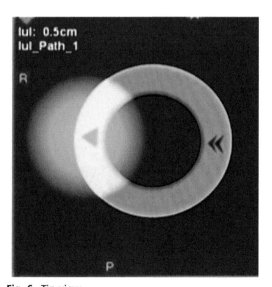

Fig. 6. Tip view.

Gildea and colleagues[130] conducted a larger prospective study involving 60 patients to determine the ability of this technology to diagnose peripheral lung lesions and mediastinal lymph nodes. The mean size of the pulmonary nodules was 22.8 ± 12.6 mm. The diagnostic yield was 74%, and diagnosis was obtained in 80.3% of all procedures (including lymph node sampling). Of interest was the lack of effect of the lesion size on the diagnostic yield. Pneumothorax occurred in 2 (3.5%) patients who had transbronchial biopsies of lesions that were in upper-lobe locations. Makris and colleagues[138] and Eberhardt and colleagues[139] also undertook prospective studies to determine the yield of EMN for diagnosing PPN. The diagnostic yield was found to be 67.0% and 62.5%, respectively, and was independent of lesion size. Both studies concluded that EMN can be used as a stand-alone procedure (without fluoroscopy) without compromising diagnostic yield.

It has also been established by a prospective randomized trial that the combination of R-EBUS and EMN improves the diagnostic yield of FB in PPN without compromising safety. In this particular study, Eberhardt showed that combined EBUS/EMN had a significantly higher diagnostic yield of 88% compared with that of EBUS (69%) and EMN (59%) alone. The improved yield of the joint procedure ascribed to combining the ability of EBUS to directly visualize the peripheral lung lesions with the precise navigation capabilities of EMN. The overall pneumothorax rate was 6.0% (7 patients) and 6.3% (5 patients) when EMN was used. Four of the 7 patients required a chest tube placement. Although this combination provides a higher diagnostic yield compared with either one of them alone, the issues of cost and training need to be addressed.[118]

Studies evaluating EMN with imaging modalities, such as PET-CT, as well as with the rapid on-site evaluation of cytology specimens have shown this combination to be safe and highly effective.[136,137]

A distinct advantage for EMN when compared with other bronchoscopic techniques is that the efficacy of the technique is not necessarily impacted by the size of the lesion, with several studies showing a similar diagnostic accuracy for lesions smaller or larger than 2 cm. Akin to conventional TBLB, lesions in which a bronchus leads to the abnormality (bronchus sign) have a significantly higher yield than those without a visible airway to the lesion.[133]

In summary, EMN is a useful tool to aid in the diagnosis of PPN, especially in combination with other novel technologies like R-EBUS. However, EMN systems are still limited in general application by their high capital cost and training necessary for optimal system use. The greatest experience and yield with these technologies has occurred in centers of excellence. It remains to be seen if similar results will be reproducible in less experienced centers; hence, recommendations for its routine use cannot be made at this time.[140]

ULTRATHIN BRONCHOSCOPE
Basis

The size (5.7 mm) of the conventional bronchoscope limits it from being advanced beyond a segmental or subsegmental bronchus. This limitation frequently translates into difficulty advancing endobronchial accessories to the more distant bronchi. Ultrathin bronchoscope by virtue of its smaller diameter (2.8–3.5 mm) can be inserted beyond the sixth-generation bronchi, offering the bronchoscopist an opportunity to get closer to the peripheral target (**Fig. 7**). Their maneuverability aids negotiation through a peripheral bronchus at an obtuse angle. A site that is typically difficult to approach with the conventional bronchoscope, such as the medial part of the lung apex, can be easily reached with an ultrathin bronchoscope. There is also an increased likelihood of discovering an endobronchial lesion that may have been beyond the scope of the conventional bronchoscope.[141–143]

Yield

There are no randomized controlled trials comparing the diagnostic yield of ultrathin bronchoscopy with the conventional modalities. Across the studies,

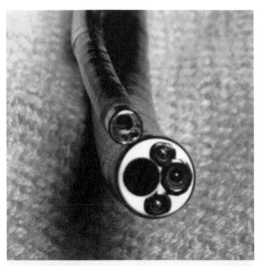

Fig. 7. Ultrathin bronchoscope compared with a standard bronchoscope.

the overall diagnostic yield of an ultrathin broncho-scope for small peripheral lesions (less than 30 mm in size) is variable, ranging from 57% to 81%.[141,144,145] Early studies were conducted using an ultrathin bronchoscope with a 1.2-mm working channel, using it as an adjunct to conventional bronchoscopy. In 17 patients with PPN, Rooney and colleagues[146] performed TBBx with standard bronchoscopy under fluoroscopic guidance, fol-lowing the same bronchial route to the lesion as established by the ultrathin bronchoscope. Their diagnostic yield was 65% (11 out of 17) in all patients examined and 70% (7 out of 10) in patients with le-sions less than 30 mm in size. Yamamoto and colleagues,[147] while studying this modality in 35 pa-tients with PPN, pointed out that sufficient material could not always be obtained with the miniaturized instruments that are introduced through a 1.2-mm working channel. Oki and colleagues[141] studied an ultrathin bronchoscope with a larger 1.7-mm work-ing channel in 118 patients with localized peripheral pulmonary lesions. They reported a cumulative yield of 69%, with a yield of 57% in lesions less than 20 mm.

Combinations of ultrathin bronchoscope with other advanced modalities, especially those that can assist in navigating to the region of interest, have also been reported. Shinagawa and col-leagues[148] reported the utility of the ultrathin bronchoscope in combination with virtual bron-choscopic guidance for small peripheral lesions. Although they found the technique effective with a diagnostic yield of 65.4%, difficulties in navi-gating to the target were encountered because of the limp nature of the scope and difficulty to control it in the peripheral lung. A follow-up study by the same investigators evaluating the factors related to diagnostic sensitivity of the ultrathin bronchoscope highlighted the usefulness of the CT artery sign. Based on the premise that the pul-monary artery and the bronchus are next to each other in the periphery of the lung, they used pul-monary artery as a substitute for the traditional bronchus sign in peripheral areas where bronchi are not visualized.[145] Newer virtual bronchoscopy systems also offer navigational assistance by dis-playing the subsequent airway branching as the ultrathin bronchoscope is advanced and by rotating images as the scope is rotated to pre-serve the orientation. Using such navigation, Asano and colleagues[144] reported a diagnostic yield of using the ultrathin bronchoscope of up to 81.6% for PPN.

Innovative technology has led to the development of a thin 1.4-mm R-EBUS probe that is compatible with an ultrathin bronchoscope.[113] Diagnostic yield of R-EBUS–TBBx using the ultrathin bronchoscope

has been reported to be comparable with the guide-sheath method, with the added advantage of a significantly shorter procedural time.[106]

Recently, a hybrid tracking system that uses EM and image-based techniques has been reported to improve the accuracy and stability of the ultrathin bronchoscope.[149]

Despite all the available literature, to date, no randomized controlled trial has confirmed that ultrathin bronchoscope in isolation increases the diagnostic yield of standard bronchoscopy. Akin to other advanced techniques, its future probably lies in combination with other modalities, espe-cially the ones that can assist navigation in the complex 3D world of peripheral airways.

VIRTUAL BRONCHOSCOPIC NAVIGATION
Basis

Virtual bronchoscopy (VB), as the name suggests, is a simulation of actual bronchoscopy by the application of 3D display techniques to the air-ways. VB navigation (VBN) is a method in which virtual bronchoscopic images of the bronchial path to a peripheral lesion are generated and used as a guide to navigate the bronchoscope.[150] The amount of detail displayed in VBN depends on the CT quality from which the images are gener-ated. The advent of multi-detector CT imaging has facilitated detailed and accurate 3D recon-struction. Concerns regarding misalignment of vir-tual and real images as a result of the rotation of the bronchoscope do exist. To circumvent these, VBN systems that allow automatic synchronization of virtual and actual images for reliable navigation have been developed.[115,144,151]

Yield

VBN being primarily an imaging modality defining the track to a lesion has been tested in conjunction with various other techniques, including CT-guided ultrathin bronchoscopy, x-ray fluoroscopic bron-choscopy, and R-EBUS with a GS (R-EBUS–GS).

VBN with CT-Guided Ultrathin Bronchoscopy

CT guidance allows visualization of lesions that cannot be observed with fluoroscopy.[152,153] Combining VBN with CT-guided ultrathin bron-choscopy, Asano and colleagues[154] found that the ultrathin bronchoscope could be successfully guided along the planned path toward the lesion in 30 out of 36 (83.3%) PPN. A subsequent study by the same investigators in smaller lesions that were less than 3 cm revealed an even higher yield. The investigators were able to guide the broncho-scope to the expected path in 33 out of 36

(94.7%), with a diagnostic yield of 81.6%.[144] Despite a similar combination of technologies, Shinagawa and colleagues[155] reported a lower diagnostic yield of 70.4% in lesions less than 2 cm in diameter, with a higher percentage of benign cases deemed as the cause of a relatively lower diagnostic yield. Overall, although the diagnostic yield is considered acceptable, the concerns of radiation exposure caused by CT imaging are, however, the primary deterrent for this combination.

VBN with X-ray Fluoroscopy

To date, only 1 study by Tachihara and colleagues[156] has looked at this combination in 96 PPN less than or equal to 30 mm in size. Their overall yield was 62.5%, with diagnostic rates being 35.0%, 61.4%, and 94.7% for lesions less than or equal to 10 mm, 10 to 20 mm, and more than 20 mm, respectively.

VBN with EBUS

Three studies have assessed the diagnostic yield of combining VBN with EBUS for PPN. Asahina and colleagues,[120] using VBN with R-EBUS–GS, reported an overall diagnostic yield of 63.3% (19 out of 30) in PPN less than or equal to 30 mm in diameter. Asano and colleagues[115] reported an 84.4% (27 out of 32) diagnostic yield for peripheral lesions using VBN and EBUS-GS with a thin bronchoscope. A recent prospective, multicenter, randomized trial demonstrated that VBN-assisted R-EBUS–GS significantly improved the diagnostic yield of small (less than 30 mm) PPN to 80.4%, which was 13% higher than in the non-VBN–assisted group.[109]

In addition to the diagnostic purposes, VBN has also found an application in providing guidance for therapeutic procedures by marking the location of the lesion as well as the resection range for fluoroscopic-assisted thoracoscopic surgery.[157,158] Beyond all this, VBN can and does serve an important educational purpose for illustratively teaching the bronchial branching pattern.

CT FLUOROSCOPY
Basis

Conventional bronchoscopic TBBx of pulmonary nodules is performed under x-ray fluoroscopy. This 2D technique has a limited capacity in terms of visualization and localization of PPN and, hence, does not guarantee accurate access to a peripheral lesion. CT fluoroscopy, with its 3D capabilities, has been demonstrated to be potentially useful in guiding bronchoscopic procedures for small peripheral lesions.[145,152]

Yield

Case series using CT fluoroscopy for peripheral lesions have reported a diagnostic sensitivity of 62% to 67% for PPN. Using ultrathin bronchoscopy with CT guidance has resulted in diagnostic yields ranging from 65.4% to as high as 78.4%.[145,148,159,160] However, most studies had no comparator group, so the incremental value cannot be calculated except by extrapolation using historical control subjects.

A retrospective study by Tsushima and colleagues[81,161] compared patients who had undergone conventional bronchoscopy from 1999 to 2001 to those patients who had undergone CT-guided bronchoscopy from 2001 to 2003. After stratification for size, CT scan–guided bronchoscopy was found to be significantly superior for lesions less than 15 mm in diameter. Ost and colleagues[81] conducted the first and only prospective randomized trial comparing CT scan–guided bronchoscopy with conventional bronchoscopy for the diagnosis of lung cancer in PPN and mediastinal lymph nodes. Contrary to popular belief and prior data, the sensitivity for diagnosing malignancy with CT-guided bronchoscopy versus conventional bronchoscopy for peripheral lesions was not significantly different (71% vs 76%, respectively; $P = 1.0$).

Radiation exposure for patients and operators remains a major handicap whenever CT guidance is used. Mean CT fluoroscopy exposure time has been measured at 228 to 240 seconds per procedure.[81,162] To this end, the use of a dedicated low-dose CT protocol was recently demonstrated to reduce radiation doses considerably.[159]

Combination of Techniques and Diagnostic Approach

The discussion thus far has focused primarily on the independent modalities that have enhanced the various components of standard bronchoscopy. The availability of advanced CT scanners has permitted not just the sharper and detailed evaluation of lesions but also the generation of high-quality virtual bronchoscopic images of road maps to PPN. Navigational guidance has taken a giant leap by incorporating the science of electromagnetism. The ultrathin scopes have allowed bronchoscopists to charter unforeseen territory in human airways. R-EBUS has added a degree of certainty in what was frequently a best-guess technique for localization of nodules during bronchoscopic sampling. Because many of these techniques are exclusive of one another in terms of what they offer and achieve, it is not unreasonable to expect that a combination of technologies is likely to result in cumulative benefits. Hergott and Tremblay[30] classified the novel bronchoscopic modalities into 3 different categories:

Maneuverability techniques: ultrathin bronchoscopy, EMN with steerable probe component, and bihinged curette that can be inserted through the GS to maneuver into specific airways
Road map techniques: VB and EMN
Confirmation of navigation techniques: fluoroscopy, CT fluoroscopy, R-EBUS

It could be surmised that an ideal combination would include at least one component from each category to provide the best results. We are beginning to see some early literature validating the higher yield of combining these technologies. The works of Eberhardt and colleagues[118] as well as the recent meta-analysis by Wang Memoli and colleagues[40] are both pointers in this direction.

Before committing to making blanket recommendations for any of these technologies, a few facts warrant reinforcement:

1. To date, none of the new techniques either alone or in combination have consistently matched the yield of TTNA for PPN.
2. Time-tested conventional bronchoscopic techniques, when used together, still have a diagnostic yield of 63% in lesions larger than 2 cm
3. A major burden of PPN comes from developing economies where logistic and health infrastructure limitations weigh heavily in medical decision making. In many of these settings, mass access to modern innovations in bronchoscopy, in terms of equipment and trained personnel, may be a long time coming.

As more scientific data becomes available, the challenge ahead lies in prudently incorporating these modalities into algorithms for diagnosing PPN in a cost-effective manner. For patients with a very low probability of cancer, watchful waiting is still the best option. For those with a very high probability of cancer who are surgical candidates, operative resection is preferred. For patients with an intermediate probability of cancer, the decision of TTNA versus a bronchoscopic approach has to be carefully deliberated in each case, weighing the risk-to-benefit ratio for each approach. As is lucidly pointed out by Ost and Gould,[163] at the end of the day, patient preferences may have the biggest say because the absolute difference in outcomes between strategies may not be large.

SUMMARY

From the preceding discussion, it can be safely inferred that the search for an ideal modality for the diagnosis of PPN is still going on. Major strides have been made in bronchology, and technological advancements promise a future that is likely to witness many more innovations. The challenge lies not just in understanding the science behind these ideas and innovations but also in incorporating these in diagnostic pathways that can be consistently applied across different landscapes. Although available evidence and recommendations are presented, the authors appreciate that recommendations, by their very nature, cannot encompass all possible scenarios that occur in day-to-day clinical practice. The final decision for using a modality, alone or in combination, may be based not just on what technique works best but also on expertise that is available and affordable.

REFERENCES

1. Wahidi MM, Govert JA, Goudar RK, et al. Evidence for the treatment of patients with pulmonary nodules: when is it lung cancer? ACCP evidence-based clinical practice guidelines (2nd edition). Chest 2007;132(Suppl 3):94S–107S.
2. Henschke CI, McCauley DI, Yenkelevitz DF, et al. Early lung cancer action project: overall design and findings from baseline screening. Lancet 1999;354(9173):99–105.
3. The National Lung Screening Trial Research Team. Reduced lung-cancer mortality with low-dose computed tomographic screening. N Engl J Med 2011;365(5):395–409.
4. Schreiber G, McCrory DC. Performance characteristics of different modalities for diagnosis of suspected lung cancer: summary of published evidence. Chest 2003;123(Suppl 1):115S–28S.
5. Gould MK, Fletcher J, Iannettoni MD, et al. Evaluation of patients with pulmonary nodules: when is it lung cancer?: ACCP evidence-based clinical practice guidelines (2nd edition). Chest 2007; 132(Suppl 3):108S–30S.
6. Good CA, Wilson TW. The solitary circumscribed pulmonary nodule; study of seven hundred five cases encountered roentgenologically in a period of three and one-half years. J Am Med Assoc 1958;166(3):210–5.
7. Travis WD, Brambilla E, Noguchi M, et al. International association for the study of lung cancer/American Thoracic Society/European Respiratory Society international multidisciplinary classification of lung adenocarcinoma. J Thorac Oncol 2011;6(2):244–85.
8. Hain SF, Curran KM, Beggs AD, et al. FDG-PET as a "metabolic biopsy" tool in thoracic lesions with

indeterminate biopsy. Eur J Nucl Med 2001;28(9): 1336–40.

9. Chang CY, Tzao C, Lee SC, et al. Incremental value of integrated FDG-PET/CT in evaluating indeterminate solitary pulmonary nodule for malignancy. Mol Imaging Biol 2010;12(2):204–9.

10. MacMohan H, Austin JH, Gamsu G, et al. Guidelines for management of small pulmonary nodules detected on CT scans: a statement from the Fleischner Society. Radiology 2005;237(2): 395–400.

11. Pieterson RH, Hansen HJ, Dirksen A, et al. Lung cancer screening and video-assisted thoracic surgery. J Thorac Oncol 2012;7(6):1026–31.

12. Chen S, Zhou J, Zhang J, et al. Video-assisted thoracoscopic solitary pulmonary nodule resection after CT-guided hookwire localization: 43 cases report and literature review. Surg Endosc 2011; 25(6):1723–9.

13. Mullan BF, Stanford W, Barnhart W, et al. Lung nodules: improved wire for CT-guided localization. Radiology 1999;211(2):561–5.

14. Suzuki K, Nagal K, Yoshida J, et al. Video-assisted thoracoscopic surgery for small indeterminate pulmonary nodules: indications for preoperative marking. Chest 1999;115(2):563–8.

15. Eichfeld U, Dietrich A, Ott R, et al. Video-assisted thoracoscopic surgery for pulmonary nodules after computed tomography-guided marking with a spiral wire. Ann Thorac Surg 2005;79(1):313–6.

16. Bellomi M, Veronesi G, Trifiro G, et al. Computed tomography-guided preoperative radiotracer localization of nonpalpable lung nodules. Ann Thorac Surg 2010;90(6):1959–64.

17. Leong S, Ju H, Marshall H, et al. Electromagnetic navigation bronchoscopy: a descriptive analysis. J Thorac Dis 2012;4(2):173–85.

18. Andrade RS. Electromagnetic navigation bronchoscopy-guided thoracoscopic wedge resection of small pulmonary nodules. Semin Thorac Cardiovasc Surg 2010;22(3):262–5.

19. Hur J, Lee HJ, Nam JE, et al. Diagnostic accuracy of CT fluoroscopy-guided needle aspiration biopsy of ground-glass opacity pulmonary lesions. AJR Am J Roentgenol 2009;192(3):629–34.

20. Yamauchi Y, Izumi Y, Nakatsuka S, et al. Diagnostic performance of percutaneous core needle lung biopsy under multi-CT fluoroscopic guidance for ground-glass opacity pulmonary lesions. Eur J Radiol 2011;79(2):e85–9.

21. Hur J, Lee HJ, Byun MK, et al. Computed tomographic fluoroscopy-guided needle aspiration biopsy as a second biopsy technique after indeterminate transbronchial biopsy results for pulmonary lesions: comparison with second transbronchial biopsy. J Comput Assist Tomogr 2010; 34(2):290–5.

22. Lacasse Y, Wong E, Guyatt GH, et al. Transthoracic needle aspiration biopsy for the diagnosis of localised pulmonary lesions: a meta-analysis. Thorax 1999;54(10):884–93.

23. Birchard KR. Transthoracic needle biopsy. Semin Intervent Radiol 2011;28(1):87–97.

24. Klein JS, Zarka MA. Transthoracic needle biopsy. Radiol Clin North Am 2000;38(2):235–66.

25. Quon D, Fong TC, Mellor J, et al. Pulmonary function testing in predicting complications from percutaneous lung biopsy. Can Assoc Radiol J 1988; 39(4):267–9.

26. Ng YL, Patsios D, Roberts H, et al. CT-guided percutaneous fine-needle aspiration biopsy of pulmonary nodules measuring 10 mm or less. Clin Radiol 2008;63(3):272–7.

27. Wallace MJ, Krishnamurthy S, Broemeling LD, et al. CT-guided percutaneous fine-needle aspiration biopsy of small (< or =1-cm) pulmonary lesions. Radiology 2002;225(3):823–8.

28. Kothary N, Lock L, Sze DY, et al. Computed tomography-guided percutaneous needle biopsy of pulmonary nodules: impact of nodule size on diagnostic accuracy. Clin Lung Cancer 2009; 10(5):360–3.

29. Rivera MP, Mehta AC. American College of Chest Physicians. Initial diagnosis of lung cancer: ACCP evidence-based clinical practice guidelines (2nd edition). Chest 2007;132(Suppl 3): 131S–48S.

30. Hergott CA, Tremblay A. Role of bronchoscopy in the evaluation of solitary pulmonary nodules. Clin Chest Med 2010;31(1):49–63.

31. Moore EH. Percutaneous lung biopsy: an ordering clinician's guide to current practice. Semin Respir Crit Care Med 2008;29(4):323–34.

32. Ohno Y, Hatabu H, Takenaka D, et al. CT-guided transthoracic needle aspiration biopsy of small (< or = 20 mm) solitary pulmonary nodules. AJR Am J Roentgenol 2003;180(6):1665–9.

33. Khan KA, Zaidi S, Swan N, et al. The use of computerised tomography guided percutaneous fine needle aspiration in the evaluation of solitary pulmonary nodules. Ir Med J 2012;105(2):50–2.

34. Hasanovic A, Rekhtman N, Sigel CS, et al. Advances in fine needle aspiration cytology for the diagnosis of pulmonary carcinoma. Patholog Res Int 2011;2011:897292.

35. Wiener RS, Schwartz LM, Woloshin S, et al. Population-based risk for complications after transthoracic needle lung biopsy of a pulmonary nodule: an analysis of discharge records. Ann Intern Med 2011;155(3):137–44.

36. Yeow KM, Su IH, Pan KT, et al. Risk factors of pneumothorax and bleeding: multivariate analysis of 660 CT-guided coaxial cutting needle lung biopsies. Chest 2004;126(3):748–54.

37. Geraghty PR, Kee ST, McFarlane G, et al. CT-guided transthoracic needle aspiration biopsy of pulmonary nodules: needle size and pneumothorax rate. Radiology 2003;229(2):475–81.

38. Khan MF, Straub R, Moghaddam SR, et al. Variables affecting the risk of pneumothorax and intrapulmonal hemorrhage in CT-guided transthoracic biopsy. Eur Radiol 2008;18(7):1356–63.

39. Wu CC, Maher MM, Shephard JO. Complications of CT-guided percutaneous needle biopsy of the chest: prevention and management. AJR Am J Roentgenol 2011;196(6):W678–82.

40. Wang Memoli JS, Nietert PJ, Silvestri GA. Meta-analysis of guided bronchoscopy for the evaluation of the pulmonary nodule. Chest 2012; 142(2):385–93.

41. De Los Reyes A, Kundey SM, Wang M. The end of the primary outcome measure: a research agenda for constructing its replacement. Clin Psychol Rev 2011;31(5):829–38.

42. Tsuboi E, Ikeda S, Tajima M, et al. Transbronchial biopsy smear for diagnosis of peripheral pulmonary carcinomas. Cancer 1967;20(5):687–98.

43. Ono R, Loke J, Ikeda S. Bronchofiberscopy with curette biopsy and bronchography in the evaluation of peripheral lung lesions. Chest 1981;79(2): 162–6.

44. Bandoh S, Fujita J, Tojo Y, et al. Diagnostic accuracy and safety of flexible bronchoscopy with multiplanar reconstruction images and ultrafast Papanicolaou stain: evaluating solitary pulmonary nodules. Chest 2003;124(5):1985–92.

45. Oswald NC, Hinson KF, Canti G, et al. The diagnosis of primary lung cancer with special reference to sputum cytology. Thorax 1971;26:623–7.

46. Hattori S, Matsuda M, Nishihara H, et al. Early diagnosis of small peripheral lung cancer–cytologic diagnosis of very fresh cancer cells obtained by the TV-brushing technique. Acta Cytol 1971;15: 460–7.

47. Zavala DC. Diagnostic fiberoptic bronchoscopy: techniques and results of biopsy in 600 patients. Chest 1975;68:374–8.

48. Kvale PA, Bode FR, Kini S. Diagnostic accuracy in lung cancer; comparison of techniques used in association with flexible fiberoptic bronchoscopy. Chest 1976;69:752–7.

49. Stringfield JT, Markowitz DJ, Bentz RR, et al. The effect of tumor size and location on diagnosis by fiberoptic bronchoscopy. Chest 1977;72:474–6.

50. Radke JR, Conway WA, Eyler WR, et al. Diagnostic accuracy in peripheral lung lesions: factors predicting success with flexible fiberoptic bronchoscopy. Chest 1979;76:176–9.

51. McDougall JC, Cortese DA. Transbronchoscopic lung biopsy for localized pulmonary disease. Semin Respir Dis 1981;3:30–4.

52. Wallace JM, Deutsch AL. Flexible fiberoptic bronchoscopy and percutaneous needle lung aspiration for evaluating the solitary pulmonary nodule. Chest 1982;81:665–71.

53. Pilotti S, Rilke F, Gribaudi G, et al. Cytologic diagnosis of pulmonary carcinoma on bronchoscopic brushing material. Acta Cytol 1982;26:655–60.

54. Lam WK, So SY, Hsu C, et al. Fibreoptic bronchoscopy in the diagnosis of bronchial cancer: comparison of washings, brushings and biopsies in central and peripheral tumours. Clin Oncol 1983; 9:35–42.

55. Cox ID, Bagg LR, Russell NJ, et al. Relationship of radiologic position to the diagnostic yield of fiberoptic bronchoscopy in bronchial carcinoma. Chest 1984;85:519–22.

56. Naidich DP, Sussman R, Kutcher WL, et al. Solitary pulmonary nodules: CT-bronchoscopic correlation. Chest 1988;93:595–8.

57. Mori K, Yanase N, Kaneko M, et al. Diagnosis of peripheral lung cancer in cases of tumors 2 cm or less in size. Chest 1989;95:304–8.

58. Wagner ED, Ramzy I, Greenberg SD, et al. Transbronchial fine-needle aspiration: reliability and limitations. Am J Clin Pathol 1989;92:36–41.

59. Gay PC, Brutinel WM. Transbronchial needle aspiration in the practice of bronchoscopy. Mayo Clin Proc 1989;64:158–62.

60. Rennard SI, Albera C, Carratu L, et al. Clinical guidelines and indications for bronchoalveolar lavage (BAL): pulmonary malignancies. Eur Respir J 1990;3:956–7.

61. Mak VH, Johnston ID, Hetzel MR, et al. Value of washings and brushings at fibreoptic bronchoscopy in the diagnosis of lung cancer. Thorax 1990;45:373–6.

62. Popp W, Rauscher H, Ritschka L, et al. Diagnostic sensitivity of different techniques in the diagnosis of lung tumors with the flexible fiberoptic bronchoscope: comparison of brush biopsy, imprint cytology of forceps biopsy, and histology of forceps biopsy. Cancer 1991;67:72–5.

63. Buccheri G, Barberis P, Delfino MS. Diagnostic, morphologic, and histopathologic correlates in bronchogenic carcinoma: a review of 1,045 bronchoscopic examinations. Chest 1991;99:809–14.

64. Pirozynski M. Bronchoalveolar lavage in the diagnosis of peripheral, primary lung cancer. Chest 1992;102:372–4.

65. Utz JP, Patel AM, Edell ES. The role of transcarinal needle aspiration in the staging of bronchogenic carcinoma. Chest 1993;104:1012–6.

66. Torrington KG, Kern JD. The utility of fiberoptic bronchoscopy in the evaluation of the solitary pulmonary nodule. Chest 1993;104:1021–4.

67. de Gracia J, Bravo C, Miravitlles M, et al. Diagnostic value of bronchoalveolar lavage in

peripheral lung cancer. Am Rev Respir Dis 1993; 147:649–52.

68. Debeljak A, Mermolja M, Sorli J, et al. Bronchoalveolar lavage in the diagnosis of peripheral primary and secondary malignant lung tumors. Respiration 1994;61:226–30.

69. Castella J, Buj J, Puzo C, et al. Diagnosis and staging of bronchogenic carcinoma by transtracheal and transbronchial needle aspiration. Ann Oncol 1995;6:S21–4.

70. Sing A, Freudenberg N, Kortsik C, et al. Comparison of the sensitivity of sputum and brush cytology in the diagnosis of lung carcinomas. Acta Cytol 1997;41:399–408.

71. Wongsurakiat P, Wongbunnate S, Dejsomritrutai W, et al. Diagnostic value of bronchoalveolar lavage and postbronchoscopic sputum cytology in peripheral lung cancer. Respirology 1998;3:131–7.

72. Bilaceroglu S, Kumcuoglu Z, Alper H, et al. CT bronchus sign-guided bronchoscopic multiple diagnostic procedures in carcinomatous solitary pulmonary nodules and masses. Respiration 1998;65:49–55.

73. Aristizabal JF, Young KR, Nath H. Can chest CT decrease the use of preoperative bronchoscopy in the evaluation of suspected bronchogenic carcinoma? Chest 1998;113:1244–9.

74. Reichenberger F, Weber J, Tamm M, et al. The value of transbronchial needle aspiration in the diagnosis of peripheral pulmonary lesions. Chest 1999;116:704–8.

75. Gasparini S, Zuccatosta L, Zitti P, et al. Integration of TBNA and TCNA in the diagnosis of peripheral lung nodules: influence on staging. Ann Ital Chir 1999;70:851–5.

76. Baaklini WA, Reinoso MA, Gorin AB, et al. Diagnostic yield of fiberoptic bronchoscopy in evaluating solitary pulmonary nodules. Chest 2000;117:1049–54.

77. Baba M, Iyoda A, Yasufuku K, et al. Preoperative cytodiagnosis of very small-sized peripheral-type primary lung cancer. Lung Cancer 2002;37:277–80.

78. Trkanjec JT, Peros-Golubicic T, Grozdek D, et al. The role of transbronchial lung biopsy in the diagnosis of solitary pulmonary nodule. Coll Antropol 2003;27:669–75.

79. Kawaraya M, Gemba K, Ueoka H, et al. Evaluation of various cytological examinations by bronchoscopy in the diagnosis of peripheral lung cancer. Br J Cancer 2003;89:1885–8.

80. Sawabata N, Yokota S, Maeda H, et al. Diagnosis of solitary pulmonary nodule: optimal strategy based on nodal size. Interact Cardiovasc Thorac Surg 2006;5(2):105–8.

81. Ost D, Shah R, Anasco E, et al. A randomized trial of CT fluoroscopic-guided bronchoscopy vs conventional bronchoscopy in patients with suspected lung cancer. Chest 2008;134(3):507–13.

82. Roth K, Hardie JA, Andreassen AH, et al. Predictors of diagnostic yield in bronchoscopy: a retrospective cohort study comparing different combinations of sampling techniques. BMC Pulm Med 2008;8:2.

83. van't Westeinde SC, Horeweg N, Vernhout RM, et al. The role of conventional bronchoscopy in the work-up of suspicious CT screen detected pulmonary nodules. Chest 2012;142(2):377–84.

84. Aoshima M, Chonabayashi N. Can HRCT contribute in decision-making on indication for flexible bronchoscopy for solitary pulmonary nodules and masses? J Bronchol 2001;8:161–5.

85. Gaeta M, Pandolfo I, Volta S, et al. Bronchus sign on CT in peripheral carcinoma of the lung: value in predicting results of transbronchial biopsy. AJR Am J Roentgenol 1991;157(6):1181–5.

86. Popovich J Jr, Kvale PA, Eichenhorn MS, et al. Diagnostic accuracy of multiple biopsies from flexible fiberoptic bronchoscopy. A comparison of central versus peripheral carcinoma. Am Rev Respir Dis 1982;125(5):521–3.

87. Lee R, Ost D. Advanced bronchoscopic techniques for diagnosis of peripheral pulmonary lesions. In: Beamis JF Jr, Mathur P, Mehta AC, editors. Interventional pulmonary medicine, 2nd edition (Lung biology in health and disease, vol. 230). New York: Informa Healthcare; 2010. p. 186–99.

88. Sheski FD, Mathur PN. Endobronchial ultrasound. Chest 2008;133(1):264–70.

89. Yasufuku K. Current clinical applications of endobronchial ultrasound. Expert Rev Respir Med 2010;4(4):491–8.

90. Kurimoto N, Miyazawa T, Okimasa S, et al. Endobronchial ultrasonography using a guide sheath increases the ability to diagnose peripheral pulmonary lesions endoscopically. Chest 2004; 126(3):959–65.

91. Kikuchi E, Yamazaki K, Sukoh N, et al. Endobronchial ultrasonography with guide-sheath for peripheral pulmonary lesions. Eur Respir J 2004;24(4):533–7.

92. Chao TY, Chien MT, Lie CH, et al. Endobronchial ultrasonography-guided transbronchial needle aspiration increases the diagnostic yield of peripheral pulmonary lesions: a randomized trial. Chest 2009;136(1):229–36.

93. Herth FJ, Ernst A, Becker HD. Endobronchial ultrasound-guided transbronchial lung biopsy in solitary pulmonary nodules and peripheral lesions. Eur Respir J 2002;20(4):972–4.

94. Steinfort DP, Khor YH, Manser RL, et al. Radial probe endobronchial ultrasound for the diagnosis of peripheral lung cancer: systematic review and meta-analysis. Eur Respir J 2011;37(4):902–10.

95. Paone G, Nicastri E, Lucantoni G, et al. Endobronchial ultrasound-driven biopsy in the diagnosis of peripheral lung lesions. Chest 2005;128(5):3551–7.

96. Eberhardt R, Ernst A, Herth FJ. Ultrasound-guided transbronchial biopsy of solitary pulmonary nodules less than 20 mm. Eur Respir J 2009;34(6):1284–7.

97. Dooms CA, Verbeken EK, Becker HD, et al. Endobronchial ultrasonography in bronchoscopic occult pulmonary lesions. J Thorac Oncol 2007;2(2):121–4.

98. Huang CT, Ho CC, Tsai YJ, et al. Factors influencing visibility and diagnostic yield of transbronchial biopsy using endobronchial ultrasound in peripheral pulmonary lesions. Respirology 2009; 14(6):859–64.

99. Ostendorf U, Scherff A, Khanavkar B, et al. Diagnosis of peripheral lung lesions by EBUS-guided TBB in routine practice. Pneumologie 2011; 65(12):730–5.

100. Shinagawa N, Nakano K, Asahina H, et al. Endobronchial ultrasonography with a guide sheath in the diagnosis of benign peripheral diseases. Ann Thorac Surg 2012;93(3):951–7.

101. Steinfort DP, Vincent J, Heinze S, et al. Comparative effectiveness of radial probe endobronchial ultrasound versus CT-guided needle biopsy for evaluation of peripheral pulmonary lesions: a randomized pragmatic trial. Respir Med 2011; 105(11):1704–11.

102. Herth FJ, Eberhardt R, Becker HD, et al. Endobronchial ultrasound-guided transbronchial lung biopsy in fluoroscopically invisible solitary pulmonary nodules: a prospective trial. Chest 2006;129(1): 147–50.

103. Lin CY, Lan CC, Wu YK, et al. Factors that affect the diagnostic yield of endobronchial ultrasonography-assisted transbronchial lung biopsy. J Laparoendosc Adv Surg Tech A 2012;22(4):319–23.

104. Ishida M, Suzuki M, Furumoto A, et al. Transbronchial biopsy using endobronchial ultrasonography with a guide sheath increased the diagnostic yield of peripheral pulmonary lesions. Intern Med 2012; 51(5):455–60.

105. Boonsarngsuk V, Raweelert P, Juthakarn S. Endobronchial ultrasound plus fluoroscopy versus fluoroscopy-guided bronchoscopy: a comparison of diagnostic yields in peripheral pulmonary lesions. Lung 2012;190(2):233–7.

106. Oki M, Saka H, Kitagawa C, et al. Randomized study of endobronchial ultrasound-guided transbronchial biopsy: thin bronchoscopic method versus guide sheath method. J Thorac Oncol 2012;7(3):535–41.

107. Kuo CH, Lin SM, Chung FT, et al. Echoic features as predictors of diagnostic yield of endobronchial ultrasound-guided transbronchial lung biopsy in peripheral pulmonary lesions. Ultrasound Med Biol 2011;37(11):1755–61.

108. Fujita Y, Seki N, Kurimoto N, et al. Introduction of endobronchial ultrasonography (EBUS) in bronchoscopy clearly reduces fluoroscopy time: comparison of 147 cases in groups before and after EBUS introduction. Jpn J Clin Oncol 2011; 41(10):1177–81.

109. Ishida T, Asano F, Yamazaki K, et al, Virtual Navigation in Japan Trial Group. Virtual bronchoscopic navigation combined with endobronchial ultrasound to diagnose small peripheral pulmonary lesions: a randomised trial. Thorax 2011;66(12): 1072–7.

110. Roth K, Eagan TM, Andreassen AH, et al. A randomised trial of endobronchial ultrasound guided sampling in peripheral lung lesions. Lung Cancer 2011;74(2):219–25.

111. Eckardt J, Olsen KE, Licht PB. Endobronchial ultrasound-guided transbronchial needle aspiration of undiagnosed chest tumors. World J Surg 2010;34(8):1823–7.

112. Disayabutr S, Tscheikuna J, Nana A. The endobronchial ultrasound-guided transbronchial lung biopsy in peripheral pulmonary lesions. J Med Assoc Thai 2010;93(Suppl 1):S94–101.

113. Oki M, Saka H, Kitagawa C, et al. Endobronchial ultrasound-guided transbronchial biopsy using novel thin bronchoscope for diagnosis of peripheral pulmonary lesions. J Thorac Oncol 2009; 4(10):1274–7.

114. Fielding DI, Robinson PJ, Kurimoto N. Biopsy site selection for endobronchial ultrasound guide-sheath transbronchial biopsy of peripheral lung lesions. Intern Med J 2008;38(2):77–84.

115. Asano F, Matsuno Y, Tsuzuku A, et al. Diagnosis of peripheral pulmonary lesions using a bronchoscope insertion guidance system combined with endobronchial ultrasonography with a guide sheath. Lung Cancer 2008;60(3):366–73.

116. Yamada N, Yamazaki K, Kurimoto N, et al. Factors related to diagnostic yield of transbronchial biopsy using endobronchial ultrasonography with a guide sheath in small peripheral pulmonary lesions. Chest 2007;132(2):603–8.

117. Yoshikawa M, Sukoh N, Yamazaki K, et al. Diagnostic value of endobronchial ultrasonography with a guide sheath for peripheral pulmonary lesions without x-ray fluoroscopy. Chest 2007; 131(6):1788–93.

118. Eberhardt R, Anantham D, Ernst A, et al. Multimodality bronchoscopic diagnosis of peripheral lung lesions: a randomized controlled trial. Am J Respir Crit Care Med 2007;176(1):36–41.

119. Chung YH, Lie CH, Chao TY, et al. Endobronchial ultrasonography with distance for peripheral pulmonary lesions. Respir Med 2007;101(4):738–45.

120. Asahina H, Yamazaki K, Onodera Y, et al. Transbronchial biopsy using endobronchial ultrasonography with a guide sheath and virtual bronchoscopic navigation. Chest 2005;128(3): 1761–5.

121. Yang MC, Liu WT, Wang CH, et al. Diagnostic value of endobronchial ultrasound-guided transbronchial lung biopsy in peripheral lung cancers. J Formos Med Assoc 2004;103(2):124–9.

122. Shirakawa T, Imamura F, Hamamoto J, et al. Usefulness of endobronchial ultrasonography for transbronchial lung biopsies of peripheral lung lesions. Respiration 2004;71(3):260–8.

123. Mizugaki H, Shinagawa N, Kanegae K, et al. Combining transbronchial biopsy using endobronchial ultrasonography with a guide sheath and positron emission tomography for the diagnosis of small peripheral pulmonary lesions. Lung Cancer 2010;68(2):211–5.

124. Kurimoto N, Murayama M, Yoshioka S, et al. Analysis of the internal structure of peripheral pulmonary lesions using endobronchial ultrasonography. Chest 2002;122(6):1887–94.

125. Huang Y, Chen ZX, Ren HY, et al. Differential diagnosis of malignant and benign peripheral pulmonary lesions based on two characteristic echo features of endobronchial ultrasonography. Nan Fang Yi Ke Da Xue Xue Bao 2012;32(7):1016–9.

126. Becker HC, Herth F, Ernst A, et al. Bronchoscopic biopsy of peripheral lung lesions under electromagnetic guidance. A pilot study. J Bronchol 2005;12:9–13.

127. Schwarz Y, Mehta AC, Ernst A, et al. Electromagnetic navigation during flexible bronchoscopy. Respiration 2003;70(5):516–22.

128. Schwarz Y, Greif J, Becker HD, et al. Real-time electromagnetic navigation bronchoscopy to peripheral lung lesions using overlaid CT images: the first human study. Chest 2006;129(4):988–94.

129. Hautmann H, Schneider A, Pinkau T, et al. Electromagnetic catheter navigation during bronchoscopy: validation of a novel method by conventional fluoroscopy. Chest 2005;128(1):382–7.

130. Gildea TR, Mazzone PJ, Karnak D, et al. Electromagnetic navigation diagnostic bronchoscopy: a prospective study. Am J Respir Crit Care Med 2006;174(9):982–9.

131. Pearlstein DP, Quinn CC, Burtis CC, et al. Electromagnetic navigation bronchoscopy performed by thoracic surgeons: one center's early success. Ann Thorac Surg 2012;93(3):944–9.

132. Mahajan A, Patel S, Wightman R, et al. Electromagnetic navigational bronchoscopy: an effective and safe approach to diagnosing peripheral lung lesions unreachable by conventional bronchoscopy in high risk patients. J Bronchology Interv Pulmonol 2011;18(2):133–7.

133. Seijo LM, de Torres JP, Lozano MD, et al. Diagnostic yield of electromagnetic navigation bronchoscopy is highly dependent on the presence of a bronchus sign on CT imaging results from a prospective study. Chest 2010;138(6):1316–21.

134. Eberhardt R, Morgan RK, Ernst A, et al. Comparison of suction catheter versus forceps biopsy for sampling of solitary pulmonary nodules guided by electromagnetic navigational bronchoscopy. Respiration 2010;79(1):54–60.

135. Bertoletti L, Robert A, Cottier M, et al. Accuracy and feasibility of electromagnetic navigated bronchoscopy under nitrous oxide sedation for pulmonary peripheral opacities: an outpatient study. Respiration 2009;78(3):293–300.

136. Lamprecht B, Porsch P, Pirich C, et al. Electromagnetic navigation bronchoscopy in combination with PET-CT and rapid on-site cytopathologic examination for diagnosis of peripheral lung lesions. Lung 2009;187(1):55–9.

137. Wilson DS, Barlett RJ. Improved diagnostic yield of bronchoscopy in a community practice: a combination of electromagnetic navigation system and rapid on-site evaluation. J Bronchol 2007;14(4):227–32.

138. Makris D, Scherpereel A, Leroy S, et al. Electromagnetic navigation diagnostic bronchoscopy for small peripheral lung lesions. Eur Respir J 2007; 29(6):1187–92.

139. Eberhardt R, Anantham D, Herth F, et al. Electromagnetic navigation diagnostic bronchoscopy in peripheral lung lesions. Chest 2007;131(6):1800–5.

140. Haas AR, Vachani A, Sterman DH. Advances in diagnostic bronchoscopy. Am J Respir Crit Care Med 2010;182(5):589–97.

141. Oki M, Saka H, Kitagawa C, et al. Novel thin bronchoscope with a 1.7-mm working channel for peripheral pulmonary lesions. Eur Respir J 2008; 32(2):465–71.

142. Saka H, Oki M, Kumazawa A, et al. Diagnosis of pulmonary peripheral lesions using an ultrathin bronchoscope. J Jpn Soc Bronchol 2000;22:617–9.

143. Asano F, Kimura T, Shindou J, et al. Usefulness of CT-guided ultrathin bronchoscopy in the diagnosis of peripheral pulmonary lesions that could not be diagnosed by standard transbronchial biopsy. J Jpn Soc Bronchol 2002;24:80–5.

144. Asano F, Matsuno Y, Shinagawa N, et al. A virtual bronchoscopic navigation system for pulmonary peripheral lesions. Chest 2006;130(2):559–66.

145. Shinagawa N, Yamazaki K, Onodera Y, et al. Factors related to diagnostic sensitivity using an ultrathin bronchoscope under CT guidance. Chest 2007;131(2):549–53.

146. Rooney CP, Wolf K, McLennan G. Ultrathin bronchoscopy as an adjunct to standard bronchoscopy in the diagnosis of peripheral lung lesions. A preliminary report. Respiration 2002;69(1):63–8.

147. Yamamoto S, Ueno K, Imamura F, et al. Usefulness of ultrathin bronchoscopy in diagnosis of lung cancer. Lung Cancer 2004;46(1):43–8.

148. Shinagawa N, Yamazaki K, Onodera Y, et al. CT-guided transbronchial biopsy using an ultrathin

bronchoscope with virtual bronchoscopic navigation. Chest 2004;125(3):1138–43.

149. Soper TD, Haynor DR, Glenny RW, et al. In vivo validation of a hybrid tracking system for navigation of an ultrathin bronchoscope within peripheral airways. IEEE Trans Biomed Eng 2010;57(3): 736–45.

150. Asano F, Matsuno Y, Matsushita T, et al. Transbronchial diagnosis of a pulmonary peripheral small lesion using an ultrathin bronchoscope with virtual bronchoscopic navigation. J Bronchol 2002;9: 108–11.

151. Eberhardt R, Kahn N, Gompelmann D, et al. LungPoint–a new approach to peripheral lesions. J Thorac Oncol 2010;5(10):1559–63.

152. Wagner U, Walthers EM, Gelmetti W, et al. Computer-tomographically guided fiberbronchoscopic transbronchial biopsy of small pulmonary lesions: a feasibility study. Respiration 1996;63(3):181–6.

153. Kobayashi T, Shimamura K, Hanai K, et al. Computed tomography-guided bronchoscopy with an ultrathin fiberscope. Diagn Ther Endosc 1996;2(4):229–32.

154. Asano F, Matsuno Y, Takeichi N, et al. Virtual bronchoscopy in navigation of an ultrathin bronchoscope. J Jpn Soc Bronchol 2002;24:433–8.

155. Shinagawa N, Yamazaki K, Onodera Y, et al. Virtual bronchoscopic navigation system shortens the examination time–feasibility study of virtual bronchoscopic navigation system. Lung Cancer 2007; 56(2):201–6.

156. Tachihara M, Ishida T, Kanazawa K, et al. A virtual bronchoscopic navigation system under x-ray fluoroscopy for transbronchial diagnosis of small peripheral pulmonary lesions. Lung Cancer 2007; 57(3):322–7.

157. Asano F, Matsuno Y, Ibuka T, et al. A barium marking method using an ultrathin bronchoscope with virtual bronchoscopic navigation. Respirology 2004;9(3):409–13.

158. Asano F, Shindoh J, Shigemitsu K, et al. Ultrathin bronchoscopic barium marking with virtual bronchoscopic navigation for fluoroscopy-assisted thoracoscopic surgery. Chest 2004;126(5):1687–93.

159. Hautmann H, Henke MO, Bitterling H. High diagnostic yield from transbronchial biopsy of solitary pulmonary nodules using low-dose CT-guidance. Respirology 2010;15(4):677–82.

160. Matsuno Y, Asano F, Shindoh J, et al. CT-guided ultrathin bronchoscopy: bioptic approach and factors in predicting diagnosis. Intern Med 2011; 50(19):2143–8.

161. Tsushima K, Sone S, Hanaoka T, et al. Comparison of bronchoscopic diagnosis for peripheral pulmonary nodule under fluoroscopic guidance with CT guidance. Respir Med 2006;100(4):737–45.

162. White CS, Weiner EA, Patel P, et al. Transbronchial needle aspiration: guidance with CT fluoroscopy. Chest 2000;118(6):1630–8.

163. Ost DE, Gould MK. Decision making in patients with pulmonary nodules. Am J Respir Crit Care Med 2012;185(4):363–72.

Endobronchial Ablative Therapies

Joseph C. Seaman, MD[a],*, Ali I. Musani, MD, FCCP, FACP[b]

KEYWORDS

- Ablative therapy • Airway lesions • Endobronchial therapy • Bronchoscopy

KEY POINTS

- Patients with symptomatic airway lesions may receive significant clinical improvement after treatment with endobronchial ablative therapies.
- There are several airway ablative therapies—the choice of ablative technique depends on the lesion and the clinical situation.
- Blending ablative techniques together may enhance patient outcomes.
- Ablative techniques require additional training to master their use.
- Ablative techniques can be used with flexible and rigid bronchoscopy.

INTRODUCTION

A variety of benign and malignant diseases may result in endoluminal lesions. Depending on the extent and location of an endoluminal lesion, patients may exhibit significant symptoms of dyspnea, cough, postobstructive atelectasis, postobstructive pleural effusion, and hemoptysis.[1,2] Removing or decreasing the overall size of the endobronchial lesion may improve a patient's symptoms, quality of life, and life expectancy.[1–7] There are a variety of endobronchial ablative therapies available to treat endoluminal lesions.[1,2] The choice among different endobronchial ablative therapies depends on the size of the lesion, location of the lesion, characteristics of the lesion, availability of the different therapies at the practicing institution, and the training and skill of the bronchoscopist.[1] Many of the different ablative therapies are blended together to provide additional benefit.[8–10] This article presents a review of common endobronchial ablative therapies used in interventional pulmonology.

INDICATIONS AND CONTRAINDICATIONS FOR ENDOBRONCHIAL ABLATIVE THERAPIES

Endobronchial ablative therapies are indicated for endoluminal lesions, which are associated with a variety of respiratory symptoms (**Box 1**). Lesions that occupy more than 50% of the airway lumen and are associated with respiratory symptoms generally improve with ablation of the lesion.[1,11] Lesions within the lumen of the airway can lead to a chronic cough due to airway irritation and ineffective mucociliary clearance.[1,2] Altered mucociliary clearance can also lead to atelectasis and recurrent pneumonia. Endoluminal lesions can lead to abnormal airway physiology, resulting in ventilation and perfusion mismatching. Finally, lesions within the airway can be friable and associated with hemoptysis.[12]

There are few contraindications for ablation of abnormal endobronchial lesions (see **Box 1**). An absolute contraindication to endobronchial ablative therapies is the presence of extrinsic airway compression.[1,11,12] A lesion that extrinsically

Disclaimers: None.
[a] Department of Clinical Sciences, Florida State University College of Medicine, Lung Associates of Sarasota, 1921 Waldemere Street, Suite 705, Sarasota, FL 34239, USA; [b] Division of Interventional Pulmonology, Department of Pulmonary and Critical Care Medicine, National Jewish Health, 1400 Jackson Street, J 225, Denver, CO 80206, USA
* Corresponding author.
E-mail address: joey.seaman@gmail.com

chestmed.theclinics.com

compresses the airway cannot be addressed by most ablative technologies. Ablative techniques render therapy through a physical contact or interaction with the abnormal endoluminal tissue. Lesions that are associated with extrinsic airway compression of the airway lumen have normal endobronchial or endotracheal tissue. Brachytherapy is the only technique used to address lesions extrinsic to the airway.[13,14] The field of radiation effect rendered by brachytherapy includes tissues up to and beyond 1 cm from the brachytherapy catheter.[13,14]

Relative contraindications include distal airway obstructions, airway obstructions present for more than 4 weeks, obstructions longer than 4 cm, and patients who require more than 40% fraction of inspired oxygen (F_{IO_2}) during bronchoscopy.[11] Obstructions in small distal airways may be futile to treat. The amount of functional lung distal to the point of obstruction may not warrant the risk associated with attempting to ablate a lesion in a distal airway.[11] The distal airway wall is thinner than larger proximal airways. The thinner airway wall is associated with an increased risk of airway perforation.

Atelectasis and lobar collapse due to airway obstructions that have been present for more than 4 weeks may not improve with the ablation of an endoluminal lesion.[9] The pathophysiology behind persistent alveolar collapse and atelectasis after removal of an obstructing luminal lesion is not entirely known. It is assumed that prolonged alveolar collapse and atelectasis lead to loss of surfactant, abnormal mucus collection and inspissation, airway wall inflammation, and malacia, each of which contributes to the limited or no expansion of previously atelectatic lung tissue.

Long endoluminal airway lesions can be difficult to manage.[11] Extensive tumor debulking is associated with prolonged surgical times, increased risk of airway perforations, increased risk of bleeding, and residual airway wall malacia. When used alone, endobronchial ablative techniques are associated with poor outcomes and limited symptomatic improvement. Brachytherapy is a therapeutic option that may be beneficial for long or complicated airway lesions.[13,14] Using ablative therapies with airway stenting and balloon bronchoplasty may provide a suitable treatment strategy to address long airway lesions while minimizing complications.[10,12]

Endobronchial ablative therapies that generate heat, high temperatures, or electrical currents are associated with airway fires.[1,12,15] To minimize the risk of airway fires, bronchoscopists should limit the inspired oxygen concentration to no more than 40% and extend the ablative device at least 4 mm to 5 mm from the end of the bronchoscope and at least 1 cm from the end of the endotracheal tube.[11,12] To further limit the risk of airway fires, consideration could be given to the use of a rigid bronchoscope.

ENDOBRONCHIAL ABLATIVE THERAPIES

There are several types of endobronchial ablative therapies available (**Table 1**). Commonly these therapies are divided into hot and cold therapies. Hot therapies refer to light amplification by simulated emission of radiation (laser), electrocautery, and argon plasma coagulation (APC). These therapies in general use some form of heat energy transfer to provide the therapeutic intervention. Cold therapy refers to the use of cryotherapy. Additional therapies that are not classified within a hot or cold category include brachytherapy and photodynamic therapy (PDT). Brachytherapy uses the placement of radioactive material within the airway to provide therapeutic benefit. PDT refers to the use of an infused photoporphyrin molecule that is taken up by malignant tumor cells and then activated during bronchoscopy using a light source at a specific wavelength. Each of these therapies has unique risks, benefits, and indications.

Table 1
Comparison of endobronchial ablative therapies

	Laser	Electrocautery	Argon Plasma Coagulation	Cryotherapy	Brachytherapy	Photodynamic
Time to improvement	Immediate	Immediate	Immediate to days	Days to weeks	Days to weeks	Days to weeks
Control of bleeding	Excellent	Excellent	Excellent	None	None	None
Tumor specific	No	No	No	No	Yes	Yes
Depth of penetration	Variable, dependent on power settings	Variable, dependent on power settings	3 mm	3 mm	Variable, dependent on radiation dose	3 mm
Expense	+++	+	++	++	++++	++++

The relative expense of each therapy is represented by "+" – one "+" correlates with the least expensive therapy whereas "++++" correlates with the most expensive therapy.

LASER

Laser therapy uses light energy transmitted through fibers to desiccate endoluminal tissue.[1,12] There are several types of lasers (potassium titanyl phosphate, yttrium aluminum pevroskite, carbon dioxide, and Nd:YAG).[1] Each laser is unique in that each medium (for example, Nd:YAG) used for light generation emits light at a specific wavelength. Nd:YAG, potassium titanyl phosphate, and yttrium aluminum pevroskite lasers are commonly used during bronchoscopy given that they emit light energy transmitted through optical fibers.[12] Laser therapy is a commonly used endobronchial ablative therapy due to predictable tissue effects, precise area of treatment effect, rapid and immediate results, repeatability of treatments, and the ability to blend laser airway interventions with other airway interventions.[11,16]

Laser therapy destroys tissue through thermal activity. Thermal activity is generated as a result of the transfer of light energy to tissue.[1,11] Lasers are used in many different settings. Lasers are used to coagulate superficial bleeding lesions or to ablate endoluminal tissues.[1,11,12] At low-power settings, lasers have a shallow effect and coagulate tissue.[12] At higher-power settings, lasers penetrate deeper and result in carbonization and vaporization of tissue.[12] In addition to modifying the power settings, bronchoscopists adjust the distance from the tip of the laser fiber to modify the effect at the level of the tissue.[17] Holding the fiber 1 cm away from the lesion results in a shallow penetration whereas holding the fiber 3 mm to 4 mm away from the lesion results in deeper penetration. This variation in effect allows bronchoscopists to adjust the focus of the procedure according to the characteristics of the lesion and may provide individualized treatments for different areas of the lesion.

Laser therapy provides a precise and effective treatment. Given the ability to carbonize and vaporize tissue, the effects of laser therapy are immediate.[12] The immediate effects often result in dramatic improvements in a patient's complaints or symptoms. The tissue surrounding the target tissue is also affected. There is some degree of heat transfer to adjacent tissues. The cells within the adjacent tissue absorb heat energy. The absorption of heat energy results in some degree of thermal injury and cell death of surrounding tissue. The adjacent thermal energy and cell death are responsible for the delayed effect of laser therapy. The delayed effects of laser therapy are seen 48 to 96 hours after the bronchoscopy and result in a further improvement in airway lumen size. **Fig. 1** depicts the use of laser ablative therapy in a malignant airway obstruction. In this case, the ablative technique was followed by the placement of a fully covered self-expandable metallic stent.

Electrocautery

Electrocautery uses the flow of electricity to generate heat. Electrical current flows from the probe into the target tissue adjacent to the tip of the probe. Heat generation occurs in target tissues given the differences in resistance.[1] The heat generation results in cell death. The effects of electrocautery depend on several variables, including the nature of the lesion, current waveform properties, and the power setting, machine mode, and type of probe used.[1,12,18,19] The electrical current waveforms are adjusted to achieve different results. Waveforms with high frequency result in a cut mode whereas waveforms with a low

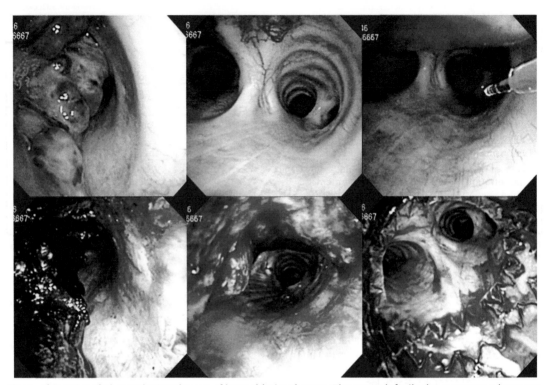

Fig. 1. This series of photos depicts the use of laser ablative therapy. The upper-left tile demonstrates a large malignant lesion in the midtrachea. The upper-middle tile depicts lower trachea and bilateral proximal mainstem bronchi that are free of malignant disease. The upper-right tile shows the laser fiber in the distal trachea. The lower-left tile depicts the midtrachea after laser ablation—note the large eschar. The lower-middle tile depicts the midtrachea after eschar débridement—note the significant improvement in airway patency. The lower-right tile depicts the midtrachea to low trachea after deployment of a fully covered self-expandable metallic stent. This is an example of blending therapies to maximize clinical benefit.

frequency result in a coagulation mode.[18,19] The frequency is modified to achieve a blended effect. High-power settings vaporize and carbonize tissue whereas low-power settings are used for coagulation.[12,18,19] Similarly, high-power settings penetrate deep into tissue whereas low-power settings have a shallow effect.[18,19] Depending on the probe used, the treatment effect is precise or more diffuse. Electrocautery results in an immediate ablative effect due to tissue carbonization and vaporization.[12,18,19] As with laser therapy, there is also a delayed effect. The delayed effect is due to the cytocidal effect of heat generation in adjacent tissue. The cost associated with electrocautery is minimal because most health care centers have electrocautery machines available.[19,20] In addition, the specialized probes and instruments can be purchased as needed, thereby decreasing lofty instrument fees.[19,20]

There are many instruments available for use with electrocautery. Common instruments include a probe, snare, knife, and forceps. The variety of instruments allows for variability in addressing

endobronchial lesions.[19] Given that most of the instruments require close proximity to the lesion treated, the probes tend to require frequent cleaning and lead to longer procedure times compared with laser therapy. **Fig. 2** depicts the use of an electrocautery knife and probe used to ablate a simple benign subglottic stenosis due to prolonged endotracheal intubation. **Fig. 3** depicts the use of an electracautery snare and probe to remove and ablate an endobronchial lesion.

Argon Plasma Coagulation

APC works similarly to electrocautery.[1] APC uses argon gas as the medium through which the electrical current flows to the tissue treated.[1,18,21] Argon gas emanates from a port on the tip of the APC catheter. The tip of the catheter has an electrode that generates an electrical current. When activated, electrical current flows from the tip of the catheter to the target tissue.

APC has superficial effects on tissue and is an excellent option for coagulation.[1,12,18,21] Given

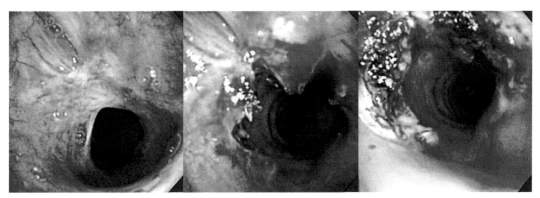

Fig. 2. The left tile depicts a narrow simple benign subglottic stenosis due to prolonged endotracheal intubation. The middle tile depicts the same lesion after electrocautery knife treatment. The incisions allow the tissue to relax and increase the size of the airway. The right tile depicts the same lesion treated with the electrocautery probe to remove the redundant stenotic tissue.

the shallow effects, it is not optimal for debulking endobronchial tissue because carbonization and vaporization are unlikely.[11] APC lacks precision because the argon gas emanates from the tip of the catheter and flows in all directions.[11,12] This nonspecific spray of gas also allows for treating lesions in unusual locations or at right angles to the tip of the probe.[18] As with laser and electrocautery, there is an immediate tissue ablative effect as well as a delayed cytocidal effect of heat transmission.

Cryotherapy

Cryotherapy refers to the use of extreme cold to treat airway lesions.[1] Cryotherapy uses a special probe through which a rapidly expanding gas (nitrous oxide or liquid nitrogen are 2 gases that are commonly used) flows to the tip of the catheter and cools it to a temperature of -40°C.[1,22] The probe is applied to the target lesion (physical contact is made with the tissue) and cooled to its target temperature.[1,22] Active cooling occurs for 30 to 60 seconds followed by a period of passive rewarming. The freeze-and-thaw cycle is repeated 2 to 3 times for maximal effect. The probe is then repositioned to treat adjacent areas.

Cryotherapy has several issues that make it less desirable than laser, electrocautery, or APC. Cryotherapy lacks precision, has a shallow treatment effect, and has no immediate effect.[1,22] Malignant tissue is particularly sensitive to cryotherapy given the water content of malignant cells whereas cartilage and normal respiratory tissue tends to be resistant to cryotherapy.[22] Maximal tissue destruction occurs 1 to 2 weeks after cryotherapy and requires repeat treatments to achieve the desired effect.[22] In addition, cryotherapy is time consuming given the multiple repeat freeze-and-thaw cycles.

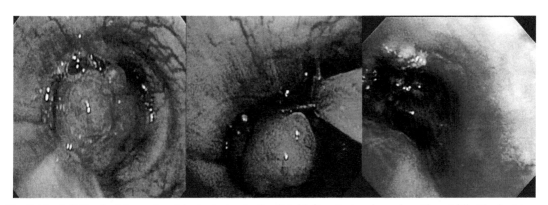

Fig. 3. The left tile depicts a polypoid mass lesion in the distal left mainstem bronchus. The middle tile depicts an electrocautery snare being placed over the polypoid mass lesion. The right tile depicts the distal left mainstem after removal of the polypoid lesion. The base of the polypoid lesion required treatment with the electrocautery probe. Patency was restored to the left mainstem.

Brachytherapy

Brachytherapy refers to the use of radiation to treat malignant lesions.[1] Typically, a bronchoscopy is performed and the target airways are identified. Then, a specialized catheter is inserted through the working channel of a standard flexible bronchoscope and placed under direct visualization or with the assistance of fluoroscopy or ultrasound.[13,14,22] Depending on the type or location of the lesion, multiple catheters may be used.[13] Once secured, radiation seeds are advanced through the catheter and into the desired location.[13,22] Once the treatment has been rendered, the probe and seeds are removed.

Brachytherapy is not used for lesions that are associated with acute complaints of dyspnea.[1,22] There are no immediate effects with radiation therapy.[1,22] Maximal effect is seen several weeks after the treatment.[22] Brachytherapy is generally used for long lesions growing into airways or lesions compressing the airways.[13,14,22] High doses of radiotherapy are delivered to selected areas, allowing for excellent treatment response. In addition, it can be offered to patients who have already received maximal external beam radiation and who are not candidates for more conventional endobronchial ablative techniques such as laser, electrocautery, or photodynamic therapy.[13,22] Brachytherapy is expensive and requires specialized facilities to render the treatments.

Photodynamic Therapy

PDT refers to the application of light energy to tissues that have been pretreated with a photosensitizer.[1,11,22,23] Patients receive an intravenous injection of a photosensitization agent (such as Photofrin) 2 to 3 days before their planned bronchoscopy.[22,23] The photosensitization agent is taken up by actively metabolizing cells and to a higher degree by malignant tissues.[22,23] A standard bronchoscope is then used to survey the airway and to advance the light probe into position.[22,23] Once in position, the light probe is activated and emits light at a specific frequency to activate the photosensitizing agent.[22,23] Once activated, the photosensitizing agent results in the generation of reactive oxygen species that damage cellular structures and leads to cell death.[22,23] PDT does not result in immediate effects.[1,11] The maximal effect is seen several days after PDT.[22,23] Patients generally undergo repeat bronchoscopy 2 to 4 days after PDT treatment to remove sloughed tissue.[22,23] PDT is repeated as necessary to reach deeper tissue as layers of malignant tissue are removed.[22,23]

COMPLICATIONS OF ENDOBRONCHIAL ABLATIVE THERAPIES

Most complications are similar to those experienced with routine flexible bronchoscopy (Table 2). Rare complications of routine bronchoscopy, such as respiratory failure, myocardial infarction, cardiac arrhythmia, and death, may occur more frequently with these advanced techniques.[15,16,24] The reason that the incidence may be increased is due to prolonged sedation given during the procedure and the need for decreased fractional inspired oxygen levels (in laser, electrocautery, and APC), which may allow transient or prolonged hypoxia during the procedure.[15,16,24] In addition, each of the endobronchial ablative therapies has unique risks specifically related to the technology of the therapy.

Airway perforation is a potential complication related to laser, electrocautery, and, to a lesser extent, APC.[1,11,12,15,16,24] These hot therapies immediate ablate and dissect tissue. With dissection

Table 2
Complications of endobronchial ablative therapies

Type of Endobronchial Therapy	Airway Perforation	Hemorrhage	Airway Fire	Air Embolism	Respiratory Failure	Myocardial Infarction, Arrhythmia	Death
Laser	Possible	Possible	Possible	Very rare	Possible	Rare	Very rare
Electrocautery	Possible	Possible	Possible	No	Possible	Rare	Very rare
APC	Unlikely	Unlikely	Possible	No	Possible	Rare	Very rare
Cryotherapy	No	No	No	No	Possible	Rare	Very rare
PDT	No	No	No	No	Possible	Rare	Very rare
Brachytherapy	No	Unlikely	No	No	Possible	Rare	Very rare

Rates of complication vary significantly among pulmonologists, airway centers, and patients. Precise estimates of risk are difficult to site as such qualitative estimates are commonly described.

into deeper levels of tissue or when the angle of the instrument is perpendicular to the airway wall, it is possible that the airway wall is perforated, leading to pneumomediastinum, pneumothorax, and hemorrhage. To reduce the risk of these severe complications, bronchoscopists should deploy the therapy parallel to the airway wall and frequently re-evaluate the tissue planes dissected to prevent dissection into deeper tissue or through the airway wall. Additionally, power settings, modes, or different instruments are used to minimize the depth of penetration and potentially reduce the risk of airway perforation.[1,11,12] Cryotherapy, PDT, and brachytherapy are unlikely to cause airway perforation because they do not actively ablate tissue and do not dissect through the airway wall.[22]

Endobronchial ablative therapies are commonly used to address bleeding endoluminal lesions; however, they also cause bleeding.[1,12,15] Electrocautery and laser are excellent therapies to address bleeding airway lesions; however, both of these therapies dissect through airway walls and into bronchial vessels, causing massive hemoptysis.[11,15] Given the shallow effects of APC, it is unlikely to cause massive bleeding.[1,18,21] Cryotherapy, PDT, and brachytherapy are unlikely to cause massive hemoptysis because they do not actively ablate or dissect through tissue.[22] PDT and brachytherapy are associated with delayed hemoptysis due to mucosal tissue breakdown and ulceration as a result of the therapy.[22]

Airway fires are a potentially catastrophic complication of laser, electrocautery, and APC ablative therapies. If high oxygen levels are present within the airway during activation of these technologies, the bronchoscope, endotracheal tube, or the tissue itself could be ignited.[11,12] To limit this dreaded complication, oxygen concentration should be kept to below 40% and preferably below 30% as long as feasibly possible.[11,12] If optimal oxygen levels cannot be

---

Box 2
Practical considerations of endobronchial ablative therapies

Hot therapies (laser, electrocautery, and APC)

- FIO_2 must stay below 40% to reduce the risk of airway fires.
- When advanced airways are needed, a laryngeal mask airway instead of an endotracheal tube should be considered to reduce the risk for airway fires.
- Using a rigid bronchoscope should be considered, when available and appropriate to the situation, to reduce the risk for airway fires.
- Ideal interventions often are associated with immediate clinical improvement.

Electrocautery and APC

- Due to the electrical current, caution should be used in patients with pacemakers.
- Wide array of specialized intruments that allow for unique interventions (for electrocautery).
- Electrocautery achieves similar results to laser and is more economical.

Cryotherapy

- Results are delayed.
- It is able to be performed with any inspired level of oxygen.
- It is time consuming.

Photodynamic therapy

- Associated with intense photosensitivity to sunlight.
- Results may take days to weeks.
- Repeat bronchoscopy is required to remove sloughed tissue.
- Applicable only in patients with tumors that have significant blood flow.

Brachytherapy

- Additional radiation may be delivered to areas that have received maximal external beam radiation.
- It can be delivered to long lesions or lesions that are external to and compressing the airway.
- It is expensive and requires special facilities.

achieved, then the procedure should be aborted and an alternate ablative technique used. In addition, the tip of the laser fiber or the electrocautery instrument should be at least 1 cm away from the end of the bronchoscope and several centimeters away from the endotracheal tube. Limiting the use of endotracheal tubes may reduce the risk of airway fires. Laryngeal mask airways, which remain above the vocal cords, provide excellent ventilation and control of the airway while limiting ignitable material in the airway. Finally, in high-risk airways, consideration is given to the use of a metallic rigid bronchoscope as an alternative to a flexible bronchoscope, thus further limiting the presence of ignitable material in the airway.

Air embolism is a rare complication of laser therapy. The cause is believed a result of bronchial wall blood vessel disruption in the setting of positive pressure ventilation and the use of a gas cooled laser fiber.[25,26] Air embolism can result in cerebral infarction. This complication is limited by using noncontact laser fibers and non–gas-cooled fibers.[25,26]

PRACTICAL CONSIDERATIONS OF ENDOBRONCHIAL ABLATIVE THERAPIES

Endobronchial ablative therapies are used to treat several malignant and nonmalignant airway lesions. Choosing among the different endobronchial ablative therapies can be difficult. Optimal therapy depends on the type of lesion, location of the lesion, whether a lesion is malignant or benign, amount of inspired oxygen needed to maintain safe oxygen saturations, availability of the ablative therapies, training and experience of the practitioner rendering the therapy, and whether immediate effects are desired (**Box 2**).

Laser and electrocautery result in immediate relief of airway stenosis and are commonly deployed in patients who have critical airway narrowing and require immediate intervention.[12,19,20] These airway interventions are commonly used in conjunction with other advanced airway techniques (such as balloon bronchoplasty and stenting) to enhance airway patency and to improve the duration of effect.[10] Although there are different technologies, they achieve similar results.[19,20] In addition, electrocautery is more economical because most health care institutions have the necessary electrocautery device and are only required to purchase new probes or instruments.[20]

Using endobronchial ablative therapies in practice requires additional training. Additional training

is necessary to determine the optimal therapy for patients as well as to use the therapy safely, limit complications, and manage complications if they occur. The knowledge gained through additional training maximizes patient benefit while reducing risks to patients.

SUMMARY

There are many endobronchial ablative therapies. Each endobronchial therapy is unique and has distinct risks and benefits associated with its use. Patients with endoluminal disease may receive significant benefit through endobronchial intervention, and patients with benign airway disease may receive lifelong relief. The choice of optimal endobronchial ablative therapy depends on several patient factors and technical issues. The decision to blend the ablative techniques with other airway interventions should be considered and depends on the clinical situation. Bronchoscopists using endobronchial ablative therapies should be experienced and well trained with the therapy used.

REFERENCES

1. Bolliger CT, Mathur PN, Beamis JF, et al. ERS/ATS statement on interventional pulmonology. Eur Respir J 2002;19:356–73.

2. Amjadi K, Voduc N, Cruysberghs Y, et al. Impact of interventional bronchoscopy on quality of life in malignant airway obstruction. Respiration 2008;76:421–8.

3. Galluccio G, Lucantoni G, Battistoni P, et al. Interventional endoscopy in the management of benign tracheal stenoses: definitive treatment at long-term follow-up. Eur J Cardiothorac Surg 2009;35:429–34.

4. Chhajed PN, Baty F, Pless M, et al. Outcome of treated advanced non-small cell lung cancer with and without central airway obstruction. Chest 2006;130:1803–7.

5. Litle VR, Christie NA, Fernando HC, et al. Photodynamic therapy for endobronchial metastases from nonbronchogenic primaries. Ann Thorac Surg 2003;76:370–5.

6. Hujala K, Sipila J, Grenman R. Endotracheal and bronchial laser surgery in the treatment of malignant and benign lower airway obstructions. Eur Arch Otorhinolaryngol 2003;260:219–22.

7. Boyd M, Rubio E. The utility of interventional pulmonary procedures in liberating patients with malignancy-associated central airway obstruction from mechanical ventilation. Lung 2012;190:471–6.

8. Santos RS, Raftopoulos Y, Keenan RJ, et al. Bronchoscopic palliation of primary lung cancer: single

or multimodality therapy? Surg Endosc 2004;18: 931–6.

9. Chella A, Ambroqi MC, Ribechini A, et al. Combined Nd-YAG laser/HDR brachytherapy versus Nd-YAG laser only in malignant central airway involvement: a prospective randomized study. Lung Cancer 2000;27:169–75.

10. Hann CC, Prasetyo D, Wright GM. Endobronchial palliation using Nd:YAG laser is associated with improved survival when combined with multimodal adjuvant treatments. J Thorac Oncol 2007;2:59–64.

11. Folch E, Mehta AC. Airway interventions in the tracheobronchial tree. Semin Respir Crit Care Med 2008;29:441–52.

12. Bolliger CT, Sutedja TG, Strausz J, et al. Therapeutic bronchoscopy with immediate effect: laser, electrocautery, argon plasma coagulation and stents. Eur Respir J 2006;27:1258–71.

13. Klopp AH, Eapen GA, Komaki RR. Endobronchial brachytherapy: an effective option for palliation of malignant bronchial obstruction. Clin Lung Cancer 2006;8:203–7.

14. Ung YC, Yu E, Falkson C, et al. The role of high-dose-rate brachytherapy in the palliation of symptoms in patients with non-small-cell lung cancer: a systematic review. Brachytherapy 2006;5:189–202.

15. Cavaliere S, Venuta F, Foccoli P, et al. Endoscopic treatment of malignant airway obstructions in 2,008 patients. Chest 1996;110:1536–42.

16. Cavaliere S, Foccoli P, Farina PL. Nd:YAG laser bronchoscopy. A five-year experience with 1,396 applications in 1,000 patients. Chest 1988;94:15–21.

17. Breen DP, Dutau H. Endobronchial laser treatment: an essential tool in therapeutic bronchoscopy. Eur Respir Mon 2010;48:149–60.

18. Tremblay A, Marquette CH. Endobronchial electrocautery and argon plasma coagulation: a practical approach. Can Respir J 2004;11:305–10.

19. Wahidi MM, Unroe MA, Adlakha N, et al. The use of electrocautery as the primary ablation modality for malignant and benign airway obstruction. J Thorac Oncol 2011;6:1516–20.

20. Boxem T, Muller M, Venmans B, et al. Nd-YAG laser vs bronchoscopic electrocautery for palliation of symptomatic airway obstruction: a cost-effectiveness study. Chest 1999;116:1108–12.

21. Sheski FD, Mathur PN. Endobronchial electrosurgery: argon plasma coagulation and electrocautery. Semin Respir Crit Care Med 2004;25:367–74.

22. Vergnon JM, Huber RM, Moghissi K. Place of cryotherapy, brachytherapy, and photodynamic therapy in therapeutic bronchoscopy of lung cancers. Eur Respir J 2006;28:200–18.

23. Jones BU, Helmy M, Brenner M, et al. Photodynamic therapy for patients with advanced non-small-cell carcinoma of the lung. Clin Lung Cancer 2001;3:37–41.

24. Brutinel WM, Cortese DA, McDougall JC, et al. A two-year experience with the neodymium-YAG laser in endobronchial obstruction. Chest 1987;91: 159–65.

25. Ross DJ, Mohsenifar Z, Potkin RT, et al. Pathogenesis of cerebral air embolism during neodymium-YAG laser photoresection. Chest 1988;94:660–2.

26. Tellides G, Ugurlu BS, Kim RW, et al. Pathogenesis of systemic air embolism during bronchoscopic Nd:YAG laser operations. Ann Thorac Surg 1998; 65:930–4.

Rigid Bronchoscopy

Hervé Dutau, MD[a],*, Thomas Vandemoortele, MD, FRCPC[b],
David P. Breen, MB, BA, BCh[c]

KEYWORDS

- Interventional pulmonology • Interventional bronchoscopy • Rigid bronchoscopy
- Flexible bronchoscopy • Airway stenting • Airway obstruction • Airway stenosis

KEY POINTS

- The rigid bronchoscope is the instrument of choice in most bronchoscopic therapeutic procedures.
- The rigid bronchoscope is not only a tool to visualize the airway but also a therapeutic instrument in itself or in association with other endoscopic techniques.
- Most of the scientific associations agree on this point.
- Rigid bronchoscopy requires training and a dedicated facility or easy access to an operating room with anesthetic support.
- Rigid bronchoscopy is mandatory in airway stenting when using silicone stents, which still represent the gold standard. Interventional bronchoscopy is a minimally invasive option in a variety of cases, and can occasionally represent a bridge to definitive surgical management.
- If there are surgical contraindications, endoscopic techniques are acceptable definitive palliation interventions.

HISTORICAL BACKGROUND

Gustav Killian first described rigid bronchoscopy for therapeutic airway indications in Freiburg (Germany) in 1895. The first reported procedure involved the removal of a pork bone from the bronchus of a farmer using a rigid esophagoscope. Killian continued to experiment with rigid tubes in both cadavers and patients and, in 1898, described the successful removal of foreign bodies (FBs) in 3 more cases. The technique was further advanced by the discovery of the anesthetizing effect of locally applied cocaine. At the same time, on the other side of the Atlantic Ocean, Chevalier Jackson was instrumental in developing the modern rigid bronchoscope. In 1904, he developed an endoscope with a small light at the distal end. He pioneered endobronchial treatment of the complications of tuberculosis, which was the leading cause of airway disease during the first half of the twentieth century. He is also credited with the first reported endoluminal mechanical resections of endobronchial tumors. Other significant historical advances included the optical telescope by Broyles and the solid rod lens optical system by Hopkins.[1] Modern bronchoscopy benefited from the vision of Shigeto Ikeda, a Japanese pulmonologist, who developed the flexible bronchoscope using optic fibers,[1] which transformed the diagnostic work-up for lung cancer and visualization of the bronchial tree. It is less invasive, does not require, general anesthesia, and provides superior visualization of small peripheral airways. The rigid bronchoscope was regarded as obsolete and

Conflict of Interest: Consultant for Novatech, La Ciotat, France (H. Dutau); none (T. Vandemoortele, D.P. Breen).
[a] Department of Thoracic Oncology, Pleural Diseases and Interventional Pulmonology, North University Hospital, Chemin des Bourrely, Marseille 13015, France; [b] Department of Pulmonology, Hôpital Notre-Dame, Centre Hospitalier de l'Université de Montréal (CHUM), 1560 Sherbrooke Street East, Montreal, Quebec H2L 4M1, Canada; [c] Department of Respiratory Medicine, Galway University Hospitals, Newcastle Road, Galway, Ireland
* Corresponding author.
E-mail address: herve.dutau@mail.ap-hm.fr

Clin Chest Med 34 (2013) 427–435
http://dx.doi.org/10.1016/j.ccm.2013.04.003
0272-5231/13/$ – see front matter © 2013 Elsevier Inc. All rights reserved.

chestmed.theclinics.com

was virtually abandoned in favor of the flexible bronchoscope. Few endoscopists were exposed to the technique and adequate training became a rarity.

However, some European physicians continued to use the rigid system for the treatment of airway diseases, including Jean-François Dumon, who is regarded as a pioneer in interventional pulmonary medicine. He was one of the first bronchoscopists[2–5] to use laser therapy in the airway and standardized its use.[6,7] Another major advance was the invention of a dedicated silicone stent for the trachea and bronchi.[8] Before the era of the Dumon stents, the only available option for reestablishing patency of the trachea after surgery was the Montgomery T tube, which required a tracheotomy for placement.[9] The combination of laser debulking of the endoluminal component and postresection endotracheal stent placement when there is concurrent extrinsic compression allowed immediate and lasting palliation of malignant central airway obstruction, which allowed pulmonologists to treat central airway diseases that had formerly been considered either untreatable or treatable only via extensive, and often prohibitively dangerous, surgical procedures.

RIGID BRONCHOSCOPY EQUIPMENT

The modern rigid bronchoscope is a straight, hollow stainless steel tube that has not significantly changed from the equipment developed by Chevalier Jackson.[10] It is available in various lengths and diameters ranging from 5 mm to 13.5 mm. The barrel wall is 2 to 3 mm thick and the internal diameter is uniform throughout. The distal end of most bronchoscopes is beveled, allowing atraumatic passage through the vocal cords. The bevel can also be used to core out an endobronchial tumor and to corkscrew the bronchoscope through tight stenoses.[10,11] Slits in the distal wall of the bronchoscope allow contralateral ventilation during intubation of a main bronchus. The tracheoscope is shorter in length than the bronchoscope and has no ventilation slits. The proximal end of the bronchoscope consists of a central opening and various side ports for connection of jet ventilation or conventional ventilation devices as well as a source of illumination. The EFER-Dumon rigid bronchoscope, as manufactured by EFER Endoscopy (La Ciotat, France) has a universal proximal head that can be connected to all the bronchoscope barrels (**Fig. 1**). In addition, the various barrel sizes are color coded. Other manufacturers of rigid bronchoscopy equipment include the Texas rigid integrated bronchoscope (**Fig. 2**) from Richard Wolf (Knittlingen,

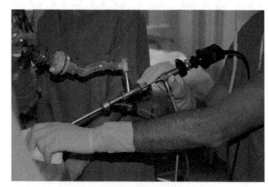

Fig. 1. The EFER rigid bronchoscope.

Germany), the Karl Storz Rigid Bronchoscope (Tuttlingen, Germany) (**Fig. 3**), and, soon, the Dutau-Novatech rigid bronchoscope (La Ciotat, France) (**Fig. 4**). Illumination in modern rigid bronchoscopes is provided by a xenon light source with a prismatic light deflector that is attached proximally to allow full use of the bronchoscope lumen. A Hopkins rod rigid telescope is passed through the central opening of the bronchoscope barrel. The bronchoscopist can either look down the eyepiece of the telescope, or a charge-coupled chip video camera can be connected to the eyepiece for visualization on a monitor, which also allows the physician to record procedures. Before the development of the flexible bronchoscope, angled telescopes were needed to view all bronchial subdivisions, but currently most endoscopists prefer to pass a flexible bronchoscope via the barrel of the rigid bronchoscope for this purpose. The Texas rigid bronchoscope is the first fully integrated rigid bronchoscope with a semiflexible endoscope inside. The theoretic benefit of the Texas system is the full inner lumen of the rigid bronchoscope. The semiflexible endoscope is attachable to a separate channel inside the tube.

Various accessory instruments, including forceps, suction catheters, laser fibers, and stent delivery systems, are used during rigid bronchoscopy by passage via the proximal opening.

RIGID BRONCHOSCOPY TECHNIQUE

After induction of anesthesia, the patient's head is partially extended and the bronchoscope is

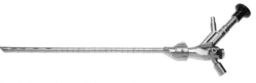

Fig. 2. The Texas rigid bronchoscope.

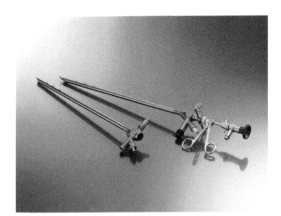

Fig. 3. The Storz rigid bronchoscope.

introduced in the midline with the bevel anteriorly (see **Fig. 4**).[10] Care should be taken to avoid trauma to the patient's upper teeth during intubation by protection with the bronchoscopist's finger or the use of a protective guard. The bronchoscope is advanced under the epiglottis and rotated 90° to allow atraumatic passage through the vocal cords. Once the trachea is entered, the bronchoscope is rotated back 90° and advanced to the lower trachea. To enter one side of the bronchial tree, the patient's head is rotated toward the contralateral shoulder. When using the tracheoscope, thinner diameter bronchoscope barrels can be inserted through the lumen of the tracheoscope. There is therefore no need to remove the tracheoscope or to reintubate the patient. A flexible bronchoscope can also be passed through the lumen of the rigid bronchoscope to allow inspection of distal airways. In addition, the flexible scope is essential for airway toileting and specimen collection. Both bronchoscopes are often used by interventional pulmonologists during therapeutic bronchoscopy. An alternative technique of intubation involves the use of a laryngoscope to lift the epiglottis anteriorly and guide the passage of the bronchoscope to the level of the vocal cords.

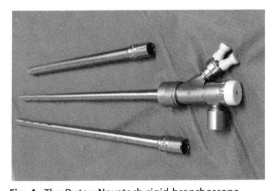

Fig. 4. The Dutau-Novatech rigid bronchoscope.

RIGID BRONCHOSCOPY INDICATIONS

The rigid bronchoscope is an invaluable tool in interventional bronchoscopy.[12–14] With maximal safety and under general anesthesia, it allows adequate ventilation of the patient through a side port; efficient suctioning of blood, secretions, pus, and smoke via large suction catheters; and the use of accessory instruments (laser probes, cryoprobes, rigid forceps, and so forth).[10]

It also allows therapeutic interventions such as dilation of stenoses or extrinsic compression, and mechanical coring and debulking of endoluminal tumors using the distal sharp bevel to rapidly recanalize the airway.[15] In addition, an FB can safely be removed using the rigid forceps. The rigid bronchoscope is the instrument of choice in cases of acute respiratory failure secondary to endoluminal obstruction, because it allows a rapid procedure while maintaining airway patency and adequate ventilation. Because of the obvious anatomic limitations, its use is not suitable for upper lobe disease. A rigid bronchoscope is required for silicone stent placement using a dedicated rigid loading system.

Treatment of central airway obstruction with a flexible bronchoscope alone is not generally recommended, particularly in the case of tracheal lesions. Its small working channel may not be sufficient to prevent airway flooding in cases of massive bleeding. Biopsy forceps have a small diameter and can only sample small tumoral fragments, leading to long and fastidious procedures.[1] In an attempt to overcome this, metallic snares or baskets have been developed to remove large pieces of tumors or FBs.[10] Rigid and flexible bronchoscopy remain complementary techniques, and most pulmonologists use both instruments concurrently during interventions. Flexible bronchoscopy is an important tool with easy maneuverability that allows exploration and clearing of the peripheral airways. In addition, flexible bronchoscopy is the only tool available for the treatment of upper lobe obstruction. A variety of tools (laser, thermocoagulation, argon plasma coagulation, and cryoprobes) can be introduced in its working channel.

FBs

The use of rigid bronchoscopy versus flexible bronchoscopy has been widely debated in the literature.[16–18] The rigid bronchoscope provides excellent access to the subglottic airways and passage of the rigid grasping forceps. Optical forceps allow direct visualization of the FB and optically guided grasping. As an alternative, a rigid telescope and a forceps can be used coaxially through the bronchoscope (**Fig. 5**). During the

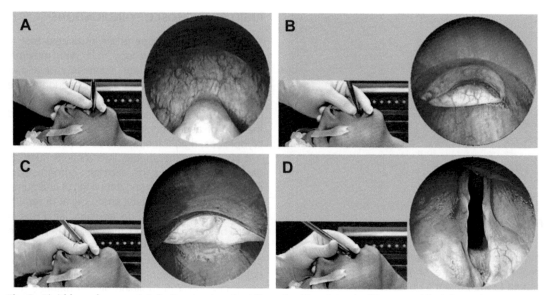

Fig. 5. Rigid bronchoscopy intubation landmarks: (*A*) uvula, (*B*) epiglottis, (*C*) arytenoids, (*D*) vocal cords.

extraction procedure, it is crucial not to push the FB distally with the bronchoscope, the forceps, or the suction catheter. If blood and secretions are present proximally to the FB, these should be cleared by careful suctioning. The optical forceps is then advanced in the bronchial axis, a few millimeters proximal to the FB. For smooth and rounded FBs, the key is to grip the largest volume of the FB. In this setting, the smooth forceps (FB forceps) are preferred to the sharp alligator forceps. The forceps' cups are opened maximally and the forceps is advanced under visual control taking care not to push the FB downwards. The FB is then gently but securely gripped. Both forceps and FB are pulled up, a few millimeters distal to the tip of the bronchoscope, and then the instruments and FB are withdrawn en bloc from the trachea. Alligator forceps are used for grasping sharp or irregular FBs. In case of large, hard FBs, such as pistachio shells, breaking the FB into 2 or 3 fragments may help extraction. In contrast, vigorous grasping of friable FBs, such as peanuts, should be avoided, because it may result in maceration and distal wedging of small fragments. Heavy FBs, such as metallic FBs, tend to move distally because of gravity; in this setting, it may be helpful to place the patient in the Trendelenburg position. During the last step of extraction, the FB can be lost accidentally, either because it is blocked in the narrow glottic area or because there was some inappropriate coaxial movement between the bronchoscope and the forceps, causing the tip of the bronchoscope to push the FB out of the forceps' cups or jaws. If this occurs, the operator should first carefully inspect the oral cavity and the larynx with the laryngoscope and grasp the FB with a Magill forceps, if possible, before reintubating the trachea with the bronchoscope. Once the FB is removed, the trachea is reintubated with the rigid bronchoscope and the airways are carefully reexamined, ideally with a fiberoptic bronchoscope passed through the rigid tube, to rule out another FB or residual fragments.[19]

Silicone Stent Placement

The main purpose of stents designed for use in the central airways (trachea, mainstem bronchi, and, in select cases, lobar bronchi) is to restore patency of the airway to as close a normal caliber as possible. Any endoluminal disorder responsible for debilitating symptoms such as dyspnea and associated with a significant reduction in airway luminal diameter (greater than 50%) may be an indication for a silicone airway stent.[20,21]

Five major indications have been established[20]:

1. Extrinsic compression from tumors or lymph nodes
2. Stabilization of airway patency after endoscopic removal of intraluminally growing cancer
3. Treatment of benign strictures
4. Stabilization of collapsing airways (malacia and polychondritis)
5. Treatment of fistulas (eg, stump dehiscences or tracheoesophageal fistulas)

Endoluminally growing tumors should be treated initially by laser resection, for example, and then a stent should be placed if it is still necessary. Treating benign lesions requires particular caution, because stents may cause harm in the long run, even if early benefit is noted.[21] In general, only removable stents should be used for these indications until a multidisciplinary team has determined inoperability.[21]

Airway stents are generally divided into 2 types: the silicone stents and the metallic stents.[21] The Dumon stent (Tracheobronxane, Novatech, La Ciotat, France) remains the reference standard because it is the most commonly placed stent worldwide. This airway stent has a simple design consisting of a silicone tube with small studs on the external surface to reduce the risk of migration.[8] They have become, de facto, the gold standard for the treatment of benign and malignant stenoses over the past 10 years.[21] There are 2 specific designs: straight and Y shaped (for disease involving the carina).[22] Stents are available in various lengths and diameters to accommodate both pediatric[23] and adult anatomy. For irregularly shaped stenoses (ie, those with marked reduced central airway caliber compared with the extremities), specialized hourglass-shaped stents are available.[24] These hourglass-shaped stents are particularly useful in cases of short benign tracheal disease. Dumon stents are ideally inserted through a dedicated rigid bronchoscope (**Fig. 6**). The commercialized introducer set includes a loading tool and a pusher. A Dumon stent can be repositioned, removed, and replaced at any time with ease using standard grasping rigid forceps.

Malignant Airway Stenosis

Bronchial obstruction is frequently encountered during the course of bronchial carcinoma: more than 30% of bronchial carcinomas present with central airway obstruction.[25]

Such obstructions may lead to specific complications, including reduced survival and decreased quality of life.[26] However, most patients die from general complications caused by their primary intrathoracic disease or extrathoracic extension, and only about 35% from local complications (severe hemoptysis, lung infections, or asphyxia).[26] Given that oncologic treatments do not generally result in prompt improvement in patients' symptoms,[27,28] endoscopic treatments are necessary adjuncts to the tailored management of patients at all stages of the disease (neoadjuvant, adjuvant, and palliative). In addition, bronchial obstruction-related complications (atelectasis, respiratory insufficiency or distress, repeated infections) are likely to interfere with optimal oncologic treatments, such as chemotherapy or radiotherapy. Malignant airway obstruction is often classified based on the type of airway involvement.[29] Airway involvement can be intrinsic, limited to endoluminal involvement, an extrinsic compression, or a mixed condition with both tumor within the airway (ie, intrinsic), and external compression of the airway (ie, extrinsic).[14,29] In summary,[14,29] purely intrinsic involvement can often be managed with debulking techniques to remove the endoluminal tumor. The rigid bronchoscope is then the instrument of choice. Three steps can be described. The first is coagulation and devascularization of the tumor, the second is mechanical coring, and the third is coagulation of the tumoral base (**Fig. 7**). This technique is called laser (or electrocautery, or argon plasma)-assisted mechanical debulking (**Fig. 8**). On occasions, a stent may be placed as a bridge to chemoradiotherapy or alternatively may be considered as a permanent solution when the risk of local recurrence is high. Extrinsic compression without intraluminal disease is readily treated with dilation followed by stenting. Mixed (intrinsic and extrinsic) obstruction is usually managed with both debulking and stent insertion. Benefits noted after successful bronchoscopic treatment of obstruction usually last for 2 to 3 months.[30] Benefit duration after stent placement is generally reported to be around 4 months before tumoral stent overgrowth,[31] but this duration can be increased with the use of effective oncologic treatments (ie, chemotherapy and/or radiotherapy).[32]

Other indications for endobronchial treatment include endobronchial metastases (eg, esophageal, thyroid, renal cell carcinoma, colon, and melanoma) or alternatively low-grade primary tumors (eg, adenoid cystic carcinomas, typical or atypical carcinoids).

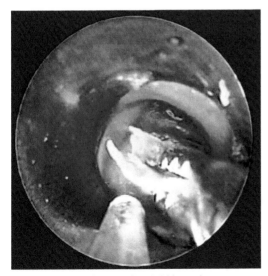

Fig. 6. FB removal using the rigid bronchoscope.

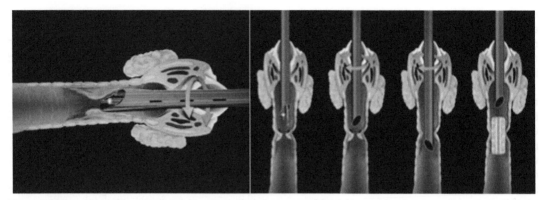

Fig. 7. Silicone stent placement with the rigid bronchoscope. The arrow explain the necessary rotation of the rigid bronchoscope during the dilation of a tracheal benign stenosis.

Benign Airway Stenosis

Postintubation or posttracheostomy tracheal stenosis

Despite the decreasing incidence of postintubation or posttracheostomy tracheal stenosis (PITTS), management of such conditions remains challenging. Even if surgical repair (sleeve resection) is the best definitive solution, approximately 50% of patients present with acute respiratory distress prompting emergent less invasive endoscopic treatments as a bridge to surgery or as definitive treatment in cases with contraindications to surgery.[33] Moreover, tracheal stenosis can recur after tracheal sleeve resection.

PITTS can be divided into 2 different types: the weblike PITTS (disease of the tracheal mucosa sparing the cartilaginous rings) and the complex PITTS (involving deterioration of the cartilaginous support).[34] The weblike PITTS is generally successfully treated by radial mucosal incisions followed by mechanical dilation.[35] The success rate is close to 90% after 1 to 3 sessions.[36] For the

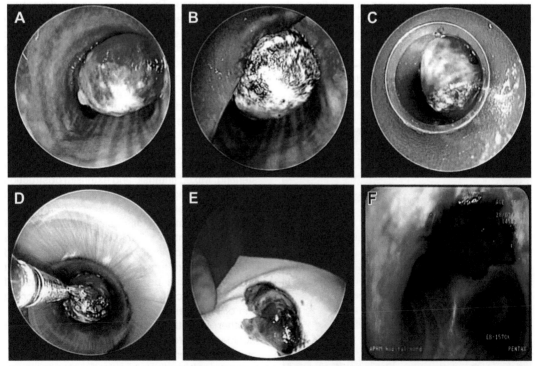

Fig. 8. The various stages of laser-assisted mechanical debulking. (*A*) A tumor obstructing the trachea, (*B*) coagulation of the lesion with laser, (*C*) mechanical resection using the bevel of the rigid bronchoscope, (*D, E*) removal of a large piece of tumor with a rigid forceps, (*F*) carbonization of the tumor base with laser.

complex PITTS, mechanical dilation alone is usually not sufficient.[34] In cases of surgical contraindication, the next step is the placement of a stent to maintain the long-term patency of the tracheal lumen and prevent recurrence.[34]

The choice of stent is important. Self-expandable metallic stents (SEMS) have been shown to make potentially operable PITTS inoperable because of the severe complications associated with the technique.[37] These prompted the US Food and Drug Administration to publish recommendations to limit the use of SEMS in benign tracheal stenosis.[38] Silicone stents are more suitable because of their easy removal, and are not likely to jeopardize a future surgery. Long-term results (no recurrence after stent removal at 1 year) vary from 40% when the stent is placed for 6 months, up to 70% when the stent remains in place for 18 months.[34,36,39,40] In addition, silicone stents require surveillance and may present complications like migrations, granulations, and/or mucus obstructions that can affect the quality of life of the patient.[41] Migration is probably the most challenging complication in this indication, with an incidence ranging from 11% to 17.5%,[33] especially when the stenosis is close to the vocal cords. This complication can be reduced by the use of a dedicated hourglass silicone stent[24] or by external fixation.[42,43] Endoscopic techniques represent, in about 50% of cases, an efficient treatment of PITTS, but many questions remain regarding its long-term efficacy and its impact on quality of life compared with surgery.

Bronchial stenosis following lung transplantation

Improvement in surgical techniques, immunosuppressive regimen, and postoperative care have resulted in improved clinical outcomes, because airway complication rates have decreased, presently ranging from 5% to 30% with an associated mortality of 2% to 3%.[44–49]

Several endoscopic interventions may allow effective management of lung transplantation (LT)–related airway complications. Such procedures include cryotherapy, laser photoresection, balloon bronchoplasty, electrocautery, brachytherapy, airway dilation using rigid bronchoscope, and stent placement.[50] Stent placement is usually considered for bronchomalacia, bronchial stenosis, combined stenosis and malacia, or bronchial dehiscence when these conditions are responsible for respiratory symptoms, persistent decline in lung function, or postobstructive complications such as mucus retention and/or infection. Although many studies have previously described management of LT-related airway complications with SEMS, few data are available with regard to the use of silicone stents for this indication. Stent placement can result in mucosal ischemia, and restenosis is a common finding. Although the overall results (survival and clinical outcome) favor stent placement, a high rate of stent-related problems such as scarring, mucus plugging, bacterial colonization, and migration have to be accepted with currently available stents. It is advisable to select a stent that can be removed if necessary without causing further tissue damage. Our group recently published a retrospective study on Dumon stent placement in anastomotic stenosis after LT.[51] These stents could be removed definitively in 70% of the patients without further recurrence.[51]

ANESTHESIA

Rigid bronchoscopy brings together a unique set of conditions that result in a significant challenge for the anesthetist and endoscopist alike.[52,53] This includes the necessity of both specialties to share the same airway during the procedure. In addition, the underlying disease often significantly compromises the airway. Also, most patients are of advanced age and have multiple pulmonary and nonpulmonary comorbidities that complicate the management of the case.

All cases should be assessed preoperatively to address any reversible conditions that may adversely affect the outcome of the procedure. This assessment should address the cardiovascular and pulmonary systems. All imaging should be reviewed to document the location of the obstruction and assess how this will interfere with ventilation. In addition, performing routine blood tests including coagulation and arterial gases may be beneficial. However, most patients present as emergent cases, and there is therefore no time to perform an in-depth preoperative assessment.

In the setting of rigid bronchoscopy, general anesthesia is required and various techniques have been used, including spontaneous ventilation with manual assistance, jet ventilation, inhalation ventilation, and mechanical ventilation. In the case of an obstructed airway, jet ventilation carries an increased risk for barotrauma if expiration is obstructed. To address this potential complication, the Richard Wolf company has developed the Hemer rigid bronchoscope with a measuring tube connected to the bronchoscope lumen allowing measurement of inspiratory and expiratory pressures, as well as oxygen and carbon dioxide concentrations. In general, anesthesia is induced using a combination of a benzodiazepine, such as midazolam, and an opiate, such as remifentanil. Anesthesia is maintained using different techniques, frequently chosen based on the experience of the anesthetist. These techniques include target-controlled infusion devices, simple infusion devices, and topping up according to the desired level of sedation. There is insufficient evidence to recommend one technique rather than another and the choice of anesthetic agent and mode of ventilation is often made after discussion between the anesthetists and endoscopists at individual centers. Irrespective of the technique used, it is imperative that members of the team have a good working relationship, because both the anesthetist and endoscopist need to work in unison during the procedure.[52,53]

SUMMARY

The rigid bronchoscope is the instrument of choice in most bronchoscopic therapeutic procedures. The rigid bronchoscope is not only a tool to visualize the airway but also a therapeutic instrument in itself or in association with other endoscopic techniques. Most of the scientific associations (European Respiratory Society, American Thoracic Society, American College of Chest Physicians) agree on this point. Rigid bronchoscopy requires training and a dedicated facility or easy access to an operating room with anesthetic support. Moreover, rigid bronchoscopy is mandatory in airway stenting when using silicone stents, which still represent the gold standard. Interventional bronchoscopy is a minimally invasive option in a variety of cases, and can occasionally represent a bridge to definitive surgical management. If there are surgical contraindications, endoscopic techniques are acceptable definitive palliation interventions.

REFERENCES

1. Becker HD, Marsh BR. History of the rigid bronchoscope. In: Bolliger CT, Mathur PN, editors. Interventional bronchoscopy, vol. 30. Basel (Switzerland): Karger, Prog Respir Res; 2000. p. 2–15.
2. Toty L, Personne C, Colchen A, et al. Bronchoscopic management of tracheal lesions using the YAG laser. Thorax 1981;36:175–8.
3. Dumon JF, Reboud E, Garbe L, et al. Treatment of tracheobronchial lesions by laser photoresection. Chest 1982;81:278–84.
4. Unger M. Bronchoscopic utilisation of the Nd YAG laser for obstructive lesions of the trachea and bronchi. Surg Clin North Am 1984;64:931–8.
5. Kvale PA, Eichenhorn MS, Radke JR, et al. Yag laser photoresection of lesions obstructing the central airways. Chest 1985;87:283–8.
6. Dumon JF, Reboud E, Garbe L, et al. Treatment of tracheobronchial lesions by laser photoresection. Chest 1982;81:278–84.
7. Dumon JF, Shapshay S, Bourcereau J, et al. Principles for safety in application of Nd-YAG laser in bronchology. Chest 1984;86:163–8.
8. Dumon JF. A dedicated tracheobronchial stent. Chest 1990;97:328–32.
9. Montgomery WW. Silicone tracheal canula. Ann Otol Rhinol Laryngol 1980;89:521–9.
10. Plekker D, Koegelenberg CF, Bolliger CT. Different techniques of bronchoscopy. Eur Respir Mon 2010; 48:1–17.
11. Ayers ML, Beamis JF Jr. Rigid bronchoscopy in the twenty first century. Clin Chest Med 2001;21: 355–64.
12. Bolliger CT, Mathur PN, Beamis JF, et al. ERS/ATS statement on interventional pulmonology. European Respiratory Society/American Thoracic Society. Eur Respir J 2002;19:356–73.
13. Ernst A, Silvestri GA, Johnstone D. Interventional pulmonary procedures. Guidelines from the American College of Chest Physicians. Chest 2003;123: 1693–717.
14. Ernst A, Feller-Kopman D, Becker H, et al. Central airway obstruction: state of the art. Am J Respir Crit Care Med 2004;169:1278–97.
15. Seijo LM, Sterman DH. Interventional pulmonology. N Engl J Med 2001;344:740–9.
16. Delage A, Marquette CH. Airway foreign bodies: clinical presentation, diagnosis and treatment. Eur Respir Mon 2010;48:135–48.
17. Martinot A, Closset M, Marquette CH, et al. Indications for flexible versus rigid bronchoscopy in children with suspected foreign-body aspiration. Am J Respir Crit Care Med 1997;155:1676–9.
18. Prakash UB, Midthun DE, Edell ES. Indications for flexible versus rigid bronchoscopy in children with suspected foreign-body aspiration. Am J Respir Crit Care Med 1997;156:1017–9.
19. Kim IG, Brummitt WM, Humphry A, et al. Foreign body in the airway: a review of 202 cases. Laryngoscope 1973;83:347–54.
20. Wood DE, Liu YH, Vallieres E, et al. Airway stenting for malignant and benign tracheobronchial stenosis. Ann Thorac Surg 2003;76:167–74.
21. Freitag L. Airway stents. In: Strausz J, Bolliger CT, editors. Interventional pulmonology, vol. 18. Eur Respir Mon 2010;48:190–217.
22. Dutau H, Toublanc B, Lamb C, et al. Use of the Dumon Y-stent in the management of malignant diseases involving the carina: a retrospective review of 86 patients. Chest 2004;126:951–8.
23. Fayon M, Donato L, de Blic J, et al. The French experience of silicone tracheobronchial stenting in children. Pediatr Pulmonol 2005;39:21–7.
24. Vergnon JM, Costes F, Polio JC. Efficacy and tolerance of a new silicone stent for the treatment of benign tracheal stenosis: preliminary results. Chest 2000;118:422–6.

25. Minna JD, Higgins GA, Glatstein EJ. Cancer of the lung. In: De Vita VT, Hellman S, Rosenberg SA, editors. Cancer principles and practice of oncology. 3rd edition. Philadelphia: JB Lippincott; 1989. p. 591–705.

26. Stanley K. Prognostic factors for survival in patients with inoperable lung cancer. J Natl Cancer Inst 1980;65:25–32.

27. Parrat E, Pujol JL, Gautier V, et al. Chest tumor response during lung cancer chemotherapy. Computed tomography versus fiberoptic bronchoscopy. Chest 1993;103:1495–510.

28. Cherry KG, Moran E, Sassoon CS, et al. Effect of radiation therapy on bronchial obstruction due to bronchogenic carcinoma. Chest 1989;95:582–4.

29. Vergnon JM. Les traitements endoscopiques du cancer bronchique. Rev Mal Respir 2008;25. 3S160–6.

30. Mohsenifar Z, Jasper A, Koerner S. Physiologic assessment of lung function in patients undergoing laser photoresection of tracheobronchial tumors. Chest 1988;93:65–9.

31. Vergnon JM, Costes F, Bayon MC, et al. Efficacy of tracheal and bronchial stent placement on respiratory functional tests. Chest 1995;107:741–6.

32. Han CC, Prasetyo D, Wright GM. Endobronchial palliation using Nd:YAG laser is associated with improved survival when combined with multimodal adjuvant treatments. J Thorac Oncol 2007;2:59–64.

33. Baignee PE, Marquette CH, Ramon P, et al. Endoscopic treatment of post-intubation tracheal stenosis. A propos of 58 cases. Rev Mal Respir 1995;12: 585–92.

34. Brichet A, Verkindre C, Dupont J, et al. Multidisciplinary approach to management of post-intubation tracheal stenoses. Eur Respir J 1999; 13:888–93.

35. Mehta AC, Lee FY, Cordasco EM, et al. Concentric tracheal and subglottic stenosis. Management using Nd-YAG laser for mucosal sparing followed by gentle dilatation. Chest 1993;104:673–7.

36. Galluccio G, Lucantoni G, Battistoni P, et al. Interventional endoscopy in the management of benign tracheal stenoses: definitive treatment at long-term follow up. Eur J Cardiothorac Surg 2009;35:429–33.

37. Gaissert HA, Grillo HC, Wright CD, et al. Complication of benign tracheobronchial strictures by self-expanding metal stents. J Thorac Cardiovasc Surg 2003;126:744–7.

38. FDA. US Food and Drug Administration. FDA public health notification: complications from metallic tracheal stents in patients with benign airway disorders. 2005. Available at: www.fda.gov/MedicalDevices/Safety/AlertsandNotices/PublicHealthNotifications/UCM062115. Accessed July 29, 2005.

39. Martinez-Ballarin JL, Diaz-Jimenez JP, Castro MJ, et al. Silicone stents in the management of benign tracheobronchial stenoses. Tolerance and early results in 63 patients. Chest 1996;103:626–9.

40. Cavaliere S, Bezzi M, Toninelli C, et al. Management of post-intubation tracheal stenoses using the endoscopic approach. Monaldi Arch Chest Dis 2007;67:71–2.

41. Bolliger CT, Probst R, Tschopp K, et al. Silicone stents in the management of inoperable tracheobronchial stenoses. Indications and limitations. Chest 1993;104:1653–9.

42. Miwa K, Takamori S, Hayashi A, et al. Fixation of silicone stents in the subglottic trachea: preventing stent migration using a fixation apparatus. Ann Thorac Surg 2004;78:2188–90.

43. Colt H, Harrel J, Neuman T, et al. External fixation of subglottic tracheal stents. Chest 1994;105:1653–7.

44. Mulligan MS. Endoscopic management of airway complications after lung transplantation. Chest Surg Clin N Am 2001;11:907–15.

45. Alvarez A, Algar J, Santos F, et al. Airway complications after lung transplantation: a review of 151 anastomoses. Eur J Cardiothorac Surg 2001;19: 381–7.

46. Shennib H, Massard G. Airway complications in lung transplantation. Ann Thorac Surg 1994;57: 506–11.

47. Colt HG, Janssen JP, Dumon JF, et al. Endoscopic management of bronchial stenosis after double lung transplantation. Chest 1992;102:10–6.

48. Ruttmann E, Ulmer H, Marchese M, et al. Evaluation of factors damaging the bronchial wall in lung transplantation. J Heart Lung Transplant 2005;24:275–81.

49. de Hoyos AL, Patterson GA, Maurer JR, et al. Pulmonary transplantation. Early and late results. The Toronto Lung Transplant Group. J Thorac Cardiovasc Surg 1992;103:295–306.

50. Santacruz JF, Mehta AC. Airway complications and management after lung transplantation: ischemia, dehiscence, and stenosis. Proc Am Thorac Soc 2009;6:79–93.

51. Dutau H, Cavailles A, Sakr L, et al. Silicone stent placement for the management of anastomotic airway complications in lung transplant recipients: a retrospective study: short and long terms outcome. J Heart Lung Transplant 2010;29:658–64.

52. Lorx A, Valkó L, Pénzes I. Anaesthesia for interventional bronchoscopy. In: Strausz J, Bolliger CT, editors. Interventional pulmonology, vol. 48. Plymouth (United Kingdom): European Respiratory Society Monograph; 2010. p. 18–32.

53. Sarkiss M. Anesthesia for bronchoscopy and interventional pulmonology: from moderate sedation to jet ventilation. Curr Opin Pulm Med 2011;17: 274–8.

Bronchial Thermoplasty
A Novel Therapy for Severe Asthma

Ajay Sheshadri, MD, Mario Castro, MD,
Alexander Chen, MD*

KEYWORDS

- Bronchial thermoplasty • Severe asthma • Airway remodeling • Airway smooth muscle

KEY POINTS

- Traditional asthma controller medications are often unsuccessful in controlling the symptoms of patients with severe asthma.
- Bronchial thermoplasty presents a novel therapy in which radiofrequency energy is used to decrease bronchoconstriction by a reduction in airway smooth muscle.
- Current clinical evidence suggests that bronchial thermoplasty may be effective in reducing asthma exacerbations and improving asthma symptoms.
- Long-term data suggest that bronchial thermoplasty is safe and a disease modifier with persistence of effect.

INTRODUCTION

Asthma is an airway disease characterized by chronic inflammation, bronchial hyperreactivity, and variable airflow obstruction triggered by a variety of stimuli, including allergens and infections. The prevalence of asthma has been steadily rising in the United States and in 2010 was estimated to affect 8.4% of the population, or 25.7 million people.[1] Health care costs from asthma in the United States are estimated at $56 billion annually.[2] Every year, more than 50% of asthma patients experience exacerbations of asthma, which are characterized by cough, wheezing, chest tightness, and dyspnea.[3] These symptoms are usually reversible, either spontaneously or with treatment, yet those patients who experience frequent exacerbations may have an accelerated decline in lung function as compared with those who do not.[4–6] Importantly, those with severe asthma, as defined by recent National Heart, Lung, and Blood Institute guidelines, often experience the most frequent exacerbations and account for most health care use costs in asthma.[7]

Typical pharmacotherapy for asthma includes short-acting β2-agonists (SABA), long-acting β2-agonists (LABA), leukotriene modifiers, inhaled corticosteroids (ICS), and oral corticosteroids (OCS). The American Thoracic Society has defined patients with severe, refractory asthma as those who require OCS greater than 50% of the year or high-dose inhaled steroids with the goal of obtaining

Disclosures: A. Sheshadri has no professional or financial interests to disclose. A. Chen has lectured for Asthmatx/Boston Scientific. M. Castro served as consultant or on the advisory board for Genentech, IPS, Medimmune, NKT Therapeutics, and Schering. He lectured for Asthmax/Boston Scientific, Boehringer Ingelheim, Genentech, GSK, Merck, and Pfizer. His University received industry-sponsored grants from Amgen, Asthmatx/Boston Scientific, Ception/Cephalon, Genentech, GSK, Kalbios, MedImmune, Merck, Novartis, and Sanofi-Aventis. His University received grant monies from the NIH and the ALA and received royalties from Elsevier.

Division of Pulmonary and Critical Care Medicine, Department of Internal Medicine, Washington University at St. Louis School of Medicine, Campus Box 8052, 660 South Euclid, St Louis, MO 63110-1093, USA
* Corresponding author.
E-mail address: achen@dom.wustl.edu

Clin Chest Med 34 (2013) 437–444
http://dx.doi.org/10.1016/j.ccm.2013.03.003
0272-5231/13/$ – see front matter © 2013 Elsevier Inc. All rights reserved.

asthma control.[8] However, for many patients, even this aggressive anti-inflammatory therapy may not be sufficient to achieve adequate control of symptoms. Currently, the only agent approved for add-on therapy for severe allergic asthma that is uncontrolled on inhaled or oral corticosteroids is the anti-Immunoglobulin E monoclonal antibody omalizumab. Omalizumab requires biweekly dosing for some patients, is expensive, and provides control only in a subset of asthma patients with allergic disease. New therapies are needed to address the unmet need of patients with severe asthma for whom these therapies are not effective.

AIRWAY SMOOTH MUSCLE IN ASTHMA

The smooth muscle within the walls of airways, or airway smooth muscle (ASM), has been postulated to play a role in multiple normal processes in the healthy airway, including regulation of bronchomotor tone, immunomodulation, and extracellular matrix deposition, although some also claim that it is a vestigial structure without a real salutary function.[9] However, ASM mass is considerably increased in asthma when compared with healthy controls and these same processes contribute to the chronic inflammation and airway remodeling present in severe asthma.[10] In addition, there is substantial hypertrophy and hyperplasia of ASM cells in fatal asthma as compared with nonfatal asthma.[11] This increase in ASM mass contributes to the bronchoconstriction, airway inflammation, and airway remodeling seen in severe asthma. It follows that a reduction in ASM in patients with asthma would potentially alleviate the amount of bronchoconstriction present in the airway and perhaps decrease airway remodeling.

Radiofrequency (RF) energy has safely been used to treat a variety of clinical conditions, including lung cancer,[12] hepatocellular carcinoma,[13] and cardiac conduction abnormalities.[14] Early studies in canines showed that RF at low energies could be safely performed in large airways to reduce ASM mass.[15] This intervention also reduced airway hyperresponsiveness (AHR) within 1 week, and the effect lasted up to 3 years. This rapid loss of sensitivity to cholinergic agents may be due to immediate disruption of actin-myosin filaments, although subsequent loss of ASM mass may be due to cellular necrosis or apoptosis.[16] Large airways account for most of the airway resistance in humans, and therefore, pose a viable target for ablation of ASM in patients with asthma.[17] The application of RF energy to ablate smooth muscle in the large airways of patients with asthma is called bronchial thermoplasty (BT)

and is performed using the Alair Bronchial Thermoplasty System (Boston Scientific, Inc, Natick, MA, USA).

THE ALAIR BRONCHIAL THERMOPLASTY SYSTEM

The Alair Bronchial Thermoplasty System comprises the Alair Controller System (**Fig. 1**), which includes the RF controller, a footswitch, and a return electrode, and the Alair catheter (**Fig. 2**), which contains an expandable 4-arm array and a handle with depressible actuator. The flexible catheter is 1.5 mm in diameter, sterile, disposable, and designed to be introduced in the working channel of a bronchoscope (ideally 4.9–5.2 mm outer diameter) with a working channel of at least 2.0 mm. Larger bronchoscopes may preclude the access to smaller airways, which should be treated.[18] The distal tip of the catheter has an expandable 4-arm array, which is designed to make contact with the walls of airways 3 to 10 mm in diameter. The proximal end of the catheter connects to the controller, which also has inputs for the return gel-electrode (typically placed on the patient's back or thigh) and the footswitch. The depressible actuator is located on the handle at the end of the catheter and controls expansion and collapse of the electrode array. Pressing and releasing the footswitch once triggers the delivery of RF energy through the electrode array on the catheter to the airway wall for 10 seconds, constituting an "activation." The Controller System monitors power, impedance, and duration and delivers an appropriate amount of RF energy to the airways.[15] The bronchoscopist can also press and release the footswitch a second time to terminate the delivery of energy at any time.

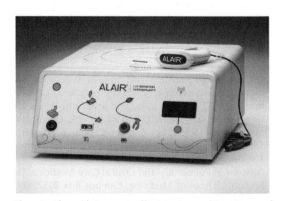

Fig. 1. The Alair controller system. (*Courtesy of* Boston Scientific Corporation, Inc, Natick, MA; with permission.)

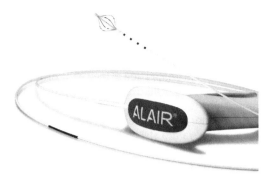

Fig. 2. The Alair catheter with expandable 4-arm array. Black markings are measured at 5-mm intervals from the tip. (*Courtesy of* Boston Scientific Corporation, Inc, Natick, MA; with permission.)

PREPROCEDURE ASSESSMENT

The Food and Drug Administration has approved the Alair Bronchial Thermoplasty System for the treatment of severe persistent asthma in patients 18 years and older (Alair package insert). Selection criteria are outlined in **Box 1** and are adapted from inclusion and exclusion criteria from the Asthma Intervention Research 2 (AIR2) trial, discussed later.[19] A thorough clinical assessment of the patient is imperative before performing BT. To perform BT safely, any potential patient must have stable asthma symptoms without an increase in rescue inhaler usage and no recent exacerbations or infections in the 2 weeks preceding the procedure. If a patient meets these criteria, he or she should receive prednisone at 50 mg/d for the 3 days before the procedure, the day of the procedure, and the day after the procedure to minimize inflammation after BT. On the day of the procedure, the patient's postbronchodilator forced expiratory volume in 1 second (FEV_1) should be within 10% of his or her documented baseline and oxygen saturation should be greater than 90%.[18]

Before the procedure, patients should receive a short-acting bronchodilator and an anti-sialogogue, typically atropine (0.4–0.6 mg IV/IM) or glycopyrrolate (0.2–0.4 mg IV/IM). Albuterol or another SABA should be administered by nebulizer (2.5–5.0 mg) or by metered-dose inhaler (4–8 puffs). A topical anesthetic should be used to numb the posterior pharynx and larynx before the procedure according to institutional practice.

Moderate sedation should be used during the procedure according to institutional guidelines. The authors prefer midazolam and fentanyl because of their rapid onset of action, ease of titration, and ease of reversal if necessary. Other institutions have used propofol, and some perform BT under general anesthesia. The amount of sedation given during BT can often be much higher than

Box 1
Inclusion and exclusion criteria for bronchial thermoplasty

Inclusion criteria

- Adults ages 18–65
- Severe persistent asthma (symptoms throughout the day, symptoms most nights, SABA use several times per day, normal activities are extremely limited by disease)
- Currently using regularly scheduled high-dose ICS and LABA
- Positive methacholine bronchoprovocation test (PC_{20} <8 mg/mL)
- Prebronchodilator FEV_1 $\leq$60% predicted at baseline OR postbronchodilator FEV_1 >65% predicted
- Nonsmoker for at least 1 year OR <10 pack-year smoking history if current smoker

Exclusion criteria

- History of life-threatening asthma requiring intubation
- Intensive care unit admission for asthma in past 24 months without intubation
- $\geq$3 hospitalizations for asthma exacerbations in the last 12 months
- >3 lower respiratory tract infections requiring antibiotics in the last 12 months
- >4 pulses of OCS in the last 3 months
- Known sensitivity to medications required to perform bronchoscopy
- Patients with a pacemaker, internal defibrillator, or other implantable electronic device.

Adapted from Castro M, Rubin AS, Laviolette M, et al. Effectiveness and safety of bronchial thermoplasty in the treatment of severe asthma: a multi-center, randomized, double-blind, sham-controlled clinical trial. Am J Respir Crit Care Med 2010;181:116–24.

during typical bronchoscopy due to the fact that the procedure often lasts 45 minutes to 1 hour. During the procedure, topical anesthesia is paramount to suppress the cough reflex. The authors initially use 3 aliquots of 2 mL 1% lidocaine at the level of the vocal cords, followed by 2 mL aliquots of 1% lidocaine along the trachea, on the carina, and down each main stem bronchus. Additional 2 mL aliquots of 1% lidocaine are used as needed during the procedure to anesthetize treated airways. Oxygen supplementation should not exceed 40% Fio_2 to prevent the theoretical concern of airway ignition. The decision for managing the airway during BT is based on the preference of the bronchoscopist. The authors typically use no endotracheal tube or a laryngeal mask airway in those with narrowing of oropharynx. Other institutions have used an endotracheal tube and general anesthesia.

PERFORMING BRONCHIAL THERMOPLASTY

BT should be performed by an experienced bronchoscopist in conjunction with an asthma specialist. Airways are treated in 3 separate sessions, each 3 weeks apart: the right lower lobe is treated in the first session, the left lower lobe in the second session, and both upper lobes in the final session. The right middle lobe is not treated because of concerns of airway collapse secondary to right middle lobe syndrome.[20] In each session, the airway tree is carefully visualized, and the bronchoscopist devises a plan for systematically treating every visual airway in region being treated. In general, the bronchoscopist works from distal to proximal airways and methodically works from a bronchopulmonary segment to immediate adjacent segments across the lobe until all visible

airways that are 3 mm or greater in diameter are treated once and only once. Each activation is recorded on a diagram of the tracheobronchial tree (**Fig. 3**). The lobar segmental airways are typically the last airways treated due to their ease of access. In the second and third sessions, the previously treated lobe is examined to ensure adequate healing from the previous session. If the previously treated airways are still inflamed or have copious mucous secretions, the BT session may need to be postponed and the secretions removed.

After the session has been meticulously planned, treatment of the airways with BT can commence. The catheter is inserted into the chosen airway and should always be kept in bronchoscopic vision. The bronchoscopist should take care not to kink the catheter, which could impede the deployment of the electrode array. Once the catheter has been positioned, the actuator is depressed until all 4 arms of the electrode array are visualized to be in contact with the airway wall (**Fig. 4**). The bronchoscopist can then press and release the footswitch for the delivery of RF

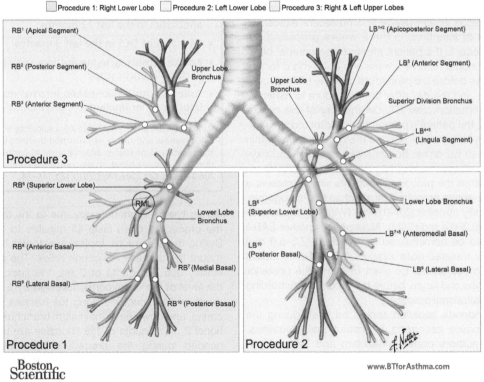

Fig. 3. Diagram of the tracheobronchial tree used for planning BT and recording activations. LB, left bronchus; RB, right bronchus; RML, right middle lobe. (*Courtesy of* Boston Scientific Corporation, Inc, Natick, MA. Netter illustration from www.netterimages.com. © Elsevier Inc. All rights reserved.)

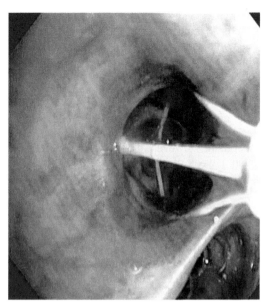

Fig. 4. The Alair catheter with deployed array in a subsegmental airway.

energy, and the Controller System will play an audible cue. Care should be taken not to overexpand the electrode array, which may cause an array arm to invert instead of expand. The array may be cleaned to remove any mucus that accumulates to facilitate positioning of the catheter. If the electrode array does not make adequate contact with the airway wall, the Controller System will play a different audible cue, advising the

bronchoscopist to make subtle changes with array positioning to ensure adequate contact. If the array is dislodged (eg, by a strong cough), the system will automatically abort the activation. Once the Controller System delivers the RF energy, the actuator may be released and the catheter drawn proximally 5 mm, as noted by the marks on the catheter shaft. Activations should be adjacent to each other along the airway but not overlapping (**Fig. 5**). All planned airways are treated in this fashion until the session is complete. A typical session lasts 45 minutes to 1 hour and involves up to 100 activations.

POSTPROCEDURE ASSESSMENT

After the BT procedure is complete, the patient should be monitored as per normal institutional postbronchoscopy guidelines. Patients may take longer to recover because of the greater amount of sedation typically required for BT, again due to the fact that BT often takes longer than typical bronchoscopy. Lung sounds should be auscultated immediately after the procedure and again before discharge. After patients recover from sedation, post-BT spirometry measurements are performed. Patients must have a postbronchodilator FEV_1 of 80% of their preprocedure measurement to be considered for discharge. Serial measurements are sometimes needed due to delayed recovery. Patients may need to be admitted for observation if recovery from BT is delayed; **Box 2** lists criteria for hospital admission. Once

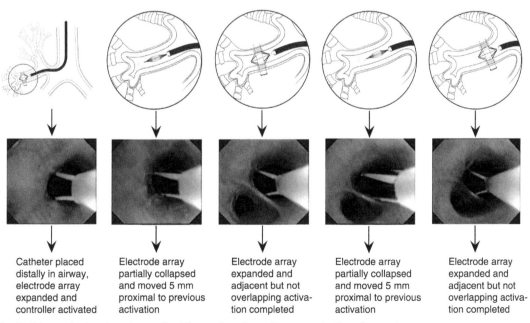

| Catheter placed distally in airway, electrode array expanded and controller activated | Electrode array partially collapsed and moved 5 mm proximal to previous activation | Electrode array expanded and adjacent but not overlapping activation completed | Electrode array partially collapsed and moved 5 mm proximal to previous activation | Electrode array expanded and adjacent but not overlapping activation completed |

Fig. 5. Schematic showing the method for performing adjacent activations in an airway.

Box 2
Hospital admission criteria

- Severe or persistent cough at end of monitoring period
- Failure of postbronchodilator FEV_1 to return to within 20% of preprocedure level at end of monitoring period
- Persistent oxygen saturation <90% at end of monitoring period
- Persistent tachycardia >130 bpm at end of monitoring period
- Unexpected altered mental status during or after procedure
- Hemoptysis >50 mL during 4-hour postrecovery period
- Excessive requirement of bronchodilator during monitoring period
- Absence of companion or caregiver to assist on the day of treatment

---

patients are discharged after BT is performed, they should be notified that they may experience worsening symptoms of asthma and should take prednisone as prescribed. Patients often experience more coughing, wheezing, chest tightness and dyspnea in the 24 to 48 hours following BT, but these usually improve within 1 week after BT and can be treated with bronchodilators and, if needed, systemic corticosteroids. A clinical provider should maintain close follow-up with the patient by phone at 24 hours, 48 hours, and 1 week to assess clinical symptoms. A clinic visit is typically scheduled 2 to 3 weeks after a BT treatment for follow-up as well as to assess clinically in anticipation of subsequent BT treatments.[18]

CLINICAL EVIDENCE FOR BRONCHIAL THERMOPLASTY

The first trial of BT in humans was performed to determine the safety of the procedure in 8 subjects who were scheduled to undergo lung resection for suspected or proven lung cancer.[21] All subjects tolerated the therapy well and proceeded to their planned surgery. One subject showed signs of airway narrowing but was asymptomatic. When the Alair system was used to apply a temperature of 65°C to the airways, a notable reduction in ASM was observed on histopathologic specimens. Subsequently, Cox and colleagues[22] performed a prospective, nonrandomized feasibility study in 16 subjects with mild to moderate asthma to

determine the safety of the procedure in this population. All subjects had stable asthma without recent infection or exacerbation of asthma symptoms. BT was safely performed in a similar fashion to the description mentioned earlier. One subject received only 2 treatments due to recurrent infections after the second treatment. Adverse events were common shortly after the procedure, including cough, dyspnea, wheezing, and bronchospasm. However, these symptoms resolved within 1 week of the procedure, and there were no hospitalizations or emergency room visits related to asthma exacerbation within 12 weeks of the first BT treatment. Lung function did not change significantly in 2 years of treatment, but AHR improved at 12 weeks, 1 year, and 2 years as measured by methacholine bronchoprovocation challenge and subjects experienced more symptom-free days at 12 weeks.

The AIR Trial was the first randomized, controlled trial of BT and enrolled 112 patients with moderate to severe persistent asthma, who were randomized to LABA plus ICS, or BT with LABA plus ICS.[23] Subjects included were on LABA plus ICS before enrollment, had documented AHR and airway obstruction (prebronchodilator FEV_1 60%–85%) and stable asthma symptoms, but had clear worsening of asthma symptoms as measured by the Asthma Quality of Life Questionnaire (AQLQ) if LABA therapy was withdrawn for 2 weeks. The primary outcome measured was mild rate of exacerbation during periods of LABA withdrawal, as defined by reduction in morning peak expiratory flow, increased rescue medication use, or nocturnal asthma symptoms. The rate of mild exacerbations in 1 year of study in subjects in the BT arm was halved, whereas the rate of mild exacerbations in the control arm remained the same. Subjects who received BT were estimated to experience 10 fewer mild exacerbations within the first year, used less rescue medication, and had more symptom-free days. There were more adverse events in the BT arm, usually worsening of asthma control with most occurring within 1 day of a BT treatment.

The Research in Severe Asthma trial was a randomized, controlled trial in which subjects with severe persistent asthma on high-dose ICS with LABA and with AHR were randomized to receive BT or continue current therapy. Six weeks after treatment, subjects in both groups were maintained on stable doses of steroids for 16 weeks before entering a "wean phase" in which OCS and ICS doses were weaned at predetermined time points over 1 year.[24] Four of 8 subjects in the BT arm and 1 of 7 subjects in the control arm were weaned off OCS at 1 year. In addition, patients in the BT arm had improved asthma symptoms by the Asthma Control Questionnaire and AQLQ and had decreased rescue medication use and increased prebronchodilator FEV_1 as compared with the control arm. Adverse events included lobar collapse in 2 patients in the BT arm requiring therapeutic aspiration of mucus.

The most recent and largest trial of BT to date is the AIR2 trial performed by Castro and colleagues.[19] In this study, 288 adults with severe asthma on ICS and LABA with a low AQLQ score, frequent symptoms, and documented AHR by methacholine bronchoprovocation were randomized to BT or a sham procedure. Importantly, the subjects included in AIR2 had to be taking at least 1000 µg/d of beclomethasone or an equivalent ICS, which is a much higher required dose of ICS than in the original AIR trial (200 µg/d of beclomethasone or equivalent). In addition, subjects in AIR2 were all classified as severe asthmatics, as opposed to the original AIR, which also included those with moderate disease.

The sham procedure in AIR2 was identical to the BT procedure with the exception that the Alair catheter did not deliver any RF energy when the foot pedal was depressed. One hundred ninety patients were randomized to BT and 98 patients were randomized to the sham procedure. Adverse events were similar in both groups, although more patients were hospitalized in the BT arm (8.4%) as compared with the sham arm (2%). Reasons for hospitalization included worsening of asthma, segmental atelectasis, lower respiratory tract infection, hemoptysis, and low FEV_1. Although both arms experienced significant improvements in quality of life as measured by AQLQ, 79% of subjects in the BT arm reported a clinically meaningful increase of 0.5 in AQLQ as compared with 64% in the sham arm, highlighting the strength of the placebo effect in patients with severe asthma in a proper sham-controlled trial, as has been documented in sham-controlled studies in other diseases as well.[25,26] Importantly, in the year following BT or sham treatment, subjects in the BT arm had a 32% decrease in severe exacerbations, 66% decrease in days work/school days lost due to asthma symptoms, and an 84% risk reduction in emergency department visits.

The Alair Bronchial Thermoplasty System received Food and Drug Administration approval in 2010 for the treatment of severe, refractory asthma. A postapproval study is currently ongoing to measure treatment effect and safety. In addition, long-term follow-up data are available for several of the studies discussed earlier, which demonstrate the safety and persistence of the effect of BT.[27–31] Five-year follow-up data from the original AIR trial showed no increase in adverse events and stable lung function in those subjects who received BT.[28] Furthermore, 2-year follow-up from the AIR2 trial has showed that the decreased health care use and severe rates of exacerbation in subjects with BT as compared with sham treatment were maintained between year 1 and year 2.[31] Follow-up beyond year 2 is currently ongoing.

SUMMARY

Bronchial thermoplasty is a novel treatment option for patients 18 years of age and older with severe asthma for whom management with conventional pharmacotherapy has been ineffective in controlling asthma symptoms. The procedure should be performed by an experienced bronchoscopist in conjunction with an asthma specialist. Clinical studies have shown improved asthma symptoms, fewer severe exacerbations, and decreased health care use with bronchial thermoplasty. Clinical experience has shown bronchial thermoplasty to be a safe and well-tolerated procedure that presents many potential benefits to patients with severe, refractory asthma.

REFERENCES

1. Akinbami LJ, Moorman JE, Bailey C, et al. Trends in asthma prevalence, health care use, and mortality in the United States, 2001-2010. NCHS Data Brief 2012;94. Available at: http://www.cdc.gov/nchs/data/databriefs/db94.pdf. Accessed August 10, 2012.
2. Barnett SB, Nurmagambetov TA. Costs of Asthma in the United States: 2002-2007. J Allergy Clin Immunol 2011;127:145–52.
3. Akinbami LJ, Moorman JE, Liu X. Asthma prevalence, health care use, and mortality: United States, 2005-2009. National Health Statistics Report 2011; No. 32. Available at: http://www.cdc.gov/nchs/data/nhsr/nhsr032.pdf. Accessed August 10, 2012.
4. Lange P, Parner J, Vestbo J, et al. A 15-year follow-up study of ventilatory function in adults with asthma. N Engl J Med 1998;339:1194–200.
5. O'Byrne PM, Pederson S, Lamm CJ, et al. Severe exacerbations and decline in lung function in asthma. Am J Respir Crit Care Med 2009;179:19–24.
6. Bai TR, Vonk JM, Postma DS, et al. Severe exacerbations predict lung function decline in asthma. Eur Respir J 2007;30:452–6.
7. Moore WC, Bleecker ER, Curran-Evveret D, et al. Characterization of the severe asthma phenotype by the National Heart, Lung, and Blood Institute's Severe Asthma Research Program. J Allergy Clin Immunol 2007;119:405–13.

8. Proceedings of the ATS workshop on refractory asthma: current understanding, recommendations, and unanswered questions. Am J Respir Crit Care Med 2000;162:2341–51.

9. Panettieri RA, Kotlikoff MI, Gerthoffer WT, et al. Airway smooth muscle in bronchial tone, inflammation, and remodeling. Am J Respir Crit Care Med 2008;177:248–52.

10. Ebina M, Takahashi T, Chiba T, et al. Cellular hypertrophy and hyperplasia of airway smooth muscles underlying bronchial asthma: a 3-D morphometric study. Am Rev Respir Dis 1993;148:720–6.

11. James AL, Elliot JG, Jones RL, et al. Airway smooth muscle hypertrophy and hyperplasia in asthma. Am J Respir Crit Care Med 2012;185:1058–64.

12. Fernando HC, De Hoyos A, Landreneau RJ, et al. Radiofrequency ablation for the treatment of non-small cell lung cancer in marginal surgical candidates. J Thorac Cardiovasc Surg 2005;129:639–44.

13. Bruix J, Sherman M. Management of hepatocellular carcinoma. Hepatology 2005;42:1208–36.

14. Benussi S, Nascimbene S, Calori G, et al. Surgical ablation of atrial fibrillation with a novel bipolar radiofrequency device. J Thorac Cardiovasc Surg 2005; 130:491–7.

15. Danek CJ, Lombard CM, Dungworth DL, et al. Reduction of airway hyperresponsiveness to methacholine by the application of RF energy in dogs. J Appl Physiol 2004;97:1946–53.

16. Dryda P, Tazzeo T, DoHarris L, et al. Acute response of airway muscle to extreme temperature induces disruption of actin-myosin interaction. Am J Respir Cell Mol Biol 2011;44:213–21.

17. Despas PJ, Leroux M, Macklem PT. Site of airway obstruction as determined by measuring maximal expiratory flow breathing air and a helium-oxygen mixture. J Clin Invest 1975;55:1090–9.

18. Mayse ML, Laviolette M, Rubin AS, et al. Clinical pearls for bronchial thermoplasty. J Bronchol 2007; 14:115–23.

19. Castro M, Rubin AS, Laviolette M, et al. Effectiveness and safety of bronchial thermoplasty in the treatment of severe asthma: a multi-center, randomized, double-blind, sham-controlled clinical trial. Am J Respir Crit Care Med 2010;181:116–24.

20. Banyai A. The middle lobe syndrome and its quasi-variants. Chest 1974;65:135.

21. Miller JD, Cox G, Vincic L, et al. A prospective feasibilty study of bronchial thermoplasty in the human airway. Chest 2005;127:1999–2006.

22. Cox G, Miller JD, McWilliams A, et al. Bronchial thermoplasty for asthma. Am J Respir Crit Care Med 2006;173:965–9.

23. Cox G, Thomson NC, Rubin AS, et al. Asthma control during the year after bronchial thermoplasty. N Engl J Med 2007;356:1327–37.

24. Pavord ID, Cox G, Thomson NC, et al. Safety and efficacy of bronchial thermoplasty in symptomatic, severe asthma. Am J Respir Crit Care Med 2007;176: 1185–91.

25. Linde K, Streng A, Jürgen S, et al. Acupuncture for patients with migraine: a randomized controlled trial. JAMA 2005;293:2118–25.

26. Leon MB, Kornowski R, Downey WE, et al. A blinded, randomized placebo-controlled trial of percutaneous laser myocardial revascularization to improve angina symptoms in patients with severe coronary disease. J Am Coll Cardiol 2005;46:1812–9.

27. Cox G, Laviolette M, Rubin A, et al. Long term safety of bronchial thermoplasty (BT): 3 year data from multiple studies. Am J Respir Crit Care Med 2009; 179:A2780.

28. Cox G, Laviolette M, Rubin A, et al. 5-year safety of bronchial thermoplasty demonstrated in patients with moderate to severe asthma: Asthma Intervention Research (AIR) trial. Am J Respir Crit Care Med 2010;181:A6839.

29. Thomson NC, Rubin AS, Niven RM, et al. Long-term (5 year) safety of bronchial thermoplasty: Asthma Intervention Research (AIR) trial. BMC Pulm Med 2011;11:8.

30. Pavord I. 5-year safety of bronchial thermoplasty demonstrated in patients with severe refractory asthma: Research in Severe Asthma (RISA) trial. Am J Respir Crit Care Med 2011; 183:A6382.

31. Castro M, Rubin AS, Laviolette M, et al. Two-year persistence of fffect of bronchial thermoplasty (BT) in patients with severe asthma: AIR2 trial. Chest 2010;138:768A.

Bronchoscopic Lung Volume Reduction

Michael J. Simoff, MD[a],*, Javier I. Diaz-Mendoza, MD[a],
Ahmed Y. Khan, MD[b], Rabih I. Bechara, MD[c]

KEYWORDS

- Obstructive lung disease • Lung volume reduction • Bronchoscopic lung volume reduction

KEY POINTS

- The management of obstructive lung disease, particularly emphysematous lung disease, is aggressively being pursued.
- The patient populations that will experience the greatest benefit with lung volume reduction are those that would be the worst candidates for surgical intervention.
- Identifying a bronchoscopic approach that has a true impact on this patient population will be a major accomplishment in the management of patients with chronic obstructive pulmonary disease.
- Resurgence in work on the physiologic improvements in patients successfully treated with these techniques should identify better parameters that can be used in addition to quality-of-life scores to mark successful interventions.

INTRODUCTION

Over the past decade, since the publication of the original National Emphysema Treatment Trial (NETT) results in the *New England Journal of Medicine*,[1] the concept of a procedural intervention in patients with emphysema has grown. Chronic obstructive pulmonary disease (COPD) remains the third leading cause of death in the United States (Centers for Disease Control and Prevention National Center for Health Statistics, Deaths: Preliminary Data for 2008).[2] As such, the potential for an intervention that can help control morbidity and improve quality of life could have extensive application throughout the world.

The goal of surgery was the removal of 25% to 30% of the diseased lung. The reported 90-day mortality of 7.9% in the surgical group versus the 1.3% mortality in the medical control group was significant. There were also significant postoperative morbidities (air leak for longer than 7 days, prolonged hospitalization, readmission to the intensive care unit, and so forth) in the surgical group in comparison with the medical group. When subgroup analysis was completed, approximately 30% of surgical patients demonstrated clinically significant improvement in exercise capacity and quality-of-life scores.

These results were encouraging, but underscored by the fact that major surgical procedures needed for this intervention were being performed on very poor candidates. Minimally invasive techniques need to be created to allow the opportunity to provide the potential physiologic advantages to the patients that would be candidates for volume reduction surgery, but more importantly, to those patients with severe morbidities resulting from their emphysema, who are otherwise not surgical candidates and subsequently may receive the greatest benefits.

[a] Interventional Pulmonology, Pulmonary and Critical Care Medicine, Henry Ford Hospital, 2799 West Grand Boulevard, Detroit, MI 48202, USA; [b] Pulmonary and Critical Care Medicine, Emory University School of Medicine, 1365 Clifton Road, NE, Atlanta, GA 30322, USA; [c] Pulmonary and Critical Care, Cancer Treatment Centers of America/Southeastern, 600 Parkway North, Newnan, Atlanta, GA 30265; Georgia Regents University, Augusta, GA, USA
* Corresponding author.
E-mail address: MSimoff1@hfhs.org

Clin Chest Med 34 (2013) 445–457
http://dx.doi.org/10.1016/j.ccm.2013.06.002
0272-5231/13/$ — see front matter © 2013 Elsevier Inc. All rights reserved.

This article highlights the work currently ongoing in the area of bronchoscopic lung volume reduction. There are tools now clinically available in some locations throughout the world, but no standardized technique exists.

ENDOBRONCHIAL BLOCKERS

The initial attempts at bronchoscopic lung volume reduction were aimed at correcting loss of elastic recoil in emphysematous lung, by blocking those airways with the most severe airflow limitation.[3–5] This therapy was used for patients with heterogeneous emphysema. The blockage was to induce resorption atelectasis in the more distal lung segments, thereby allowing expansion of healthier lung with resultant improvement in overall elastic recoil. In addition, reductions of anatomic dead space would translate into a decrease in dynamic air trapping and, thus, improved exercise inspiratory capacity. In a manner similar to lung volume reduction surgery (LVRS), the reduction of hyperinflation would provide further benefits to optimizing chest-wall dimensions and the operating length of the diaphragm.

Early endobronchial blockers were composed of silicone (**Fig. 1**) vascular balloons filled with radiopaque contrast; however, custom-built stainless-steel stents with occlusive biocompatible sponges in the center were soon constructed.[5] Unfortunately, experience with this modality of bronchial lung volume reduction (BLVR) revealed that the benefit seen in improvement of dyspnea and exercise tolerance afforded by the blockers was overshadowed by postprocedural complications. Such problems included significant and numerous issues with migration of the blockers after implantation and subsequent postobstructive pneumonia caused by accumulation of distal secretions, which necessitated repeated bronchoscopies.[3–5]

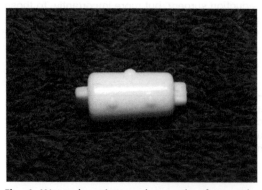

Fig. 1. Watanabe spigot and example of an endobronchial blocker. (*Courtesy of* Michael Simoff, MD.)

Ultimately, further advancements for this route of BLVR were abandoned in favor of other modalities that sought to address the issues of drainage of distal secretions and migration of the implanted devices.

ONE-WAY ENDOBRONCHIAL VALVES

The experience with endobronchial blockers highlighted what the desired characteristics of an endobronchial device aimed to reduce lung volumes should be.[5] The ideal device should cause distal atelectasis in the target lung units, be able to be implanted via flexible bronchoscopy without risk for subsequent migration, be removable if required, and should allow drainage of distal secretions while blocking airflow into airways.[5]

The intended physiologic basis for this modality is similar to that of LVRS. Despite this, only a minority of patients achieve complete collapse of the selected area distal to the implanted valves.[6–11] In the majority of patients the valves divert airflow from the segments of lung with the most severe disease to airways with less airflow limitation, thereby attempting to reduce the amount of physiologic dead space and improve dynamic airflow trapping. The 1-way valve mechanisms seek to permit drainage of secretions distal to the valve in an attempt to reduce the incidence of postobstructive pneumonia.[6–11] Two types of valve have been developed with this goal. Their clinical efficacy at achieving the desired effects has been studied over the last 10 years.

Endobronchial Valve

The valve with the largest amount of data to date is the Zephyr endobronchial valve (EBV) (Pulmonx, Redwood City, CA), formerly known as the Emphasys Zephyr EBV. This device consists of a central silicone 1-way duckbill valve attached to a nitinol (nickel-titanium alloy) self-expanding retaining frame that is wrapped in a silicone seal (**Fig. 2**).[11] After selection of a single target lobe, the Zephyr valves are implanted unilaterally in a 3-step process. The valves are removable in the event of improper positioning or complications from the valve. The valve sits flush with the carina of the segmental bifurcation when correctly positioned (**Fig. 3**).[6–8,11]

After the initial pilot studies by Toma and colleagues[11] and Yim and colleagues[5] suggested efficacy and relative safety of the procedure, several smaller studies without control arms were conducted. These case series consistently were able to demonstrate improvements in subjective scores of dyspnea, but were unable to delineate a clear improvement in traditionally measured physiologic

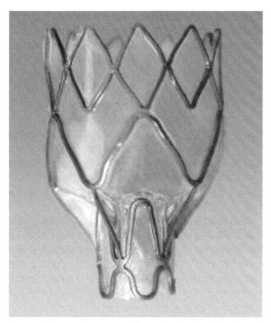

Fig. 2. The Emphasys endobronchial valve (EBV) with the central 1-way silicone duckbill valve attached to a nitinol self-expanding retaining frame that itself is wrapped in a silicone seal. (*Courtesy of* Pulmonx Inc, Redwood City, CA; Michael Simoff, MD; with permission.)

markers such as forced expiratory volume in 1 second (FEV$_1$) or distance covered in a 6-minute walk test (6MWT).[6–8]

The Endobronchial Valve for Emphysema PalliatioN Trial (VENT) study was a multicenter, prospective, double-blind trial, which enrolled 321 patients that were randomly assigned in a 2:1 ratio to unilateral therapy with a Zephyr Valve (220 patients) and standard medical management (101 patients) for their emphysema.[8] Eligibility and exclusion criteria mirrored that from the NETT

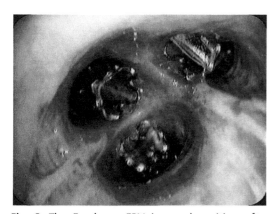

Fig. 3. The Emphasys EBV in good position after implantation in the right upper lobe. (*Courtesy of* Pulmonx Inc, Redwood City, CA; with permission.)

subgroup identified as responders. Namely, patients with heterogeneous emphysema, a FEV$_1$ of 15% to 45% of the predicted value, residual volume of more than 150% of predicted value, a body mass index (BMI) of 31.1 kg/m^2 or less for men or 32.3 kg/m^2 or less for women, a partial pressure of carbon dioxide (Paco$_2$) of less than 50 mm Hg, a partial pressure of oxygen (Pao$_2$) of more than 45 mm Hg on room air, and a postrehabilitation 6MWT distance of at least 140 m (459 ft) were enrolled. Patients were excluded if they had a carbon monoxide diffusing capacity (DLCO) of less than 20% of the predicted value, the presence of giant bullae, α1-antitrypsin deficiency, previous thoracotomy, excessive sputum, severe pulmonary hypertension, active infection, or unstable cardiac conditions.

The data obtained from the VENT study demonstrated small improvements in the primary efficacy outcomes of FEV$_1$ (4.3%; 95% confidence interval [CI] 1.4–7.2) and 6MWT (2.5%; 95% CI −1.1 to 6.1) compared with decreases in the control group at 6 months with FEV$_1$ (2.5%; 95% CI −5.4 to 0.4) and 6MWT (3.2%; 95% CI −8.9 to 2.4). Modest improvements were demonstrated in secondary efficacy measures of quality of life and dyspnea, such as the St George's Respiratory Questionnaire (SGRQ), BODE (BMI, Obstructive lung disease, Dyspnea, and Exercise tolerance) index, average daily oxygen use, and maximum workload by cycle ergometry.

A nonstatistically significant trend toward a greater rate of major complications (6.1% in the valve implant group vs 1.2% in control groups) was reported. Twelve patients developed postobstructive pneumonia with half of those requiring removal of their valves. Hemoptysis (6%), pneumothorax (4.2%), and exacerbations of COPD requiring hospital admission occurred with greater frequency in the EBV group. Six deaths occurred in the intervention arm in contrast to none in the control arm. Mortalities were not thought to be associated with the procedure or the valve implants. At the 12-month follow-up a statistically significant difference in survival benefit was not demonstrated on multivariate Cox regression analysis.

In the follow-up phase of the study, valve migration, postobstructive pneumonia distal to the valve, hemoptysis, and COPD exacerbations occurred, requiring the removal of 85 valves in 35 patients. The success rate of valve removal was 97.7%. After completion of the study another 8 patients had elective removals of the EBV attributable to adverse events. The European cohort of 171 patients demonstrated results similar to those of the United States cohort.[6] The Food and Drug Administration

(FDA) review of the study did not result in approval of the device for BLVR, because of the lack of clinically significant response seen in FEV_1.[3–16]

Further subgroup analysis of high-resolution computed tomography data revealed a correlation of clinical success with fissure integrity affording greater improvements in symptoms, measured physiologic markers, and reductions in lung volumes, resulting in expansion of the less diseased neighboring lung. Small studies with longer-term follow-up have also shown that patients who have atelectasis of the target segments show a survival benefit over other groups receiving BLVR.[7,11]

These results support theories raised in earlier studies and the experience seen with endobronchial blocker use that collateral ventilation may have a role to play in blunting the benefit and lung volume reduction that is achieved with endobronchial airway obstructive techniques. Ventilation through accessory pathways (collateral ventilation) is the likely cause of the high percentage of patients who had lobar exclusion with valve blockade but did not achieve selected atelectasis.[7,14] Further studies and new technologies are being developed to measure the amount of collateral ventilation before EBV implantation in hopes of being able to predict airway placement locations that will have a more clinically significant response to BLVR (**Fig. 4**).[14]

Intrabronchial Valve

The Spiration intrabronchial valve (IBV) (Olympus, Redmond, WA) is a self-expanding nitinol frame consisting of a central core with 5 distal anchors and 6 proximal curved radial struts.[9,10] This structure supports a polyurethane membrane, which acts as a 1-way umbrella valve when implanted against the bronchial wall (**Fig. 5**).[9,10] Aside from support, the central core also serves as a removal rod or if the device needs manipulation after initial deployment.[9,10] After selection of the target airways, appropriately sized valves are chosen. In a technique somewhat similar to that of EBV placement, the IBV is inserted via the working channel of a flexible bronchoscope on a catheter loader. Once in position the valve is deployed so it will sit flush with the carina of the segmental bronchus (**Fig. 6**).[10]

Two articles detailing experience with the placement of these valves have been published, both on the same set of patients.[9,10] One significant difference from EBV studies is the bilateral targeting and placement of these valves in the upper lobes. Similar to the trials for EBV, these trials used selection criteria that closely mirrored the NETT trial subgroup that demonstrated the greatest benefit. Patients enrolled in both studies had severe heterogeneous predominantly upper lobe emphysema with an FEV_1 of 15% to 45% predicted, total lung capacity (TLC) greater than 100% predicted, residual volume (RV) greater than 150% predicted, $Paco_2$ of less than 50 mm Hg, Pao_2 of greater than 45 mm Hg, and a postrehabilitation 6MWT distance of greater than 140 m. Exclusion criteria removed patients with an FEV_1 less than 20% predicted, DLCO less than 20% predicted, homogenous emphysema, active infection, a recent COPD exacerbation, giant bullae, pulmonary hypertension, or oxygen requirements greater than 6 L/min.

The 2 articles share 91 subjects at 11 United States and international centers. For reasons not

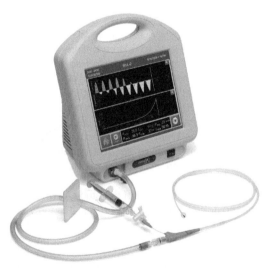

Fig. 4. The Chartis system with attached measurement catheter that is aimed to assess the presence of collateral ventilation to identify patients that will have more favorable response to treatment. (*Courtesy of* Pulmonx Inc, Redwood City, CA; with permission.)

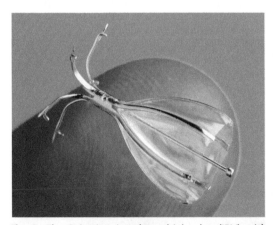

Fig. 5. The Spiration intrabronchial valve (IBV) with nitinol frame mounted silicone umbrella valve and a central core strut used to manipulate or remove the valve once deployed. (*Courtesy of* Kyle Hogarth, MD.)

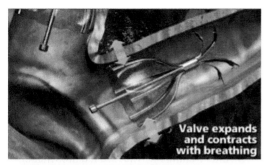

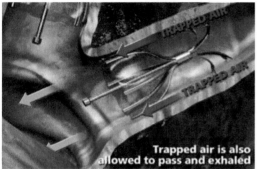

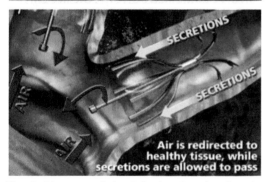

Fig. 6. Diagrams of the Spiration IBV showing the valve in good position after implantation and function, allowing drainage of secretions but blocking entry of air flow. (*Courtesy of* Kyle Hogarth, MD.)

explained in either article, 7 subjects from 2 additional centers were included in the initial article, which were not included in the later more comprehensive article. Results of both reports were similar. The pilot study, by Sterman and colleagues,[10] was a single-arm, open-label case series using a multilobar bilateral treatment approach. Primary outcomes of the study focused on safety based on the incidence of valve migration, erosion, or infection. Efficacy based on FEV$_1$, 6MWT, and SGRQ were the secondary end points. Other potential measures of efficacy included change in oxygen supplementation requirements, improvement in Medical Outcome Study Short-Form Health Survey (SF-36) scores, and improvement in the modified Medical Research Council dyspnea score.[9,10]

During the study period the protocol was changed twice. After the first third of patients were enrolled the protocol was modified to include, at the discretion of the investigator, valve treatment to the lingula in addition to the left upper lobe, with the intention to increase the amount of atelectasis achieved. Then, after enrollment of the second third of patients, the protocol was reverted to excluding the lingula from treatment with the addition of further radiographic measurements for evaluating response to the valve implants. Changes to the protocol for follow-up included cessation of a second bronchoscopy 1 month after the procedure as it was thought to be of low yield. Quantitative computed tomography (QCT) of patients for volumetric analysis of lobar volumes was added to the study protocol during the last third of the investigation as an additional marker for efficacy of treatment.[9,10]

The results of this pilot study were encouraging. No patients were lost to follow-up, although 26 patients withdrew from the study owing to adverse events associated to the valve implants. Most of the later withdrawals of patients (defined as withdrawal after 6 months postprocedure) were either related to a perceived lack of improvement by the patient or other issues such as a new diagnosis of lung cancer.[10]

As the primary end point was to evaluate safety data, a detailed analysis of all adverse events was performed. None of the deaths were determined to be procedure related. No migration or erosion was noted throughout the study. Dyspnea was seen in 8 patients on postprocedure day 3, thought to be related to implant-triggered bronchospasm. Only 2 of these patients required valve removal to alleviate the symptoms, with the remainder improving with bronchodilator treatment. Other procedure-related complications included myocardial infarction, injury to bronchi from deep valve placement, and transient hypercarbia requiring transient ventilatory overnight support. Across the course of the study, a total of 44 valves were removed for reasons of persistent bronchospasm, recurrent COPD exacerbations, pneumonia, or pneumothorax.[9,10]

A total of 11 patients developed pneumothorax, with 6 requiring chest-tube placement. Subsequent analysis revealed a higher incidence of left-sided pneumothorax in the patients who had received additional valve implants to the lingula. As in prior studies of other modalities of BLVR, a close correlation was noted between the amount of atelectasis achieved and the incidence of pneumothorax.[9,10] The suggested mechanism for this has been related to rapid atelectasis of the lung parenchyma in the presence of adhesions, tension on adjacent tissue, or overexpansion of blebs and bullae that may accompany the lung reduction. In addition, there were 3 deaths associated with pneumothorax in the study population.

In comparison with the LVRS patients in the NETT, morbidity and mortality (49.8%) were more favorable for the IBV data, which demonstrated a 5.5% 30-day morbidity for major cardiopulmonary complications.[9,10] Health-related quality of life (HRQL) measures at 6 months achieving the 4-point clinically significant threshold in the NETT patients was 60% in comparison with 55% for patients with IBV implants.[9,10] These results suggest an improved risk/benefit ratio in terms HRQL measures for IBV treatment.

On evaluation of the secondary end points of efficacy, no statistically significant change or improvement was seen in any of the measured physiologic indices such as FEV_1, TLC, RV, or 6MWT. Improvement in HRQL measures were noted in the majority of patients as measured by the SGRQ and SF-36. This population of patients with clinically significant improvement in SGRQ increased with time and remained statistically significant. Similar results of discordance between the improvements in HRQL measures and physiologic indices in the population of patients with severe emphysema have been seen in other studies of BLVR and LVRS.

It has been suggested that in this population of patients the traditional physiologic measures of FEV_1 and lung volume do not accurately predict effects of changes in regional lung volume when the obstructive defect is known to be fixed. In addition, issues with the effort-dependent variability of FEV_1 in severe emphysema owing to loss of elastic recoil could limit its utility as an outcome measure.[9]

To further investigate these proposed mechanisms, researchers used a QCT evaluation to assess changes in regional lung volume.[9] Using a previously validated quantitative volumetric computed tomography (CT) assessment tool, a statistically significant average upper lobe volume reduction of roughly 300 mL was seen 6 months posttreatment in 93% of patients. This volume reduction increased across all time points in the study period, and was accompanied by a respective increase in volume of the untreated and less severely emphysematous lung. A significant correlation was then noted between patients with improvements in their HRQL responses and QCT-assessed volume increases of greater than 10% in the nontreated lung.[9]

These observations led the investigators to postulate a third mechanism to be contributory to the improvement in HRQL scores observed. In addition to lobar atelectasis causing lung volume reduction and improvements in dynamic hyperinflation, an interlobar shift of ventilation was identified.[9] In essence, with increased ventilation to the less severely emphysematous lower lobes and shunting of airflow away from the poorly perfused lobes targeted for treatment, an improvement in the ventilation perfusion ratio was achieved. This improvement most likely represents an element of the observed improvements in dyspnea and HRQL after treatment.[9] The investigators acknowledged that the aforementioned 3 mechanisms were most likely interlinked, with each playing some role in improvements noted by the patients.[9]

At present the IBV valves are available for use in the United States with an FDA indication of humane use only for prolonged surgical air leaks, pending further studies that hope to elucidate clinically significant efficacy. A randomized controlled trial comparing the 2 valves is currently ongoing, and data from this study are yet to be reported.[17]

LUNG VOLUME REDUCTION COIL IMPLANTS

Experience with endobronchial blocker and 1-way airway valves for volume reduction have been plagued with lack of response, believed to be related to the presence of collateral ventilation.[6,8,9,14] Another approach to BLVR to overcome this challenge is the lung volume reduction coil (LVRC), an implant that physically compresses target areas in patients with severe heterogeneous emphysema to avoid the issue of collateral ventilation altogether. The RePneu Airway Coil (PneumRx, Inc, Mountain View, CA) is a nitinol wire that is preformed in a shape that compresses the lung parenchyma once deployed in the target airways (**Fig. 7**).[13,16] This approach is intended to lead to a true reduction of lung volume from the surrounding area.

The airway implants are placed under general anesthesia with flexible bronchoscopy via a rigid

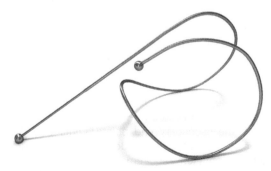

Fig. 7. The nitinol airway coil implant is seen here in its preformed shape. (*Courtesy of* PneumRX Inc, Mountain View, CA; with permission.)

bronchoscope or large endotracheal tube.[13,16] A guide wire is advanced into the target segment under fluoroscopic guidance. The length of the airway is then measured using a graduated catheter passed over the guide wire, which allows selection of the appropriate length of the LVRC implant (**Fig. 8**). After removal of the guide wire, a straightened LVRC is advanced under fluoroscopic guidance into the airway via the catheter using a grasper holding the proximal end of the implant (**Fig. 9**). Proper positioning of the implant aligns the distal tip of the LVRC 15 mm from the pleura (**Fig. 10**).[13,16] The LVRC assumes its preformed shape once the catheter is removed, thereby bending the airway and compressing the surrounding lung parenchyma. Finally, the proximal end of the LVRC is released from the grasper and the bronchoscope is removed. Repositioning or removal of the implant is performed by reversal of the procedure described earlier.[13,16]

After initial animal studies, a pilot study was conducted that enrolled 11 patients (8 with severe homogenous emphysema and 3 with severe heterogeneous disease).[13] Two procedures were performed on each patient 1 to 3 months apart. Three to 6 LVRC implants were placed during each session. Six patients received LVRC implants bilaterally, 4 had unilateral treatment, and 1 did not receive a second treatment.

The primary end point of the pilot study was safety data measured by analysis of adverse events. Herth and colleagues[13] showed in this trial that the procedure was feasible and observed adverse effects comprising initial episodes of

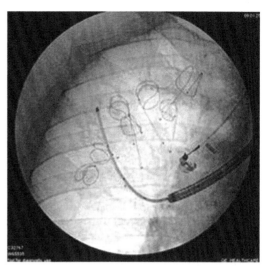

Fig. 9. Fluoroscopic guidance allows optimal positioning of the guide catheter and airway coil. Previously placed implants are also visible. (*Courtesy of* G. Deslée.)

dyspnea, cough, transient chest pain, and exacerbation of COPD that resolved with treatment. No serious adverse events occurred and none of the LVRC implants required removal during the 6-month study period. The data further suggested that in addition to improvements in HRQL, there were clinically significant improvements in pulmonary function indices such as FEV_1, forced vital capacity (FVC), and 6MWT in patients with heterogeneous disease. The study was not designed with adequate power to detect a statistical difference in efficacy data, as this was a secondary end point.

The second-generation coil was developed and used in the second LVRC study.[16] The trial focused on patients with only upper lobe predominant

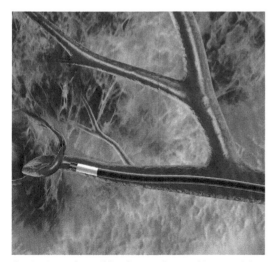

Fig. 8. Once the coil has been advanced into position, the guide catheter is withdrawn with the coil returning to its preformed shape, compressing the surrounding lung parenchyma with it. (*Courtesy of* PneumRX Inc, Mountain View, CA; with permission.)

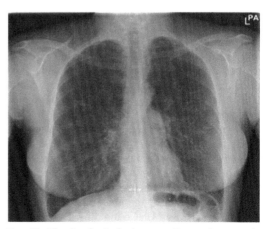

Fig. 10. The implanted airway coils can be seen in bilateral upper lobes on radiographic imaging. (*Courtesy of* D.J. Slebos.)

heterogeneous emphysema. Inclusion and exclusion criteria were almost identical to those of other BLVR studies.[16]

Once patients were identified, an assessment of the degree of emphysema was done using CT imaging. Visual assessment of sagittal reconstructions of full inspiratory thin-slice CT scans in addition to digital assessment were used to select and quantify patients with disease that was suspected to have enough destruction of upper lobe parenchyma to derive benefit from treatment, yet have enough tissue to allow LVRC placement with subsequent compression of surrounding parenchyma.[16] On completion of initial evaluations, an additional exclusion criterion was added: patients with greater than 75% destruction of their upper lobes on digital assessment were excluded.

Sixteen patients had 28 sequentially staged LVRC placement procedures. An average of 10 coils was placed per procedure. To further standardize the approach, coils were also placed in predetermined segments independent of CT findings. Bilateral implants were placed in 12 patients. Four patients received unilateral treatment because of ineligible targets contralaterally, significant clinical improvement from the initial treatment, or limitations from cardiac comorbidities.[16]

No implant migration, erosion of airways, or need to remove any of the implants occurred during the 6-month follow-up. One patient developed a pneumothorax 1 hour after the procedure, which resolved in 1 day with chest-tube decompression. In addition, 75% of patients had mild (<5 mL) hemoptysis. Transient self-limited chest pain thought to be related to pleural traction occurred in 4 patients. The frequency of COPD exacerbations and coughing were the most common issues after implantation. These events decreased to preprocedural levels after the first month. Mucosal damage, edema, and bronchoconstriction associated with the placement of the LVRC implants were postulated to be the reason for the respiratory events noted.[13,16] Nevertheless, undocumented concerns still exist for the development of pulmonary torsion, airway erosion, and infarction caused by compression of blood vessels in the target lung.

Six months postprocedure, an improvement is HRQL was seen similar to that seen in BLVR patients treated by both 1-way valves and endobronchial blockers. The almost 15-point reduction in SGRQ, however, was greater than that reported even in the favorable response subgroup of the NETT LRVS study.[13] Unlike the other BLVR device implants, this study showed a 14.9% clinically significant (P<.005) improvement in FEV_1, 13.4% improvement in FVC, 11% reduction in RV, and a

clinically relevant 84-m improvement in 6MWT distance.[16] As efficacy was again a secondary end point of this study, these results need to be interpreted with cautious optimism while awaiting further data from more adequately powered studies.

Two trials are currently ongoing to more completely address the clinical efficacy of LVRC in affecting BLVR. The larger United States study intended to recruit 315 patients has not yet started enrolling patients at the time of writing. A smaller study registered in the United Kingdom is currently ongoing whereby data are not yet available for interpretation or comment.

BRONCHOSCOPIC THERMAL VAPOR ABLATION

Bronchoscopic thermal vapor ablation (BTVA) was developed as another technique to selectively treat portions of lung that are diseased. Scarring and contraction is produced by inducing an inflammatory response to thermal injury of soft tissue as a means of lung volume reduction.[16,18–21] Animal studies have delineated the effects and extent of varying doses of treatment.

The thermal energy is delivered via bronchoscopic introduction of heated water vapor into the lung parenchyma and airways using the InterVapor system (Uptake Medical, Tustin, CA).[18–21] The system consists of a device to precisely deliver heated water vapor, a delivery handle (**Fig. 11**), and a delivery catheter with an occlusion balloon near the tip. All procedures were performed under general anesthesia with flexible bronchoscopy via a large (size 9 or 10) endotracheal tube. Two operators are needed to optimally perform this procedure, the first performing the bronchoscopy and the second manipulating the catheter system and delivery handle for the vapor therapy. Once the target segment is identified, the vapor delivery catheter is advanced into the airway with subsequent inflation of the occlusion balloon at the tip of the catheter (**Fig. 12**). The desired dose of thermal energy, using steam, is delivered to the airway. A 5-minute period between treatments is required to prevent accumulative thermal energy causing a more significant injury.

Extrapolating from the animal studies on BTVA a unilateral dose of 5 calories per gram of lung tissue treated was selected for the first pilot study in humans performed by Snell and colleagues.[21] Patients with heterogeneous upper lobe emphysema who had an FEV_1 between 15% and 45% predicted, TLC at least 100% predicted, RV greater than 150% predicted, a postrehabilitation 6MWT distance of more than 140 m, $Paco_2$ less than 50 mm Hg, and a Pao_2 greater than 45 mm Hg

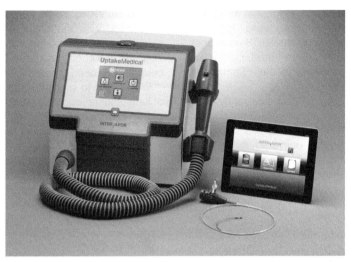

Fig. 11. The InterVapor system used to generate the steam to deliver thermal energy to the target segments. The single-patient use disposable catheter is also seen. (*Courtesy of* Uptake Medical Inc, Seattle, WA; with permission.)

were enrolled. In summary, the criteria were similar to those in studies done to evaluate other BLVR modalities.

All of the 11 patients enrolled in the pilot study received unilateral treatment to the lobe thought to have the most severe disease by the investigators.[21] No procedural complications were reported. Symptoms of nausea, cough, transient fatigue, and mild to moderate hemoptysis were noted postprocedurally. Almost 64% of patients had subsequent exacerbations of their COPD, with roughly half of these surmised to be related to infection. Two of the 7 patients with COPD exacerbations required hospitalization. Two additional patients developed pneumonitis, 1 requiring hospital admission and treatment. Atrial tachycardia and anxiety in 1 patient also required inpatient treatment. Overall, BTVR was thought to be relatively safe and, thus, a feasible procedure.[21]

Secondary end-point evaluations in this pilot study included quantitative volumetric CT

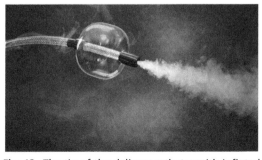

Fig. 12. The tip of the delivery catheter with inflated occlusive balloon that avoids unintended proximal delivery of steam. (*Courtesy of* Uptake Medical Inc, Seattle, WA; with permission.)

assessment.[21] A 16% volume reduction of the treated lobe was seen on chest CT analysis. The amount of volume loss noted appeared to correlate with improvements seen on SGRQ ($r = 0.83$). In conjunction with the observed target lobe volume loss, a comparable increase in the ipsilateral nontreated lobe volume of 24% was observed.[21] Total lung volume was not changed. Of the 33 segments treated with BTVA, 31 of the segmental airways showed narrowing or occlusion. Bronchoscopy repeated 6 months after the treatment did not reveal granulation tissue or airway inflammation. Improvements were seen in HRLQ with an improvement of 15.3 points on the SGRQ.[21] Pulmonary function testing, however, did not reveal any significant changes from baseline measurements of FEV_1, FVC, TLC, or RV.[21] In addition, no change was seen in 6MWT at the end of the 6-month study period.[21]

This pilot study was important in elucidating the favorable procedural safety data observed. A similar inflammatory response seen in animal studies was also noted in humans. Initially there is a blanching of the airways and an immediate chest-radiographic change that likely represents alveolar edema,[21] followed by mild nonspecific airway symptoms seen for 7 to 14 days after the procedure.[21] At 6 months, 94% of the treated airways are at least partially occluded on CT imaging, owing to fibrosis of the targeted areas.[21] The increased incidence of COPD exacerbations and cough symptoms are probably related to the induced inflammatory changes.[21]

Further studies assessing the dosimetry of thermal energy delivered have been completed. Most patients evaluated demonstrated improvement in physiologic parameters in addition to HRQL. Volumetric assessments were also improved in comparison with previous studies. Similar post-procedure complications were noted, particularly COPD exacerbations owing to the inflammatory modified response.[18–20]

Larger trials evaluating BTVA are currently under way and should be able to address any concerns on safety of the treatment. It appears that the increased thermal energy delivered in the latter studies was more effective; however, further dosimetric studies may be required to strike a balance between adverse events and efficacy.[18–21] The lack of a control arm will also need to be addressed in future studies.

BIOLOGICAL LUNG VOLUME REDUCTION

Biological lung volume reduction (BiLVR) is based on the bronchoscopic application of a fibrin hydrogel into the airways of hyperinflated areas of emphysematous lungs in order to cause scar tissue formation, which leads to a reduction of the overall lung volumes and air trapping. The first studies were performed by Ingenito and colleagues[22,23] in sheep models of emphysema, with promising results. The hydrogel contains biodegradable complexes of poly-L-lysine and chondroitin sulfate, which initiate a localized inflammatory reaction that collapses, remodels, and reduces the volume of emphysematous lung over 3 to 6 weeks.

The procedure consists in instilling fibrinogen suspension and thrombin solution into the selected subsegmental airway through a dual-lumen catheter over 10 to 15 seconds to ensure rapid polymerization of the hydrogel, followed immediately by injection of air to push the reagents peripherally.[24,25] With the recent introduction of AeriSeal (Aeris Therapeutics, Woburn, MA) as a foam sealant that is prepared at the bedside just before the procedure, the instillation may be performed through a single-lumen catheter (see **Fig. 12**).[26]

The use of BiLVR has shown to be effective in the treatment of severe upper lobe predominant emphysema[24] as well as homogeneous emphysema,[25] with significant improvement in physiologic (FEV_1 and FVC), functional (6MWT), and symptomatic (dyspnea index) parameters at 6 months. The degree of response was dose dependent and more durable with dosing of 20 mL per site when compared with only 10 mL. Patients with heterogeneous emphysema with Global Initiative for Chronic Obstructive Lung Disease (GOLD) stage III have shown the best response following this procedure.[26] All studies have also

proved BiLVR to be very safe, with no mortality associated with the procedure.[24–26] Self-limited side effects such as dyspnea, fever, radiographic infiltrate, and chest pain immediately after the procedure have been reported.[26]

In contrast to other bronchoscopic techniques of lung volume reduction, such as EBVs, the effect of BiLVR in patients with upper lobe predominant emphysema is not related to interlobar fissure integrity.[27]

The AeriSeal System has already received the approval of the European market for commercialization, although it is still considered an investigational system by the FDA. A multicenter, randomized, open-label study is currently being performed (ASPIRE trial), and results are expected by 2019.

AIRWAY BYPASS

Van Allen and colleagues[28] described "collateral ventilation" for the first time in 1930 by describing the passage of gases between different lung lobules without the existence of anatomic passageways. Later, Hogg and colleagues[29] demonstrated that collateral ventilation is greatly increased in emphysema, and that in emphysematous lungs there is lower resistance through some of the collateral channels than through the airways themselves.

Based on the results of multiple studies showing the benefits from decreasing dynamic hyperinflation in emphysematous patients by LVRS,[30] Lausberg and colleagues[31] hypothesized that creation of new exit pathways from the lung parenchyma into the airways (airway bypass) would allow the trapped gas to escape during exhalation. This study, performed in homogeneous emphysematous lungs removed at the time of lung transplantation, demonstrated a significant improvement in FEV_1 after bronchoscopic creation of 3 to 5 extra-anatomic bronchopulmonary passages in comparison with baseline values.

The Exhale Emphysema Treatment System (Bronchus Technologies, Inc, Mountain View, CA) has been used to create airway bypass in all studies since Lausberg's trial. This system comes with a Doppler transducer catheter (Exhale Doppler Probe); a Doppler processing unit to amplify the sounds of the Doppler probe; a transbronchial dilation needle for passage creation and dilation; and the Exhale drug-eluting stent, which is composed of stainless steel, paclitaxel, and silicone.

The creation of a passage requires 3 steps: first, bronchoscopic identification of a location (segmental bronchi) that is free of blood vessels

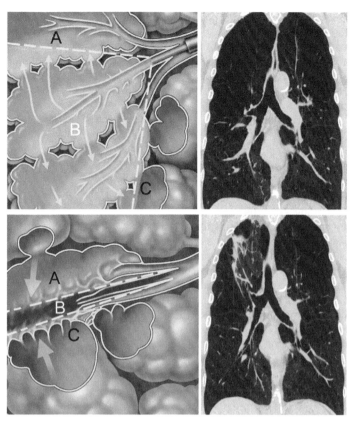

Fig. 13. Bronchoscopic instillation of the biological foam into the segmental airway will create an inflammatory reaction, leading to collapse and formation of scar tissue. (*Courtesy of* Aeris Therapeutics Inc, Woburn, MA; with permission.)

by using the Doppler probe; second, fenestration of the bronchial wall using the transbronchial needle and dilating balloon; and third, placement of the drug-eluting stent to hold the passage open (**Fig. 13**).[12] The average of implanted stents has varied from 6 to 8 per person,[12] placed during a single bronchoscopic session performed under general anesthesia and orotracheal intubation (**Fig. 14**). Serious but rare complications related to the procedure include major hemoptysis, pneumothorax with chest-tube insertion, and respiratory failure. More common complications were related to COPD exacerbations or pulmonary infections that needed hospitalization for more than 7 days.[15]

Early results from studies were promising and revealed significant improvement in different parameters at 1 month in comparison with baseline, although only improvement in RV and dyspnea scores remained significant at 6 months.[12] These results prompted the development of a multicenter, double-blind, randomized, sham-controlled trial (Exhale Airway Stents for Emphysema [EASE] trial).[15] The study recruited 315 patients with

homogeneous emphysema. Even though significant improvement in pulmonary function and dyspnea scores was found at day 1 after the procedure in the airway bypass group, these changes were not

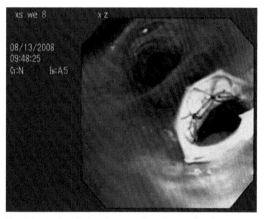

Fig. 14. An implanted stent after 6 months. (*From* Cardoso PF, Snell GI, Hopkins P, et al. Clinical application of airway bypass with paclitaxel-eluting stents: early results. J Thorac Cardiovasc Surg 2007;134:974–81; with permission. *Courtesy of* Michael Simoff, MD.)

different from those found in the sham control group at 3, 6, and 12 months' follow-up.

Based on the results of the EASE trial, the Exhale Emphysema Treatment System is currently used only for investigational purposes. Other strategies to extend the durability of its effects are currently under study.

SUMMARY

From the initial concept of surgical lung volume reduction for the treatment of emphysema, to the multiple options discussed herein, it should be evident that the management of obstructive lung disease, particularly emphysematous lung disease, is aggressively being pursued. The patient populations that will experience the greatest benefit with lung volume reduction are those that would be the worst candidates for surgical intervention. Identifying a bronchoscopic approach that has a true impact on this patient population will be a major accomplishment in the management of patients with COPD.

The use of more traditional markers of improvement (ie, increases in FEV_1 and FVC) may be the incorrect approach to evaluating the success of BLVR procedures. Resurgence in work on the physiologic improvements in patients successfully treated with these techniques should identify better parameters that can be used in addition to quality-of-life scores to mark successful interventions.

The successful use of bronchoscopic lung volume reduction may allow for better bridging for lung transplant patients as well as overall improvement the functionality of severely emphysematous patients. At present, in the United States there is no technique that is FDA approved. It is important for all physicians involved in the management of these patients to be aware of any available clinical trials and to recommend patients to them, as this is a major stem for the advancement of these technologies.

REFERENCES

1. Fishman A, Martinez F, Naunheim K, et al. A randomized trial comparing lung-volume-reduction surgery with medical therapy for severe emphysema. N Engl J Med 2003;348:2059–73.
2. Centers for Disease Control and Prevention. CDC's National Center for Health Statistics, deaths: preliminary data for 2008. 2008.
3. Ernst A, Anantham D. Endoscopic management of emphysema. Clin Chest Med 2010;31:117–26 Table of Contents.
4. Ernst A, Anantham D. Bronchoscopic lung volume reduction. Pulm Med 2011;2011:610802.
5. Hwong TM, Yim AP. New treatment modalities for end-stage emphysema. Chest Surg Clin N Am 2003;13:739–53.
6. Herth FJ, Noppen M, Valipour A, et al. Efficacy predictors of lung volume reduction with Zephyr valves in a European cohort. Eur Respir J 2012;39:1334–42.
7. Hopkinson NS, Kemp SV, Toma TP, et al. Atelectasis and survival after bronchoscopic lung volume reduction for COPD. Eur Respir J 2011;37:1346–51.
8. Sciurba FC, Ernst A, Herth FJ, et al. A randomized study of endobronchial valves for advanced emphysema. N Engl J Med 2010;363:1233–44.
9. Springmeyer SC, Bolliger CT, Waddell TK, et al. Treatment of heterogeneous emphysema using the Spiration IBV valves. Thorac Surg Clin 2009;19:247–53, ix–x.
10. Sterman DH, Mehta AC, Wood DE, et al. A multicenter pilot study of a bronchial valve for the treatment of severe emphysema. Respiration 2010;79:222–33.
11. Toma TP, Hopkinson NS, Hillier J, et al. Bronchoscopic volume reduction with valve implants in patients with severe emphysema. Lancet 2003;361:931–3.
12. Cardoso PF, Snell GI, Hopkins P, et al. Clinical application of airway bypass with paclitaxel-eluting stents: early results. J Thorac Cardiovasc Surg 2007;134:974–81.
13. Herth FJ, Eberhard R, Gompelmann D, et al. Bronchoscopic lung volume reduction with a dedicated coil: a clinical pilot study. Ther Adv Respir Dis 2010;4:225–31.
14. Herth FJ, Eberhardt R, Gompelmann D, et al. Radiological and clinical outcomes of using Chartis to plan endobronchial valve treatment. Eur Respir J 2013;41:302–8.
15. Shah PL, Slebos DJ, Cardoso PF, et al. Bronchoscopic lung-volume reduction with Exhale Airway Stents for Emphysema (EASE trial): randomised, sham-controlled, multicentre trial. Lancet 2011;378:997–1005.
16. Slebos DJ, Klooster K, Ernst A, et al. Bronchoscopic lung volume reduction coil treatment of patients with severe heterogeneous emphysema. Chest 2012;142:574–82.
17. National Institutes of Health. Implantation of endobronchial valves versus intrabronchial valves in patients with severe heterogeneous emphysema. 2011.
18. Emery MJ, Eveland RL, Eveland K, et al. Lung volume reduction by bronchoscopic administration of steam. Am J Respir Crit Care Med 2010;182:1282–91.
19. Gompelmann D, Heussel CP, Eberhardt R, et al. Efficacy of bronchoscopic thermal vapor ablation and lobar fissure completeness in patients with heterogeneous emphysema. Respiration 2012;83:400–6.
20. Snell G, Herth FJ, Hopkins P, et al. Bronchoscopic thermal vapour ablation therapy in the management

of heterogeneous emphysema. Eur Respir J 2012; 39:1326–33.

21. Snell GI, Hopkins P, Westall G, et al. A feasibility and safety study of bronchoscopic thermal vapor ablation: a novel emphysema therapy. Ann Thorac Surg 2009;88:1993–8.

22. Ingenito EP, Reilly JJ, Mentzer SJ, et al. Bronchoscopic volume reduction: a safe and effective alternative to surgical therapy for emphysema. Am J Respir Crit Care Med 2001;164:295–301.

23. Ingenito EP, Berger RL, Henderson AC, et al. Bronchoscopic lung volume reduction using tissue engineering principles. Am J Respir Crit Care Med 2003; 167:771–8.

24. Criner GJ, Pinto-Plata V, Strange C, et al. Biologic lung volume reduction in advanced upper lobe emphysema: phase 2 results. Am J Respir Crit Care Med 2009;179:791–8.

25. Refaely Y, Dransfield M, Kramer MR, et al. Biologic lung volume reduction therapy for advanced homogeneous emphysema. Eur Respir J 2010;36:20–7.

26. Herth FJ, Gompelmann D, Stanzel F, et al. Treatment of advanced emphysema with emphysematous lung sealant (AeriSeal(R)). Respiration 2011;82:36–45.

27. Magnussen H, Kramer MR, Kirsten AM, et al. Effect of fissure integrity on lung volume reduction using a polymer sealant in advanced emphysema. Thorax 2012;67:302–8.

28. Van Allen CM, Lindskog GE, Richter HG. Gaseous interchange between adjacent lung lobules. Yale J Biol Med 1930;2:297–300.

29. Hogg JC, Macklem PT, Thurlbeck WM. The resistance of collateral channels in excised human lungs. J Clin Invest 1969;48:421–31.

30. Sciurba FC, Rogers RM, Keenan RJ, et al. Improvement in pulmonary function and elastic recoil after lung-reduction surgery for diffuse emphysema. N Engl J Med 1996;334:1095–9.

31. Lausberg HF, Chino K, Patterson GA, et al. Bronchial fenestration improves expiratory flow in emphysematous human lungs. Ann Thorac Surg 2003;75: 393–7 [discussion: 398].

Malignant Pleural Effusions
A Review

Justin M. Thomas, MD, Ali I. Musani, MD*

KEYWORDS

- Malignant pleural effusions • Review • End-stage malignancies • Management

KEY POINTS

- Given the many management options for malignant pleural effusions, several different algorithms have been suggested.
- Although pleurodesis may provide permanent relief of symptoms, it also leads to more hospital days and is more costly than tunneled pleural catheters (TPCs).
- TPCs also have the benefit of providing a means to manage trapped lung, a condition not amenable to pleurodesis.
- It is important to consider the patient's overall prognosis, symptoms, functional status, and social and financial situation when selecting the modality of choice.
- It is advisable to select the most cost-effective, least invasive, and most likely modality to lead to fewer hospitalization days.

INTRODUCTION

Pleural effusions remain a significant challenge and public health problem, causing significant morbidity associated with chronic diseases. Malignant pleural effusions (MPEs), or those effusions associated with a malignancy, contribute significantly to decreased functional capacity and quality of life in patients who are victims of these malignant processes. MPEs frequently are rapid to reaccumulate and most are symptomatic, eliciting dyspnea, cough, or pain. The median length of survival for patients who are diagnosed with MPEs is 6 months.[1] So management options are focused on palliative relief of symptoms and vary from intermittent drainage to curative intent, depending on the patient's functional status, life expectancy, and social support.

INCIDENCE

The annual incidence of MPEs is estimated to be 150,000 to 175,000 in the United States[2,3] and they are believed to be present in up to 15% of patients who die with malignancies, based on 1 postmortem series.[4] In addition, exudative effusions are more often (44%–77%) associated with malignancies than any other disease process.[5,6] The most common causes of MPEs in order of most common to least common are lung cancer (most commonly adenocarcinoma), breast cancer, lymphoma, unknown primary, genitourinary, and gastrointestinal carcinomas (**Table 1**).[7–11] Lung and breast cancer account for 50% to 65% of all MPEs,[12] and 30% of patients with lung cancer develop an MPE.[13]

Disclosures: Ali I. Musani, MD has received honoraria as a consultant and a speaker, as well as a research grant from CareFusion.
Division of Pulmonary and Critical Care, Department of Medicine, National Jewish Health, 1400 Jackson Street, Denver, CO 80206, USA
* Corresponding author.
E-mail address: musania@njhealth.org

Clin Chest Med 34 (2013) 459–471
http://dx.doi.org/10.1016/j.ccm.2013.05.004
0272-5231/13/$ – see front matter © 2013 Elsevier Inc. All rights reserved.

Table 1
Most common primary tumor sites for MPEs

Primary Tumor Site	Hsu,[7] (n = 785)	Sears & Hajdu,[8] (n = 592)	Johnston,[9] (n = 472)	Chernow & Sahn,[10] (n = 96)	Salyer et al,[11] (n = 95)	Total (%)
Lung	410	112	168	32	42	764 (37.5)
Breast	101	141	70	20	11	343 (16.8)
Lymphoma	56	92	75	0	11	234 (11.5)
Gastrointestinal tract	68	32	28	13	0	141 (6.9)
Genitourinary tract	70	51	57	13	0	191 (9.4)
Other	15	88	26	5	14	148 (7.3)
Unknown primary	65	76	48	13	17	219 (10.7)

PATHOPHYSIOLOGY

Fluid collects in the pleural space (a potential space between the visceral and parietal pleural layers that normally contains only a small amount, typically 10–20 mL, of pleural fluid) when there is an abnormality of oncotic or hydrostatic pressures. For instance, in the setting of left-sided congestive heart failure, failure of the left heart to pump blood forward results in an increased pressure in the pulmonary venous system, which in turn leads to leakage of fluid from the intravascular space to the interstitial space. This fluid is then reabsorbed by the lymphatic system, which becomes overwhelmed, resulting in translocation of the fluid into to the pleural space.

MPEs are diagnosed by identifying malignant cells in pleural fluid or on pleural biopsy. However, based on autopsy studies, MPEs are present in only 60% of malignancies involving the pleura.[14,15] Most MPEs are exudative effusions, but about 5% may be transudative.[16] Paramalignant pleural effusions are those effusions associated with malignancy, but malignant cells are not recovered during pleural fluid analysis. These types of effusions arise from many different mechanisms, including obstruction of thoracic duct or bronchi by tumor, trapped lung, chemotherapy or radiation treatment, pneumonia, or pulmonary emboli.[10,17]

Malignancies that metastasize to mediastinal lymph nodes and lymphatics, such as lung and breast cancer, are the 2 leading causes of MPEs. In lung cancer, hematogenous spread of tumor cells to the visceral pleura[4] allows tumor cells to migrate across existing adhesions. Tumor cells may then obstruct stomata, which are located on the parietal pleural surface, or lymphatics further downstream in the pleural fluid absorption cascade. Breast cancer may cause an ipsilateral MPE via metastases through chest wall lymphatics or a bilateral MPE through hematogenous spread

via the liver.[18] Hodgkin lymphoma often causes lymphatic obstruction, whereas non-Hodgkin lymphoma typically has direct pleural invasion.[19]

Hemorrhagic MPEs may arise from direct tumor invasion of blood vessels or tumor-induced angiogenesis. Vascular endothelial growth factor (VEGF), a cytokine produced by many tumors that is involved in angiogenesis and vascular permeability, may be involved in pathogenesis of MPEs.[20–22] A recent study by Qian and colleagues[20] determined VEGF levels and soluble intercellular adhesion molecule-1 (sICAM-1) levels by enzyme-linked immunosorbent assay in 79 patients with lung adenocarcinoma compared with 24 patients with tuberculous effusions. These investigators found that there was a statistically significant correlation between pleural effusion VEGF levels and MPE control. Pleural effusion VEGF levels 2760 pg/mL or greater were used as a cutoff point for failure to MPE control (odds ratio = 7.06; 95% confidence interval [CI], 2.40–20.78; $P<.001$). In a multivariate analysis, pleural effusion VEGF (hazard ratio [HR], 1.16; 95% CI, 1.02–1.32) and serum sICAM-1 (HR, 1.90; 95% CI, 1.17–3.07) were confirmed as independent prognostic factors for progression-free survival. So, VEGF levels in the pleural fluid and serum sICAM-1 may be important potential survival factors in patients with lung adenocarcinoma with MPE.

Management Considerations

Although not all MPEs are symptomatic, most patients do have symptoms that limit their quality of life. Up to 90% of those experiencing symptoms have dyspnea on exertion, and up to 50% have cough or chest discomfort.[23] Because the prognosis of those with MPEs is so poor, treatment is focused on palliation of symptoms rather than cure. Many different management techniques are available for patients with MPEs, including repeated needle thoracentesis, tube thoracostomy, chemical or biological pleurodesis, pleurectomy, pleuroperitoneal shunt, and tunneled pleural catheters (TPCs). The ideal management would offer immediate and long-term relief of symptoms, have minimal side effects, lead to fewer hospitalization days, and involve a procedure requiring the least amount of time spent in the hospital and clinic, avoidance of repeat uncomfortable procedures, and the least cost.

PLEURODESIS
Mechanisms Involved in Pleurodesis

Pleurodesis is the process of obliterating the pleural space by causing extensive adhesion of the visceral and parietal pleural surfaces by means of either mechanical or chemical-induced inflammation of the pleura. Pleurodesis is used after evacuation of pleural fluid for treatment of MPEs or pneumothorax and, less commonly, some benign pleural effusions. Many different sclerosing agents are available, and they share similar mechanisms of inducing biological responses mediated by pleural mesothelial cells such as diffuse inflammation with pleural coagulation-fibrinolysis imbalance, recruitment and proliferation of fibroblasts leading to collagen production, and release of several mediators like interleukin 8, transforming growth factor β, and basic fibroblast growth factor, which contribute to the required fibrotic state.[24] It follows that in tumors such as malignant mesothelioma or extensive tumor burden of the pleura, in which normal mesothelial cells are scarce, there is a poorer response to pleurodesis.[24] Corticosteroids inhibit this response and concomitant administration of corticosteroids is associated with pleurodesis failure.[24–27] There has been debate about using low pleural fluid pH as a marker for pleurodesis failure; however, a meta-analysis[28] showed only modest value of low pH (<7.15) to predict pleurodesis failure, and thus it should be used with caution in patients with MPE being selected for this procedure.

Surgical Techniques

Medical thoracoscopy
Medical thoracoscopy, also known as pleuroscopy, has been used by physicians in Europe since 1910 to diagnose and treat pleural disease, including empyema, and is gaining popularity as a diagnostic and therapeutic tool among pulmonologists and thoracic surgeons worldwide.[17,29,30] The procedure is performed in the endoscopy unit or operating room under conscious sedation and local anesthesia, with the patient positioned in the lateral decubitus position with affected side

up and arm above the head. By not requiring general anesthesia, intubation or single-lung ventilation, this technique creates an option for patients who are otherwise poor surgical candidates and who could not tolerate single-lung ventilation. One or more trocars (5–13 mm in diameter) inserted into the pleural space between the fourth and seventh ribs in the midaxillary line are used to introduce a variety of thoracoscopes, including semirigid and rigid telescopes with a multitude of optical angle options (**Fig. 1**).[17] This technique can be used for parietal pleura biopsies, lysis of adhesions, and delivery of sclerosants to accomplish pleurodesis before a chest tube is inserted through the trocar site. Once the patient accomplishes lung reexpansion, the chest tube can be removed and the patient may return home after brief monitoring in the postanesthesia care unit. Talc pleurodesis and lung biopsy procedures require patient hospitalization for monitoring and chest tube drainage.[30] Contraindications include respiratory insufficiency requiring mechanical ventilation, intolerable hypoxemia unrelated to pleural effusion, unstable cardiovascular status, bleeding diathesis, refractory cough, or allergy to the medications used.[30] Potential complications include pneumothorax, subcutaneous emphysema, pain, fever, and rarely empyema, sepsis, and death.[31,32]

Video-assisted thoracoscopic surgery
Video-assisted thoracoscopic surgery (VATS) is similar to medical thoracoscopy in concept and equipment (although it often uses larger scopes); however, it differs in that it requires a higher level of surgical expertise and is always performed in an operating room with general anesthesia and single-lung ventilation through a double-lumen endotracheal tube. In addition to providing a means to diagnosis of the pleura and pleurodesis, VATS permits the diagnostic biopsy of lung parenchyma and select hilar lymph nodes.[17]

Decortication
MPEs with loculations or trapped lung can be managed with thoracotomy and decortication. No randomized trials reporting the effectiveness of pleurectomy or decortication for MPEs have been performed, but a review by Tan and colleagues[33] reviewed 5 case series involving 260 patients who underwent decortication for either recurrence after attempted pleurodesis or in the setting of lung trapped by tumor or a thick fibrin layer on the visceral pleura. Tan and colleagues[33] reported a perioperative mortality of up to 12.5% and a high incidence of prolonged air leak postoperatively of up to 10% to 20%. Because of its high

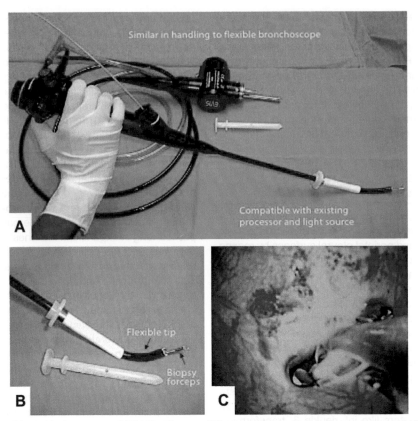

Fig. 1. (*A*) Flexible-rigid pleuroscope (LTF 160, Olympus [Olympus, Center Valley, Pennsylvania, USA]). (*B*) Pleuroscope within flexible trocar and flexible biopsy forceps (trocar: outer and inner diameters = 10 and 8 mm, respectively). (*C*) Biopsy of parietal pleura with flexible forceps. (*From* Lee P, Mathur PN, Colt HG. Advances in thoracoscopy: 100 years since Jacobaeus. Respiration 2010;79:179; with permission.)

mortality and morbidity, decortication is generally reserved for patients with significant symptoms and prolonged life expectancy and who have failed other therapeutic interventions.[17] Various forms of pleurectomy in the form of radical pleurectomy and decortication (P/D) (the process of complete parietal, visceral, and mediastinal pleurectomy, with or without removal of the pericardium or ipsilateral hemidiaphragm with curative intent), subtotal P/D (sparing pericardium and diaphragm), and extrapleural pneumonectomy (EPP) (removal of the pleura, diaphragm, pericardium, and ipsilateral lung) have been used to treat malignant mesothelioma. These procedures carry high morbidity and mortality and, when compared with supportive care and chemotherapy, have largely fallen out of favor.

Nakas and colleagues[34] compared outcomes of radical P/D (n = 51) with palliative subtotal P/D (n = 51). Radical P/D led to higher morbidity (55% vs 28%, *P* = .023) and equivalent hospital stay (12 vs 10 days, *P* = .99) compared with subtotal P/D. Maziak and colleagues[35] systematically reviewed 32 studies and found that radical P/D

had a longer median survival (14.5 vs 4.5 months) than supportive care but led to an operative mortality of 9.1%, with a complication rate of 30%. Treasure and colleagues[36] performed the MARS (Mesothelioma and Radical Surgery) trial, a randomized control multicenter trial comparing EPP (n = 24) with supportive care (n = 26) that reported an adjusted HR for overall survival between the EPP and no-EPP groups of 2.75 (95% CI, 1.21–6.26; *P* = .016). Median survival was 14.4 months (5.3–18.7) for the EPP group and 19.5 months (13.4 to time not yet reached) for the no-EPP group. No significant differences between groups were reported in the quality-of-life analyses. Because of the significant morbidity and mortality risk associated with these procedures as described earlier, P/D and EPP are discouraged except in the setting of clinical trials.[36,37]

Pleurodesis Techniques

Sclerosing agents
Many consider pleurodesis the mainstay of treatment of MPEs; however, it is associated with

multiple complications. The most common complications of chemical pleurodesis include fever and pain.[13] Other complications include empyema and local site infection, arrhythmias, cardiac arrest, myocardial infarction, and hypotension.[17] Talc is the most widely used sclerosing agent in English-speaking countries,[38] presumably because of its availability, cost, and perceived efficacy. Talc has been associated with acute respiratory distress syndrome (ARDS), acute pneumonitis, respiratory failure, and treatment-related death.[39–41] ARDS occurs in up to 9% of cases of talc pleurodesis[41]; however, this complication was associated with nongraded talc. It is believed that talc less than 10 μm in diameter may be harmful, because the pleural stomata are 8 to 10 μm in diameter and talc particles smaller than this may lead to systemic absorption of the talc and an exaggerated cytokine response.[42] There may be a decreased risk of these complications when small-particle talc (<5 μm) is removed from the preparation,[43] and in a European cohort study of 558 patients treated with 4 g of graded talc,[41] no episodes of ARDS occurred. However, more than 30% of patients with talc pleurodesis have recurrence of their MPEs by 50 days.[39] Although an optimal dose of talc for poudrage has not been established, about 5 g (8–12 mL) is usually recommended for MPEs.[44]

Although many other sclerosing agents have been used for chemical pleurodesis, including tetracycline derivatives, bleomycin, iodopovidone, silver nitrate and others, few head-to-head randomized control trials exist to help decide which agent to use. Although it may be as effective as talc with a low cost and wide availability, iodopovidone may cause the intense pleuritic pain and systemic hypotension in 6% of patients.[45] Doxycycline causes more pleuritic pain than talc.[17] According to British Thoracic Society (BTS) guidelines,[46] a recent review,[33] and Cochrane Database,[47] talc has the best rate of success in pleurodesis and is the preferred agent.

Thoracoscopic pleurodesis

Talc poudrage, or aerosolized talc, is the most widely described method of installation of talc within the pleural space. Poudrage is typically accomplished with either surgical (VATS) or medical thoracoscopy. A 24-Fr to 32-Fr chest tube should always be inserted. Graded and progressive suction should be applied and maintained until the amount of fluid aspirated per day is less than 100 mL.[44] de Campos and colleagues[48] reported on a 15-year experience with 614 consecutive patients who underwent a diagnostic or therapeutic surgical thoracoscopy under general anesthesia (with use of 3-port VATS or Carlen mediastinoscope) and showed that those with MPEs (457 patients [74.4%]) achieved a 93.4% success rate. These investigators excluded those with trapped lung and those who died within 30 days of the procedure. Another study by Aelony and colleagues[49] showed that surgical talc poudrage was successful in 88% of 25 patients with MPEs despite a low pleural pH (<7.30), a factor that has been traditionally thought of as a predictor for failed pleurodesis.

Zhang and colleagues[50] performed medical thoracoscopic talc poudrage pleurodesis on 27 patients with MPEs and achieved an overall success of pleurodesis of 96.3% (26/27), with an average duration of chest tube of 6.85 days. In either case, either with medical or with surgical thoracoscopic talc pleurodesis, although a high rate of success is achieved, prolonged hospital stays may preclude these options for patients with short life expectancy.

Chest tube pleurodesis

Talc slurry delivered through a chest tube is also an effective technique to accomplish pleurodesis. It involves the mixing of typically 4 to 5 g of talc in 50 to 100 mL of normal saline and installation of this suspension through a standard chest tube (18–24 Fr) or small-bore catheters (10–12 Fr).[51,52] This is typically followed by clamping the chest tube for 1 hour, and many investigators suggest rotating the patient to allow even distribution of the slurry[44,46] however, there has been no proven benefit with patient rotation.[53,54] Once the tube is unclamped, the tube is connected to negative 20 cm H_2O suction and removed when there is less than 100 to 150 mL drainage over 24 hours. If drainage remains greater than 250 mL per 24 hours, then the same dosage of talc may be instilled a second time. Larger chest tubes have not been shown to have lower recurrence rates over smaller chest tubes and are more uncomfortable for the patient.[55–58] Talc slurries may not accomplish complete pleurodesis and lead to loculations because they do not achieve uniform distribution and may accumulate in dependent areas of the pleural space. Dresler and colleagues[39] observed that poudrage was more successful in pleural metastatic lung and breast carcinomas, but the overall efficacy for talc poudrage versus slurry was the same in a randomized multicenter study. Mañes and colleagues[59] reported a higher rate of recurrence with talc slurry versus poudrage.

A meta-analysis of different pleurodesis techniques performed by Shaw and colleagues[47] concluded that thoracoscopic pleurodesis (TP) was more effective than tube thoracostomy pleurodesis (relative risk [RR] of nonrecurrence of effusion is 1.19 [95% CI, 1.04–1.36]) or bedside instillation (RR of nonrecurrence of effusion is 1.68 [95% CI, 1.35–2.10]).

Intrapleural fibrinolytics

The intrapleural (IP) administration of fibrinolytics has been used to manage non-MPE loculations such as that seen in empyema and complicated parapneumonic effusions. Recently, as a result of a recent study by Rahman and colleagues,[60] the combination of tissue plasminogen activator and DNase has gained a lot of attention for this indication. IP urokinase[61,62] and streptokinase[63] have been used to dissolve loculations in MPEs and have been shown to relieve dyspnea and increase pleural fluid drainage without adverse effects in this group of patients. A recent randomized control trial by Okur and colleagues[64] randomized 47 patients with MPEs to chest tube drainage with or without streptokinase (250,000 Units in 100 mL normal saline for 3 doses every 12 hours) on the second or third day of drainage. These investigators found that significantly more drainage was achieved in the fibrinolytic group (P<.001) and adequate lung reexpansion for performing talc pleurodesis was more likely in the fibrinolytic group than in the control group (96% vs 74%, P = .035).

PLEURAL DRAINAGE
Therapeutic Thoracentesis

Large-volume thoracentesis is usually the first step to both diagnosing and treating MPEs. The patient's symptomatic response to the large-volume pleural fluid removal determines whether it is prudent to proceed to more invasive techniques of either pleural drainage or pleurodesis. Up to 50% of patients with MPEs do not have symptomatic relief after thoracentesis, whether it is because of comorbid conditions, generalized deconditioning from their malignancy, or incomplete reexpansion of the lung (trapped lung). Patients with trapped lung do not have opposition of the 2 pleural surfaces and it may result from loculated pleural effusions, pleural metastases, or postobstructive collapse from endobronchial tumors. The ability to create adequate lung reexpansion radiographically after drainage is a key determinate for whether pleurodesis is a success.[65–67]

There are no absolute contraindications to thoracentesis, but caution should be advised for patients with a bleeding diathesis, positive pressure ventilation, or small amount of fluid. Risks of the procedure include bleeding, iatrogenic pneumothorax, empyema, and the development of pleural adhesions, which may limit future therapeutic options. The development of patient symptoms such as cough or chest discomfort during the thoracentesis should alert the practitioner to terminate drainage, and although there is no consensus on the amount of fluid to be drained, it is generally recommended to drain no more than 1 to 1.5 L. A risk of reexpansion pulmonary edema after large-volume thoracentesis has been described, and although the risk is low (<1%), it is associated with about 20% mortality.[68–72] Large-volume thoracentesis has been shown to be safe if the patient is asymptomatic and pleural manometry pressures remain less than negative 20 cm H_2O, yet these devices are not always readily available. Feller-Kopman and colleagues[73] reported that the symptom of cough was not associated with what is considered dangerous pleural pressure (–20 cm H_2O), and only 22% of patients with chest discomfort had pleural pressures less than –20 cm H_2O. Ideally, as much fluid as possible should be removed, allowing for the greatest symptomatic benefit for the patient and more time between interventions, in addition to providing valuable information in regards to lung reexpansion and potential for successful pleurodesis procedures in the future.

Repeated thoracentesis is a method used by practitioners treating patients with poor prognosis, poor performance status, or because of patient preference, particularly after failed pleurodesis or intercostal tube drainage.[74] It has been advocated by the BTS for palliation of breathlessness in patients with a short life expectancy. It is an ineffective way of achieving pleurodesis, because the recurrence rate at 1 month is close to 100%.[12]

TPCs

IP catheters or TPCs are soft silicone 15.5-French tubes that are inserted percutaneously as an outpatient procedure, with minimal sedation (**Fig. 2**). Patients or their home support can easily manage the drainage of the catheter typically every other day versus daily versus as needed. This strategy enables the patient with end-stage cancer to spend less time in clinics and hospitals.

TPCs are generally indicated for patients with MPEs that are associated with or without trapped lung, or 3 or fewer loculations. Often, these catheters create a spontaneous pleurodesis (SP) and, in 1 center's experience, this occurred in 42.9% of patients, with a median time to SP of 59 days.[19]

Putnam and colleagues[75] performed the first study comparing the effectiveness of TPCs with

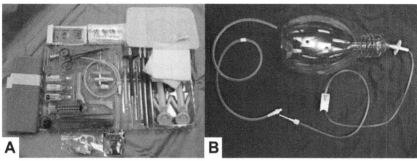

Fig. 2. (*A*) TPC PleurX kit supplied by CareFusion. (*B*) TPC with a fenestrated proximal end, silastic cuff, and 1-way valve at the distal end (*left*) and disposable vacuum bottle and drainage tubing (*right*) for insertion into the 1-way valve of the TPC.

tube thoracostomy pleurodesis in patients with symptomatic, recurrent MPEs shortly after the US Food and Drug Administration approved TPCs for management of MPEs. This was a prospective, randomized, multi-institutional study comparing TPCs (91 patients) with doxycycline pleurodesis (28 patients). The median hospitalization time was 1.0 day for the TPC group and 6.5 days for the doxycycline group. There was no statistically significant difference in symptomatic improvement in dyspnea or quality of life between the groups. There was no difference between late recurrence of effusions in patients assigned to doxycycline versus late recurrence of effusion or blockage of the catheter in the TPC patients. Forty-six percent of the patients randomized to TPCs achieved SP at a median of 26.5 days. Tremblay and colleagues[19] went on to report a series of 250 TPCs in 223 patients, most of which were inserted as an outpatient procedure, and 90.1% of the patients were successfully spared further ipsilateral pleural procedures. These investigators concluded that TPCs should be considered a first-line therapy for patients with MPEs. Warren and colleagues[76] described a series of 231 indwelling catheters in 202 patients, 210 of which were inserted as outpatients. These investigators reported that SP occurred with 58% of the catheters, and reaccumulation of pleural fluid occurred in only 5 of these 134 patients (3.8%). Van Meter and colleagues[77] reviewed 19 studies that included 1370 patients who were treated with TPCs for MPEs. These investigators reported that symptomatic improvement occurred in 95.6% of patients, and SP occurred in 45.6%. Serious complications were rare and included empyema in 2.85%. Van Meter and colleagues[77] concluded that to recommend TPC as the first-line treatment of MPEs, more prospective randomized studies comparing the TPC with pleurodesis are needed.

One of the ideal characteristics of management of MPEs, which was mentioned in the introduction, was the ability to reduce the length of hospitalization and time in the clinic for these patients. Putnam and colleagues[75] reported this earlier. A more recent study by Fysh and colleagues[78] compared the number of in-hospital days in 34 patients who elected to receive the indwelling catheter and 31 patients who elected talc pleurodesis. These investigators reported that the median number of hospital days was significantly greater in the pleurodesis group (18 days) than in the indwelling pleural catheter (IPC) group (6.5 days). Moreover, the median number of hospital days related to the effusions was significantly greater in the pleurodesis group (10 days) than in the IPC group (3 days). The patients in the IPC group also spent a smaller percentage of their remaining lives (8.0%) in the hospital, compared with the pleurodesis group (11.2%).

Another recent randomized trial by Davies and colleagues,[79] the so-called TIME2 trial (Second Therapeutic Intervention in Malignant Effusion Trial), also compared TPCs with chest tube talc slurry pleurodesis, but in an unblinded randomized control study design. A total of 108 patients were randomized from 143 patients who were initially assessed to undergo either TPC (52 patients) or talc slurry pleurodesis by tube thoracostomy. These investigators found that dyspnea improved in both groups with no significant difference in the first 42 days with a mean visual analogue scale dyspnea score (0–100 mm scale) of 24.7 in the IPC group versus 24.4 mm in the talc group (P = .96). There was a statistically significant improvement in dyspnea in the TPC group at 6 months, with a mean difference of −14.0 mm. Length of hospitalization and need for repeat pleural procedures was less in the TPC group than in the talc group (0 days vs 4 days and 6% vs 22%, respectively). There was no difference in quality of life. Forty percent of the

TPC patients versus 13% of the talc patients experienced adverse events. None of these adverse events was considered serious and they were limited to pleural infection (asymptomatic and treated with oral antibiotics), cellulitis, symptomatic fluid loculations requiring fibrinolytics, catheter site metastases, and catheter blockage. Other studies have reported similar results, and it seems that TPCs are not inferior to tube thoracostomy pleurodesis procedures and may be preferable, because TPC insertion is an outpatient procedure, thus reducing the amount of hospitalization days (a vital aspect of care in patients with a median survival of 6 months).[1]

Description of procedure

TPCs are typically placed in a bronchoscopy suite under local anesthesia with 1% to 2% lidocaine and using intravenous midazolam or fentanyl for conscious sedation as needed. A modified Seldinger technique is used to insert the TPC after ultrasonography and standard needle thoracentesis localize the effusion. A flexible wire is then introduced through the needle into the pleural cavity, followed by the creation of a 1-cm to 1.5-cm horizontal incision at that site. A second horizontal incision is made approximately 5 to 6 cm inferior or lateral to the first incision after local anesthesia is applied to the vertical tract that intersects these 2 incisions. A subcutaneous tunnel is then created with the aid of a trocar attached to the end of the TPC. The TPC is pulled through the tunnel until the polyester cuff sits 1 cm from the distal incision within the tract. A dilator with a peel-away sheath is then inserted into the thorax over the guide wire. The dilator and the guide wire are then removed. The end of the TPC is then fed through the peel-away sheath into the pleural space as the operator simultaneously peels away the sheath, with 1 finger keeping the TPC secure in the thorax. Pleural fluid (typically 1000–1500 mL or until the patient experiences pain) is then drained as simple interrupted sutures are used to close the incisions and a stay-suture secures the TPC near the inferior incision. A chest radiograph documents drainage, and evaluates for trapped lung and pneumothorax. Follow-up is typically at 2 weeks with repeat chest radiograph followed by every 4 to 8 weeks thereafter or as needed. Once drainage is less than 50 mL on 3 consecutive drainages, the catheter can then be removed, because SP has likely occurred.

Pleuroperitoneal Shunts

Pleuroperitoneal shunts (PPS) allow fluid to transfer from the pleural space into the peritoneal cavity by means of either a manual pump (Denver shunt) or passive drainage (LaVeen shunt). These shunts may be considered for patients with trapped lung who are not candidates for decortication, those who have failed chemical pleurodesis, and particularly for patients with refractory chylothorax, because it allows for recirculation of chyle. Pleuroperitoneal shunts are often complicated by shunt failure because of clotting of the catheter (up to 25% of cases with a median length of patency of 2.5 months),[80,81] shunt infections, and require manual operation, all of which have led to this management option falling out of favor and being largely supplanted by TPCs.

Genc and colleagues[82] performed 160 PPS and reported a pleurodesis success rate of 95%. Mean hospital stay in their experience was 6.2 days, with a complication rate of 14.8%, mean survival length of 7.7 months, and a greater benefit observed in patients with mesothelioma-associated effusions (10.1 months). Tsang and colleagues[83] performed 16 PPS and reported a mean hospital stay of 6.9 days, with a mean of 8.6 months before shunt failure and an overall survival length of 11 months. Schulze and colleagues[84] compared the effectiveness of PPS (N = 14) with talc pleurodesis (N = 105) in managing MPEs. These investigators reported longer operative times (55 vs 35 minutes), higher complication rates (14.3% vs 2.8%) but shorter hospital stays (8.1 vs 10.7 days) with PPS than talc pleurodesis. PPS also had lower success rates (57.1% vs 92.3%) and shorter survival lengths (4.3 ± 1.9 vs 6.7 ± 2.1 months) than talc pleurodesis.

Cost considerations

A recent cost-effective analysis of different modalities for treatment of MPEs by Puri and colleagues[85] used decision analysis to compare repeated thoracentesis (RT), TPC, bedside pleurodesis (BP), and TP. Using a base case analysis of 3-month survival, RT was the least expensive treatment ($4946), followed by TPC at $6450, BP at $11,224, and TP at $18,604. TPC was cheaper and more effective than both pleurodesis arms. The incremental cost-effectiveness ratio (ICER) (cost per quality-adjusted life-year gained over the patient's remaining lifetime) for TPC over RT was $49,978. The ICER did take into account both complications and ability to achieve pleural sclerosis with TPC. Under base case analysis for 12-month survival, BP was the least expensive treatment ($13,057), followed by TPC at $13,224, TP at $19,074, and RT at $21,377.

Future Directions

Multimodality techniques

Multimodality treatments have started to gain popularity. A recent pilot study by Reddy and colleagues[86] used a multimodality technique on patients with symptomatic MPE. These investigators used medical thoracoscopy with talc poudrage followed by drainage via TPC after the larger-bore chest tube was removed 24 hours after pleuroscopy. Reddy was able to achieve 92% successful pleurodesis and the TPC was removed at a mean of 16.7 days, with a mean length of hospitalization of only 3.2 days after procedure.

IP therapies

IP chemotherapy IP administration of chemotherapeutic agents has a promising role in the management of MPEs. Several phase I and II studies have been performed that show safety of these agents and the pharmacokinetics of various dosing regimens of 5-fluorouracil (5-FU), cisplatin, etoposide, paclitaxel, carboplatin, cytarabine, and docetaxel.[87–95] A recent phase III trial was performed by Ichinose and colleagues,[96] which compared IP cisplatin versus observation in patients who have non–small cell lung cancer with cytologically positive pleural fluid and noted a decrease in significant MPE development (8% vs 42%, $P = .008$); however, the trial was stopped prematurely because of slow enrollment. Combining chemotherapy with hyperthermotherapy has also shown some efficacy, as shown by Chen and colleagues,[97] who randomly assigned 358 patients with MPEs to either IP cisplatin and OK-432 with or without hyperthermotherapy. The hyperthermotherapy group showed both a higher overall response (93.4% vs 79.8%; $P<.05$) and better median 8.9 versus 6.2 months ($P>.05$).[97] Both groups had improved quality of life. Although IP chemotherapy has been shown to increase apoptosis of malignant cells in the pleural space,[91] achieve up to 1000 times the concentration as in plasma,[94] and provide some survival advantage,[91] larger, randomized control trials are warranted in this promising area of treatment of MPEs.

IP gene therapy Gene therapy, the process of modifying the genetic makeup of cells for therapeutic purposes, is gaining some interest in the management of MPEs. Zarogoulidis and colleagues[98] have been successful in transfecting IP tumor cells by means of injecting within the pleural space an adenoviral vector with cytosine deaminase, which converts the antifungal drug fluorocytosine (5-FC) to the antimetabolite 5-FU. This situation leads to killing of not only the transfected tumor cells but also neighboring cells through a bystander effect. Zarogoulidis and colleagues describe providing this IP therapy in 2 doses (day 1 and day 7) combined with 14 days of 5-FC 500 mg 4 times daily for 2 patients with advanced lung carcinoma (1 with non–small cell lung carcinoma and the other with small cell lung carcinoma) and MPEs. Patients had complete regression of the MPEs by computed tomography, and were complicated by neutropenia and anemia (grade III and IV). This idea of transfecting a neoplasm with cDNA encoding for an enzyme that renders tumor cells sensitive to a benign agent by converting the prodrug to a toxic metabolite is called suicide gene therapy.

Other phase I studies have had some promising results for patients with MPEs or malignant pleural mesothelioma, including IP administration of adenoviral vector transfected with interferon β (IFN-β),[99] IFN-α2b,[100] tumor suppressor p53 with or without IP chemotherapy,[101,102] A larger phase IIA study is under way at the University of Pennsylvania by Haas and colleagues[103] that involves IP administration of Ad.IFN-α2b along with chemotherapy. IP gene therapy has not been incorporated into clinical use because of the difficulty of delivering sufficient levels of the therapeutic gene to kill a large enough number of tumor cells to have an effect. Although these studies have shown some efficacy and safety, larger randomized studies are needed to determine if IP gene therapy can prove superior to standard pleurodesis or drainage methods to control effusions or prolong survival.[103]

New technology

Kriegel and colleagues[104] recently reported their 5-year experience of the use of a subcutaneous implantable pleural port (SIPP) in 137 patients. The procedure can be performed as an outpatient and involves positioning the access port within a subcutaneous compartment along the midaxillary line over the 10th to 12th ribs with the SIPP inserted between the third to fifth intercostal spaces and directed to the lung base by fluoroscopic guidance. Once placed, the patient can access the port with a Huber needle and drainage bottle to remove the pleural fluid at home. Kriegel and colleagues described an SP within 2 months in 36.8% of patients, and a median survival time of 344 days, with 1 complication of empyema, 2 with cellulites, and 3 with mechanical complications. A phase II study by Shoji and colleagues[89] describes the safe use of the SIPP to administer IP chemotherapy (5-FU and cisplatin) to 22 patients with MPEs caused by various primaries. Although more studies are needed with these devices to give a general recommendation for their use, SIPPs have the advantage of a cosmetically pleasing solution with potentially lower risk of infection than TPCs, which allows the patient to have the convenience of home drainage.

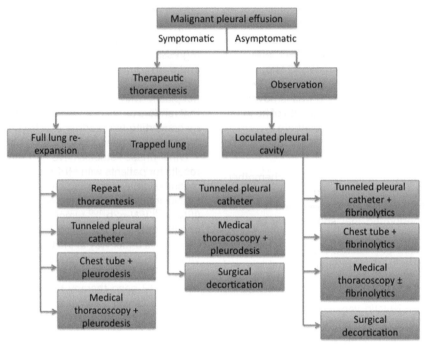

Fig. 3. Treatment algorithm for MPEs.

SUMMARY

Given the many management options for MPEs, several different algorithms have been suggested.[12] **Fig. 3** is our preferred algorithm in management of MPEs.[17] Although pleurodesis may provide permanent relief of symptoms, it also leads to more hospital days and is more costly than TPCs. TPCs also have the benefit of providing a means to manage trapped lung, a condition not amenable to pleurodesis. It is important to consider the patient's overall prognosis, symptoms, functional status, and social and financial situation when selecting the modality of choice. It is advisable to select the most cost-effective, least invasive, and most likely modality to lead to fewer hospitalization days.

REFERENCES

1. Ruckdeschel JC. Management of malignant pleural effusions. Semin Oncol 1994;22:58–63.
2. Light RW. Pleural diseases. 5th edition. Baltimore (MD): Lippincott, Williams & Wilkins; 2007.
3. Antony VB, Loddenkemper R, Astoul P, et al. Management of malignant pleural effusions. Eur Respir J 2001;18:402–19.
4. Rodriguez-Panadero F, Naranjo FB, Lopez-Mejias J. Pleural metastatic tumours and effusions. Frequency and pathogenic mechanisms in a post-mortem series. Eur Respir J 1989;2:366–9.
5. Marel M, Zrustova M, Stasny B, et al. The incidence of pleural effusion in a well-defined region: epidemiologic study in central Bohemia. Chest 1993; 104:1486–9.
6. Valdes L, Alvarez D, Valle JM, et al. The etiology of pleural effusions in an area with high incidence of tuberculosis. Chest 1996;109:158–62.
7. Hsu C. Cytologic detection of malignancy in pleural effusion: a review of 5255 samples from 3811 patients. Diagn Cytopathol 1987;3:8–12.
8. Sears D, Hajdu SI. The cytologic diagnosis of malignant neoplasms in pleural and peritoneal effusions. Acta Cytol 1987;31:85–97.
9. Johnston WW. The malignant pleural effusion. A review of cytopathologic diagnoses of 584 specimens from 472 consecutive patients. Cancer 1985;56:905–9.
10. Chernow B, Sahn SA. Carcinomatous involvement of the pleura: an analysis of 96 patients. Am J Med 1977;63:695–702.
11. Salyer WR, Eggleston JC, Erozan YS. Efficacy of pleural needle biopsy and pleural fluid cytopathology in the diagnosis of malignant neoplasm involving the pleura. Chest 1975;67:536–9.
12. Antunes G, Neville E, Duffy J, et al. BTS guidelines for the management of malignant pleural effusions. Thorax 2003;58:ii29–38.
13. Musani AI. Treatment options for malignant pleural effusion. Curr Opin Pulm Med 2009;15:380–7.
14. Meyer PC. Metastatic carcinoma of the pleura. Thorax 1966;21:437–43.

15. Light RW, Hamm H. Malignant pleural effusion: would the real cause please stand up? Eur Respir J 1997;10:1701–2.

16. Ashchi M, Golish J, Eng P, et al. Transudative malignant pleural effusions: prevalence and mechanisms. South Med J 1998;91:23–6.

17. Hsia D, Musani A. Management of malignant pleural effusions. Curr Respir Care Rep 1983;1: 73–81.

18. Fentiman I, Reubens RD, Hayward JL. Control of pleural effusions in patients with breast cancer. A randomized trial. Cancer 1983;2:737–9.

19. Tremblay A, Michaud G. Single-center experience with 250 tunneled pleural catheter insertions for malignant pleural effusions. Chest 2006;129: 362–8.

20. Qian Q, Zhan P, Sun WK, et al. Vascular endothelial growth factor and soluble intercellular adhesion molecule-1 in lung adenocarcinoma with malignant pleural effusion: correlations with patient survival and pleural effusion control. Neoplasma 2012;59: 433–9.

21. Kraft A, Weindel K, Ochs A, et al. Vascular endothelial growth factor in the sera and effusions of patients with malignant and nonmalignant disease. Cancer 1999;85:178–87.

22. Hott JW, Yu L, Antony VB, et al. Role of vascular endothelial growth factor (VEGF) in the formation of malignant pleural effusions. Am J Respir Crit Care Med 1999;159:A212.

23. Martinez-Moragon E, Aparicio J, Sanchis J, et al. Malignant pleural effusion: prognostic factors for survival and response to chemical pleurodesis in a series of 120 cases. Respiration 1998;65:108–13.

24. Rodriguez-Panadero F, Montes-Worboys A. Mechanisms of pleurodesis. Respiration 2012;83:91–8.

25. Teixeira LR, Vargas FS, Acencio MM, et al. Influence of anti-inflammatory drugs (methylprednisolone and diclofenac sodium) on experimental pleurodesis induced by silver nitrate or talc. Chest 2005;128:4041–5.

26. Teixeira LR, Wu W, Chang DS, et al. The effect of corticosteroids on pleurodesis induced by doxycycline in rabbits. Chest 2002;121:216–9.

27. Xie C, Teixeira LR, McGovern JP, et al. Systemic corticosteroids decrease the effectiveness of talc pleurodesis. Am J Respir Crit Care Med 1998; 157:1441–4.

28. Heffner JE, Nietert PJ, Barbieri C. Pleural fluid pH as a predictor of pleurodesis failure: analysis of primary data. Chest 2000;117:87–95.

29. Tassi GF, Davies RJ, Noppen M. Advanced techniques in medical thoracoscopy. Eur Respir J 2006;28:1051–9.

30. Lee P, Mathur PN, Colt HG. Advances in thoracoscopy: 100 years since Jacobaeus. Respiration 2010;79:177–86.

31. Menzies R, Charbonneau M. Thoracoscopy for the diagnosis of pleural disease. Ann Intern Med 1991; 114:271–6.

32. Colt HG. Thoracoscopy. A prospective study of safety and outcome. Chest 1995;108:324–9.

33. Tan C, Sedrakyan A, Browne J, et al. The evidence on the effectiveness of management of malignant pleural effusion: a systematic review. Eur J Cardiothorac Surg 2006;29:829–38.

34. Nakas A, Trousse DS, Martin-Ucar AE, et al. Open lung-sparing surgery for malignant pleural mesothelioma: the benefits of a radical approach within multimodality therapy. Eur J Cardiothorac Surg 2008;34:886–91.

35. Maziak DE, Gagliardi A, Haynes AE, et al. Surgical management of malignant pleural mesothelioma: a systematic review and evidence summary. Lung Cancer 2005;48:157–69.

36. Treasure T, Lang-Lazdunski L, Waller D, et al. Extrapleural pneumonectomy versus no extra-pleural pneumonectomy for patients with malignant pleural mesothelioma: clinical outcomes of the Mesothelioma and Radical Surgery (MARS) randomised feasibility study. Lancet Oncol 2011;12:763–72.

37. Zahid I, Routledge T, Bille A, et al. What is the best treatment for malignant pleural effusions? Interact Cardiovasc Thorac Surg 2011;12:818–23.

38. Lee Y, Baumann MH, Maskell NA, et al. Pleurodesis practice for malignant pleural effusion in five English-speaking countries: survey of pulmonologists. Chest 2003;124:2229–38.

39. Dresler CM, Olak J, Herndon JE 2nd, et al. Phase III intergroup study of talc poudrage vs talc slurry sclerosis for malignant pleural effusion. Chest 2005;127:909–15.

40. Rehse DH, Aye RW, Florence MG. Respiratory failure following talc pleurodesis. Am J Surg 1999;177: 437–40.

41. Janssen JP, Collier G, Astoul P, et al. Safety of pleurodesis with talc poudrage in malignant pleural effusion: a prospective cohort study. Lancet 2007; 369:1535–9.

42. Ferrer J, Villarino MA, Tura JM, et al. Talc preparations used for pleurodesis vary markedly from one preparation to another. Chest 2001;119(6): 1901–5.

43. Davies H, Lee YC, Davies RJ. Pleurodesis for malignant pleural effusion: talc, toxicity and where next? Thorax 2008;63:572–4.

44. American Thoracic Society. Management of malignant pleural effusions. Am J Respir Crit Care Med 2000;162:1987–2001.

45. Janssen J. Pleurodesis. In: Ernst A, Herth FJ, editors. Principles and practice of interventional pulmonology. New York: Springer; 2012. p. 623–30.

46. Roberts ME, Neville E, Berrisford RG, et al. Management of a malignant pleural effusion: British

Thoracic Society pleural disease guideline 2010. Thorax 2010;65(Suppl 2):ii32–40.

47. Shaw P, Agarwal R. Pleurodesis for malignant pleural effusions. Cochrane Database Syst Rev 2004;(1):CD002916.

48. de Campos JR, Vargas FS, de Campos Werebe E, et al. Thoracoscopy talc poudrage: a 15-year experience. Chest 2001;119:801–6.

49. Aelony Y, King RR, Boutin C. Malignant pleura effusions: effective pleurodesis despite low pleural pH. Chest 1998;113:1007–12.

50. Zhang W, Wang GF, Zhang H, et al. Medical thoracoscopic talc pleurodesis for malignant pleural effusion: an analysis of 27 cases. Beijing Da Xue Xue Bao 2008;40:600–2.

51. Thompson RL, Yau JC, Donnelly RF, et al. Pleurodesis with iodized talc for malignant effusions using pigtail catheters. Ann Pharmacother 1998; 32:739–42.

52. Marom EM, Patz EF Jr, Erasmus JJ, et al. Malignant pleural effusions: treatment with small-bore-catheter thoracostomy and talc pleurodesis. Radiology 1999;210:277–81.

53. Dryzer SR, Allen ML, Strange C, et al. A comparison of rotation and nonrotation in tetracycline pleurodesis. Chest 1993;104:1763–9.

54. Mager HJ, Maesen B, Verzijlbergen F, et al. Distribution of talc suspension during treatment of malignant pleural effusion with talc pleurodesis. Lung Cancer 2002;36:77–81.

55. Clementsen P, Evald T, Grode G, et al. Treatment of malignant pleural effusion: pleurodesis using a small percutaneous catheter. Respir Med 1998; 92:593–6.

56. Spiegler PA, Hurewitz AN, Groth ML. Rapid pleurodesis for malignant pleural effusions. Chest 2003;23:1895–8.

57. Parulekar W, Di Primio G, Matzinger F, et al. Use of small-bore vs. large-bore hest tubes for treatment of malignant pleural effusions. Chest 2001;120(1): 19–25.

58. Caglayan B, Torun E, Turan D, et al. Efficacy of iodopovidone pleurodesis and comparison of small-bore catheter versus large bore chest tube. Ann Surg Oncol 2008;15(9):2594–9.

59. Mañes N, Rodriguez-Panadero F, Bravo JL, et al. Talc pleurodesis: prospective and randomized study. Clinical follow-up. Chest 2000;118:131S.

60. Rahman NM, Maskell NA, West A, et al. Intrapleural use of tissue plasminogen activator and DNase in pleural infection. N Engl J Med 2011; 365:518–26.

61. Hsu LH, Soong TC, Feng AC, et al. Intrapleural urokinase for the treatment of loculated malignant pleural effusions and trapped lungs in medically inoperable cancer patients. J Thorac Oncol 2006; 1:460–7.

62. Gilkeson RC, Silverman P, Haaga JR. Using urokinase to treat malignant pleural effusions. AJR Am J Roentgenol 1999;173:781–3.

63. Davies CW, Traill ZC, Gleeson FV, et al. Intrapleural streptokinase in the management of malignant multiloculated pleural effusions. Chest 1999;115: 729–33.

64. Okur E, Baysungur V, Tezel C, et al. Streptokinase for malignant pleural effusions: a randomized controlled study. Asian Cardiovasc Thorac Ann 2011;19:238–43.

65. Hausheer FH, Yarbro JW. Diagnosis and treatment of malignant pleural effusion. Semin Oncol 1985; 12:54–75.

66. Adler RH, Sayek I. Treatment of malignant pleural effusion: a method using tube thoracostomy and talc. Ann Thorac Surg 1976;22:8–15.

67. Villanueva AG, Gray AW Jr, Shahian DM, et al. Efficacy of short term versus long term tube thoracostomy drainage before tetracycline pleurodesis in the treatment of malignant pleural effusions. Thorax 1994;49:23–5.

68. Echevarria C, Twomey D, Dunning J, et al. Does reexpansion pulmonary oedema exist? Interact Cardiovasc Thorac Surg 2008;7:485–9.

69. Sherman SC. Reexpansion pulmonary edema: a case report and a review of the current literature. J Emerg Med 2003;24:23–7.

70. Feller-Kopman D, Berkowitz D, Boiselle P, et al. Large-volume thoracentesis and the risk of reexpansion pulmonary edema. Ann Thorac Surg 2007;84:1656–61.

71. Mahfood S, Hix WR, Aaron BL, et al. Reexpansion pulmonary edema. J Thorac Imaging 1988;45:340–5.

72. Tarver RD, Broderick LS, Conces DJ Jr. Reexpansion pulmonary edema. J Thorac Imaging 1996; 11:198–209.

73. Feller-Kopman D, Walkey A, Berkowitz D, et al. The relationship of pleural pressure to symptom development during therapeutic thoracentesis. Chest 2006;129:1556–60.

74. Stretton F, Edmonds P, Marrinan M. Malignant pleural effusions. Eur J Palliat Care 1999;6:5–9.

75. Putnam JB, Light RW, Rodriguez RM, et al. A randomized comparison of indwelling pleural catheter and doxycycline pleurodesis in the management of malignant pleural effusions. Cancer 1999;86:1992–9.

76. Warren WH, Kalimi R, Khodadadian LM, et al. Management of malignant pleural effusions using the Pleur(x) catheter. Ann Thorac Surg 2008;85:1049–50.

77. Van Meter ME, McKee KY, Kohlwes RJ. Efficacy and safety of tunneled pleural catheters in adults with malignant pleural effusions: a systematic review. J Gen Intern Med 2011;26:70–6.

78. Fysh ET, Waterer GW, Kendall P, et al. Indwelling pleural catheters reduce inpatient days over

pleurodesis for malignant pleural effusion. Chest 2012;142:394–400.

79. Davies HE, Mishra EK, Kahan BC, et al. Effect of an indwelling pleural catheter vs. chest tube and talc pleurodesis for relieving dyspnea in patients with malignant pleural effusion the TIME2 randomized controlled trial. JAMA 2012;307:2383–9.

80. Reich H, Beattie EJ, Harvey JC. Pleuroperitoneal shunt for malignant pleural effusions: a one-year experience. Semin Surg Oncol 1993;9:160–2.

81. Lee KA, Harvey JC, Reich H, et al. Management of malignant pleural effusions with pleuroperitoneal shunting. J Am Coll Surg 1994;178:586–8.

82. Genc O, Petrou M, Ladas G, et al. The long-term morbidity of pleuroperitoneal shunts in the management of recurrent malignant effusions. Eur J Cardiothorac Surg 2000;18:143–6.

83. Tsang V, Fernando HC, Goldstraw P. Pleuroperitoneal shunt for recurrent malignant pleural effusions. Thorax 1990;45:369–72.

84. Schulze M, Boehle AS, Kurdow R, et al. Effective treatment of malignant pleural effusion by minimal invasive thoracic surgery: thoracoscopic talc pleurodesis and pleuroperitoneal shunts in 101 patients. Ann Thorac Surg 2001;71:1809–12.

85. Puri V, Pyrdeck TL, Crabtree TD, et al. Treatment of malignant pleural effusion: a cost-effectiveness analysis. Ann Thorac Surg 2012;94:374–80.

86. Reddy C, Ernst A, Lamb C, et al. Rapid pleurodesis for malignant pleural effusions. Chest 2011;139:1419–23.

87. Tohda Y, Iwanaga T, Takada M, et al. Intrapleural administration of cisplatin and etoposide to treat malignant pleural effusions in patients with non-small cell lung cancer. Chemotherapy 1999;45:197–204.

88. Seto T, Ushijima S, Yamamoto H, et al. Intrapleural hypotonic cisplatin treatment for malignant pleural effusion in 80 patients with non-small-cell lung cancer: a multi-institutional phase II trial. Br J Cancer 2006;95:717–21.

89. Shoji T, Tanaka F, Yanagihara K, et al. Phase II study of repeated intrapleural chemotherapy using implantable access system for management of malignant pleural effusion. Chest 2002;121:821–4.

90. Su WC, Lai WW, Chen HH, et al. Combined intrapleural and intravenous chemotherapy, and pulmonary irradiation, for treatment of patients with lung cancer presenting with malignant pleural effusion: a pilot study. Oncology 2003;64:18–24.

91. Matsuzaki Y, Edagawa M, Shimizu T, et al. Intrapleural hyperthermic perfusion with chemotherapy increases apoptosis in malignant pleuritis. Ann Thorac Surg 2004;78:1769–72.

92. Lombardi G, Nicoletto MO, Gusella M, et al. Intrapleural paclitaxel for malignant pleural effusion from ovarian and breast cancer: a phase II study with pharmacokinetic analysis. Cancer Chemother Pharmacol 2012;69:781–7.

93. Perng RP, Chen YM, Wu MF, et al. Phase II trial of intrapleural paclitaxel injection for non-small-cell lung cancer patients with malignant pleural effusions. Respir Med 1998;92:473–9.

94. Jones DR, Taylor MD, Petroni GR, et al. Phase I trial of intrapleural docetaxel through an implantable catheter in subjects with a malignant pleural effusion. J Thorac Oncol 2010;5:75–8.

95. Lerza R, Vannozzi MO, Tolino G, et al. Carboplatin and cisplatin pharmacokinetics after intrapleural combination treatment in patients with malignant pleural effusion. Ann Oncol 1997;8(4):385–91.

96. Ichinose Y, Tsuchiya R, Koike T. A prematurely terminated phase III trial of intraoperative intrapleural hypotonic cisplatin treatment in patients with resected non-small cell lung cancer with positive pleural lavage cytology: the incidence of carcinomatous pleuritis after surgical intervention. J Thorac Cardiovasc Surg 2002;123:695–9.

97. Chen WJ, Yuan SF, Yan QY, et al. Intrapleural chemo- and hyperthermotherapies for malignant pleural effusion: a randomized prospective study. Cancer Invest 2012;30:126–30.

98. Zarogoulidis P, Chatzaki E, Hohenforst-Schmidt W, et al. Management of malignant pleural effusion by suicide gene therapy in advanced stage lung cancer: a case series and literature review. Cancer Gene Ther 2012;19:593–600.

99. Sterman DH, Recio A, Carroll RG, et al. A phase I clinical trial of single-dose intrapleural IFN-beta gene transfer for malignant pleural mesothelioma and metastatic pleural effusions: high rate of antitumor immune responses. Clin Cancer Res 2007;13:4456–66.

100. Sterman DH, Haas A, Moon E, et al. A trial of intrapleural adenoviral-mediated interferon-α2b gene transfer for malignant pleural mesothelioma. Am J Respir Crit Care Med 2011;184:1395–9.

101. Zhao WZ, Wang JK, Li W, et al. Clinical research on recombinant human Ad-p53 injection combined with cisplatin in treatment of malignant pleural effusion induced by lung cancer. Ai Zheng 2009;28:1324–7.

102. Dong M, Li X, Hong LJ, et al. Advanced malignant pleural or peritoneal effusion in patients treated with recombinant adenovirus p53 injection plus cisplatin. J Int Med Res 2008;36:1273–8.

103. Haas A, Sterman DH. Novel intrapleural therapies for malignant diseases. Respiration 2012;83:277–92.

104. Kriegel I, Daniel C, Falcou MC, et al. Use of a subcutaneous implantable pleural port in the management of recurrent malignant pleurisy: five-year experience based on 168 subcutaneous implantable pleural ports. J Palliat Med 2011;14:829–34.

Bedside Ultrasound for the Interventional Pulmonologist

Kenneth E. Lyn-Kew, MD[a],*, Seth J. Koenig, MD[b]

KEYWORDS

- Ultrasound • Pleural effusion • Percutaneous tracheostomy • Thoracentesis • Lung ultrasound
- Pleural ultrasound

KEY POINTS

- Thoracic ultrasonography allows the interventional pulmonologist to both identify and characterize pleural abnormalities while providing real-time guidance for therapeutic intervention. This reduces complications and improves opportunities for pleural drainage.
- Ultrasound allows the interventional pulmonologist to accurately and safely biopsy pleural-based masses.
- Ultrasound improves the safety of percutaneous tracheostomy by identifying aberrant anatomy.

Thoracic ultrasonography is a powerful diagnostic and therapeutic tool for the interventional pulmonologist (IP). Ultrasound allows for the rapid identification, characterization, and therapeutic decision making of thoracic disorders at the point of care. Thoracic ultrasonography allows the IP to strategically place all types of chest tubes and to needle biopsy pleural-based thoracic masses. Before percutaneous tracheostomy, ultrasound defines aberrant vasculature, such as a high-riding innominate artery, and allows direct visualization of needle insertion into the trachea. Preprocedural and postprocedural assessment for pneumothorax obviates the need for chest radiography, saving time, ionizing radiation exposure, and cost allocation. Thoracic ultrasonography is easy to perform and has a steep learning curve. This article summarizes the current literature regarding thoracic ultrasonography and specifically guides the IP in use of thoracic ultrasound for practical applications. The article supplements the text with ultrasound images from real cases, with the correlation of other imaging modalities when applicable.

INTRODUCTION

Thoracic ultrasound is an ideal imaging modality for the IP. It is portable, used at point of care by the treating physician, uses no ionizing radiation, and has no inherent delay between the ordering of an imaging study and its performance. Importantly, there is no clinical dissociation between the treating physician and the physician interpreting the imaging study. Common procedures for the IP include management of pleural effusions, assessment and biopsy of pleural-based masses, and percutaneous tracheostomy. Ultrasound allows the IP to diagnose, strategize, and perform these procedures at the point of care. This requires a paradigm shift in the approach to thoracic imaging, extends the physical examination, and allows the IP to better characterize disease processes. In conjunction with clinical history,

Funding Sources: None.
Conflict of Interest: None.
[a] Department of Medicine, National Jewish Health, 1400 Jackson Street, M320, Denver, CO 80206, USA;
[b] Department of Medicine, Long Island Jewish Medical Center, Hofstra-North Shore Long Island Jewish Health System, 410 Lakeville Road, Suite 107, New Hyde Park, NY 11040, USA
* Corresponding author.
E-mail address: Lyn-KewK@NJHealth.org

Clin Chest Med 34 (2013) 473–485
http://dx.doi.org/10.1016/j.ccm.2013.04.004
0272-5231/13/$ – see front matter © 2013 Elsevier Inc. All rights reserved.

physical examination, and other imaging modalities, such as chest radiography and chest computerized tomography (CT) scan, ultrasound will undoubtedly find its place for the IP.

MACHINE REQUIREMENTS

Modern day portable ultrasound machines are capable of performing all aspects of thoracic ultrasonography. With the expense of ultrasound machines rapidly dropping and the requirement of all pulmonary and critical care training programs to teach both guided vascular access and thoracentesis, ultrasound machines should be readily accessible. A phased array transducer (3.5–5.0 MHz) with a small "footprint" designed for cardiac imaging allows for most thoracic examinations. For detailed examination of the pleural surface, for instance to determine thoracic extension of a pleural-based mass, a high-frequency (7.5–10.0 MHz) linear vascular probe is necessary. This will optimize the near field structures but sacrifices the depth of ultrasound penetration needed for examination of alveolar consolidation, pleural-based masses, and pleural effusions. Doppler capability is not a requirement for comprehensive thoracic ultrasonography but may be helpful for evaluating vascular structures when performing biopsies and during the assessment of aberrant vessels before percutaneous dilational tracheostomy.

PERFORMANCE OF THORACIC ULTRASOUND

Thoracic ultrasonography is best performed with the patient in a seated position, although for the IP this may not always be practical, as in the instance of patients receiving mechanical ventilation. A longitudinal scanning plane is preferred with the transducer indicator held in the cephalad position. Standard machine setup for thoracic ultrasonography would mean that images on the left side of the screen would be cephalad structures. Knowledge of machine controls, such as gain and depth, must be adjusted to maximize image quality.

Image acquisition begins with firm perpendicular pressure applied to the chest wall over a rib interspace. Adjacent interspaces are then examined creating a longitudinal scan line. Multiple adjacent longitudinal scan lines are performed to create a 3-dimensional model of the thorax (Fig. 1). Abnormalities identified by the IP are then focused in on and may include the use of a high-frequency linear probe.

Bone blocks the transmission of ultrasound so focal abnormalities that lie under ribs may not be seen. By angling the transducer to "look" above or below the rib space, the sonographer may reveal the area of interest. Aerated lung also blocks transmission of ultrasound such that abnormalities that do not extend to the pleural line will remain "invisible." The use of the liver or spleen as an acoustic window may allow visualization of some parenchymal abnormalities. In addition, consolidated lung and pleural effusion transmit ultrasound well and may allow visualization of the mediastinum and lung.

Although the interventionalists are usually called to perform therapeutic or diagnostic procedures, as opposed to making diagnostic decisions on patients presenting with cardiopulmonary failure, thoracic ultrasound scanning techniques remain constant. For a more detailed overview of diagnostic strategies outside of the IP specialty, excellent reviews are available.[1]

LUNG ULTRASONOGRAPHY

The integration of lung ultrasound into the physical examination, other radiologic studies, and clinical history has great practical application to the pulmonologist. Immediate diagnostic information regarding a patient's symptoms and signs of thoracic pathology become apparent without delay or clinical dissociation between the treating physician and the physician performing the examination. Acute pulmonary edema, alveolar consolidation, pneumothorax, or pleural effusions are readily apparent. Although practical skill and knowledge of the acquisition and interpretation of lung ultrasound should be learned by the IP, this article focuses on the aspects of lung ultrasound particular for the IP. These include identification of pleural-based lung masses, lung abscess, differentiation of complex pleural disease from alveolar consolidation, and determination of postprocedure pneumothorax.

Dr Daniel Lichtenstein developed the standard seminology of lung ultrasound and his original work defined all the important findings of lung ultrasonography. Although he continues to define the field of lung ultrasonography, others have validated his previous work (Fig. 2).[2–6]

Performance of lung ultrasound begins at the pleural line. With the transducer placed over an interspace, the pleural line is identified approximately 5 mm deep to the rib cortex, with rib shadows on either side (Fig. 3). The pleural line appears as a shimmering echogenic linear structure and is examined for respirophasic or cardiac movement, representing movement of the visceral pleura against the parietal pleura. This movement is called lung sliding when derived from respiratory

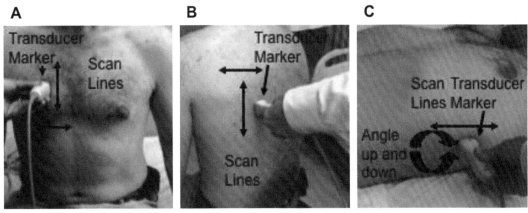

Fig. 1. Ultrasound scanning technique. (*A, B*) Anterior and posterior thoracic scanning, respectively. With firm pressure, move ultrasound probe cephalad and caudad in vertical scan line, then move medial and lateral. (*C*) Supine patient. Scan in longitudinal plane with angling posterior as to not miss a small dependent pleural effusion.

effort, or lung pulse when it results from cardiac contraction. A reduction in gain and depth will improve its visualization. The presence of lung sliding or lung pulse absolutely rules out pneumothorax at that point of examination. Multiple sites on the thorax may be rapidly examined to definitely rule out pneumothorax.[3] The absence of lung sliding suggests pneumothorax but must be considered within clinical context. For instance, prior pleurodesis may produce loss of lung sliding, a desirable sequelae for malignant pleural effusion.

We routinely search for lung sliding and lung pulse before any thoracic intervention. Providing that lung sliding or lung pulse was present before a thoracic procedure, loss of these signs is strong evidence for a procedure-associated pneumothorax. Lung point, which is defined as intermittent visualization of lung sliding from partially collapsed lung expanding to reach the pleural surface during inspiration, is diagnostic of pneumothorax.[7] This sign may allow the IP strategic placement of a chest tube just cephalad to the pneumothorax.

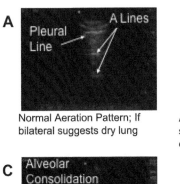

Normal Aeration Pattern; If bilateral suggests dry lung

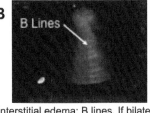

Alveolar-Interstitial edema; B lines. If bilateral suggests cardiac or noncardiac pulmonary edema; if unilateral suggests infection

Alveolar Consolidation; suggests pneumonia with clinical context.

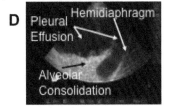

Pleural Effusion. Identify hemidiaphragm, chest wall, and anechoic space.

Fig. 2. Thoracic ultrasound patterns are illustrated. (*A*) Normal aeration pattern with A lines. (*B*) Multiple confluent B lines. These lines arise from the pleural line, move with respiration, and extend to the bottom of the screen. B lines indicate pulmonary edema. (*C*) Alveolar consolidation pattern. May be diagnostic of pneumonia or atelectasis depending on clinical circumstance. (*D*) Pleural effusion.

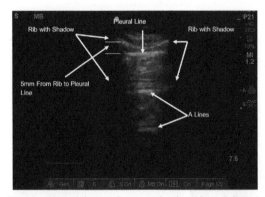

Fig. 3. Normal lung ultrasound. The pleural line is approximately 5 mm below the ribs, regardless of body habitus. There are hyperechoic rib lines on either side of the pleural line that cast shadows. Note the repetitive A line pattern. A lines are reverberation artifacts.

Differentiation of consolidated lung and complex pleural fluid may be challenging. This has obvious clinical relevance to the IP. Consolidated lung appears tissue dense, similar to the liver or spleen, and may contain sonographic air bronchograms. These are visualized as punctuate echogenic foci within consolidated lung. Movement of the air bronchograms with respiration defines a patent bronchus supplying that area of the lung (**Fig. 4**).[8]

Pleural-based masses are readily assessed using ultrasound.[9] They are typically hypoechoic and surrounded by aerated lung. For estimating size, the examiner will have to move the transducer both medial and lateral and to adjacent rib interspaces. Small masses may be visualized by angling the transducer to "look" under the ribs. Local extension of tumor and chest wall invasion

are readily detectable by ultrasonography and require use of a high-frequency linear probe. Ultrasonography is more accurate than chest CT for detection of chest wall invasion.[10] Masses and lung abscesses may also be visualized within the lung. A peripheral lung abscess that abuts the pleural surface will be easily detected. Its appearance is heterogeneous, typically with hyperechoic and irregular borders. Internally, the abscess will appear heterogeneous with relatively anechoic or hypoechoic areas interspersed with more echogenic foci, corresponding to both air and tissue necrosis (**Figs. 5–7**).

Alveolar consolidation pattern may be seen with ultrasound and may be caused by airway obstruction, parenchymal disease, or as a consequence of pleural effusion. When caused by pleural effusion, the degree of atelectasis is proportional to the size of the effusion. With large pleural effusions, the atelectatic lung appears to float with dynamic movement due to respiration and cardiac pulsation (**Fig. 8**).

Although many disease processes will be initially picked up by chest CT with subsequent referral to the IP, lung ultrasound allows the IP to confirm the diagnosis, determine and carry out diagnostic and therapeutic procedures, and follow disease regression without the use of ionizing radiation. Lung ultrasonography is not without limitation. Parenchymal lesions surrounded by aerated lung are not visible with lung ultrasound, such as small lung nodules or masses not abutting the pleural surface.

PLEURAL ULTRASONOGRAPHY

Ultrasonography is an easy-to-use modality that allows the IP to both identify and characterize

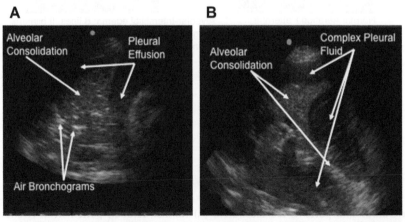

Fig. 4. Alveolar consolidation patterns. (*A*) Simple alveolar consolidation with pleural effusion. Notice air bronchograms within the consolidation. (*B*) More complex alveolar consolidation. Notice complex, septated pleural effusion surrounding alveolar consolidation.

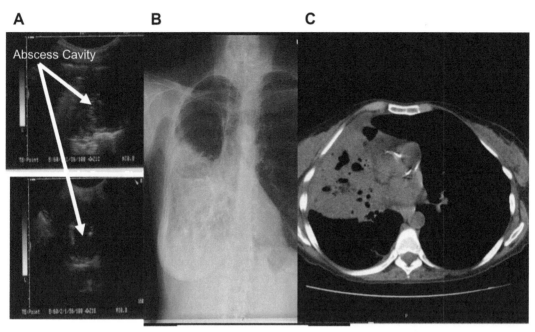

Fig. 5. Lung abscess. (*A*) Lung ultrasound showing rounded pleural-based anechoic space with punctate white foci. This represents air within the cavity. Real-time ultrasound revealed loss of lung sliding suggesting pleurodesis. (*B*) Chest radiograph. (*C*) Chest CT corresponding to the lung ultrasound.

pleural abnormalities while providing real-time guidance for therapeutic intervention. Scanning tactics and equipment requirements are identical to those of lung ultrasound. Pleural fluid is identified as anechoic or relatively hypoechoic, compared with the liver as reference, within the hemithorax. Free-flowing fluid is found in a dependent manner, whereas loculated fluid may appear anywhere within the hemithorax. Typical anatomic boundaries that define a pleural effusion are the chest wall, the hemidiaphragm, and the visceral pleura. Identification of the hemidiaphragm is crucial and requires visualization of either the liver or spleen. The visceral pleural is identified

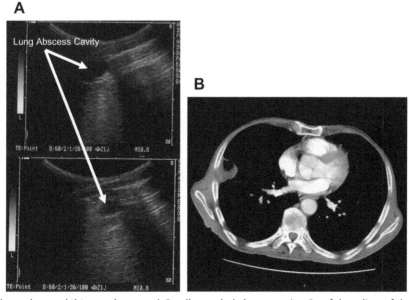

Fig. 6. Small lung abscess. (*A*) Lung ultrasound. Small rounded abscess cavity. Careful angling of the transducer is essential to fully examine the abnormality. (*B*) Corresponding chest CT.

A   B

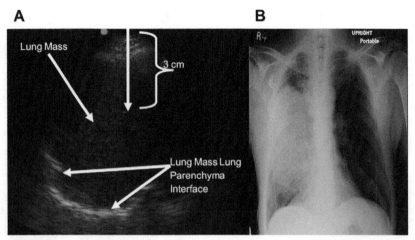

Fig. 7. Lung mass. (*A*) Lung ultrasound of a lung mass. Hypoechoic area with interface with normal lung parenchyma. Measurement from chest wall indicated at 3 cm where biopsy cutting needle was inserted. (*B*) Corresponding chest radiograph.

to avoid inadvertent iatrogenic pneumothorax. Because of respiratory and cardiac function, pleural fluid is associated with dynamic findings that include diaphragmatic movement, movement of the atelectatic lung, and shifting tissue elements (**Figs. 9** and **10**).

Ultrasonography allows both characterization of pleural fluid as well as the size of the effusion. Although accurate volumetric analysis is possible, it is rarely necessary, and estimation qualitatively as small, moderate, or large is sufficient; however, an inversion or straightening of the hemidiaphragm under load from a pleural effusion has been correlated with dyspnea. Characterization of pleural fluid anomalies, such as septations, with ultrasound is superior to standard chest radiography and chest CT.[11,12] Pleural fluid complexity, such as loculations and mobile echogenic material within the effusion, suggest an exudative process.[13] However, an anechoic effusion may be

either transudative or exudative, and will depend on clinical history and pleural fluid analysis. Pleural ultrasound may reveal a specific diagnosis, such as a malignant pleural effusion with metastatic foci along the hemidiaphragm or a lung mass revealed in the lung made atelectatic by surrounding pleural fluid (**Fig. 11**).

Most pleural effusions are readily identified by ultrasonography and when the cardinal ultrasound features of pleural effusions are observed, misidentification is unlikely (**Fig. 12**). However, obesity, heavy musculature, and soft tissue edema may degrade ultrasound image quality. This leaves

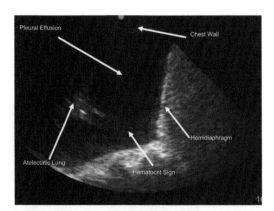

Fig. 9. Lung ultrasound of a large pleural effusion with anatomic boundaries outlined. Ultrasound confirmation of a pleural effusion should have cardinal features visualized, including chest wall, hemidiaphragm, and anechoic space (denoting pleural effusion). Notice atelectatic lung, which has dynamic motion with the respirocardiac cycle. Hematocrit sign illustrates higher-density material in a more dependent location.

Fig. 8. Lung ultrasound of a large pleural effusion with compressive atelectasis. When viewed in real time the lung appears to float with dynamic movement due to both cardiac and respiratory function.

A **B**

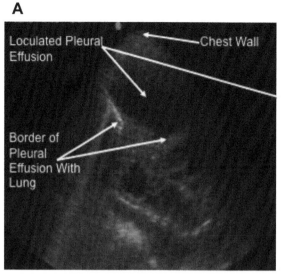 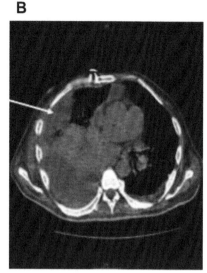

Fig. 10. Lung ultrasound showing a small anterolateral loculated pleural effusion. (*A*) Ultrasound of pleural effusion does not include hemidiaphragm. Careful ultrasound scanning must be done to identify hemidiaphragm below this loculated pleural effusion. (*B*) CT image provided for comparison.

the examiner unable to clearly identify the chest wall, hemidiaphragms, or the visceral pleura. Highly echogenic pleural fluid, as in empyema or hemothorax, may make a confident diagnosis difficult. This may require expertise in thoracic ultrasound.

PROCEDURAL GUIDANCE USING ULTRASOUND
Thoracentesis and Placement of Chest Tubes

Thoracic ultrasonography for pleural drainage reduces complications, such as pneumothorax,

and decreases the rate of "dry" taps, as well as minimizing missed opportunities for fluid analysis when only standard chest radiography is used for pleural fluid detection.[14] Importantly, ultrasound allows targeted placement of chest tubes for complex pleural disease and aids in determination of when surgical intervention may be necessary.

Regardless of the intervention, the IP should seek unequivocal identification of pleural fluid. The best site, angle, and depth of needle insertion is sought to avoid organ puncture. This requires that the patient be in the position that the procedure will be performed. Any significant deviation

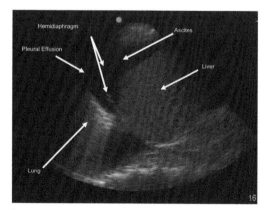

Fig. 11. Lung ultrasound showing a lung mass surrounded by atelectatic lung. There is a relatively anechoic space, corresponding to the lung mass, which is surrounded by atelectatic lung. Notice normal lung interface with atelectatic lung. Patient had an endobronchial lesion in bronchus leading to that segment. There is a small pleural effusion.

Fig. 12. Lung ultrasound showing a pleural effusion and ascites. Careful attention to the location of the hemidiaphragm and proper ultrasound transducer orientation will eliminate misidentification of an anechoic space.

in patient position after image acquisition may result in inadvertent visceral laceration or a poorly positioned drainage catheter. The angle and position of the transducer during image acquisition must be replicated with needle insertion. Depth of needle insertion may be calculated using the ultrasound image in "freeze" position and use of the caliper function on most ultrasound machines (**Fig. 13**). Significant chest wall edema and obesity may result in underestimation of depth required to reach pleural fluid. Pressing firmly on the chest wall may create a significant compression artifact. Color Doppler may be used to interrogate the intercostal space before needle insertion to avoid aberrant vasculature. Although reasonable, there are no published data to support this practice and the authors do not routinely use this practice. Before needle insertion, lung sliding should be sought. The loss of lung sliding postprocedure is good evidence of iatrogenic pneumothorax. The authors do not routinely do chest radiographs following simple thoracentesis and use ultrasound to evaluate success of pleural drainage and for pneumothorax.

Ultrasound allows the IP to both locate a safe site and trajectory for needle insertion and aids in drainage device selection. Access to pleural fluid via needle insertion allows for either simple thoracentesis or wire insertion that allows a variety of pleural drainage devices to be inserted. With careful attention to the trajectory of needle insertion, real-time imaging of needle insertion is of unproven benefit, is not routinely performed, and may be technically difficult. Ultrasound allows the IP to localize the wire within the pleural fluid and

assess its position (**Fig. 14**). Small-bore or large-bore chest tubes, tunneled indwelling pleural catheters, and introducers for medical thoracoscopy are safely placed with ultrasound guidance.

Free-flowing, anechoic effusions may be best managed with simple thoracentesis and fluid analysis, whereas an echodense, septated effusion may require larger indwelling catheters. The use of tissue plasminogen activator with or without DNase may be reasonable with complex effusions where septations appear mobile. However, thick, immobile septations may require surgical intervention (see **Fig. 14**).

Ultrasound allows for assessment of the success of pleural drainage and to follow progression or resolution of pleural disease. Standard chest radiographs are suboptimal and serial chest CTs expose the patient to significant ionizing radiation and increase health care costs.

Transthoracic Biopsy of Pleural-Based Masses

Ultrasound allows the IP to accurately and safely biopsy pleural-based masses by needle aspiration or cutting biopsy needle.[15] Careful assessment of the pleural chest wall interface is facilitated using a high-frequency linear ultrasound probe and chest wall invasion by malignant tumors is accurately assessed. Precise measurement of the depth for needle placement and angle of trajectory is mandatory. Once a lesion is identified via ultrasound, the examiner should scan through each intercostal space, as well as medial and lateral within each space, to accurately determine dimensions and a safe site for needle insertion.

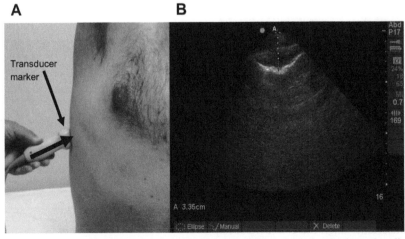

Fig. 13. Ultrasound scanning technique. (*A*) Ultrasound probe angle defined by the lateral wall of the patient and the ultrasound probe. Needle insertion must replicate that of ultrasound image. Note large black arrow denoting angle that needle must follow. (*B*) Small lateral pleural-based fluid collection. Use of caliper function defines distance of needle insertion. In this patient, needle insertion past 3.35 cm may cause iatrogenic visceral lung laceration.

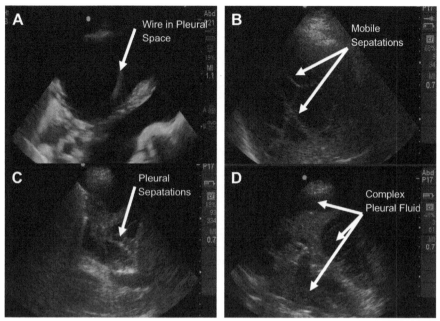

Fig. 14. Pleural effusion characterization and chest tube wire localization. (*A*) Large malignant pleural effusion with wire seen within anechoic space. (*B, C*) Complex septated pleural effusion. On real-time imaging, septations appeared mobile, prompting chest tube drainage. (*D*) Complex pleural disease. Simple aspiration revealed pus. Real-time imaging showed immobile septations within alveolar consolidation. Patient referred for definitive surgical pleural drainage.

Respirophasic movement of the mass should be sought to determine the degree of displacement, as small masses may be challenging to biopsy, unless the patient makes a breath hold. Color Doppler of the area to be biopsied may avoid puncture of vasculature. In our experience, real-time guidance of needle placement is not necessary for transthoracic puncture of pleural-based masses.

Lung Abscess: Microbiologic Diagnosis and Drainage

Ultrasonography may aid in microbiological diagnosis or therapeutic drainage of pleural-based lung abscess.[16] Ultrasound scanning technique is similar to that of pleural-based masses. However, with lung abscess puncture there is potential to soil the pleural space. Careful examination of the pleural surface for the absence of lung sliding is good evidence for pleural symphysis. This is common with lung abscess, as local inflammation causes pleurodesis. Using a high-frequency linear ultrasound probe, the examiner increases the resolution of the pleural line and seeks unequivocal evidence of pleurodesis. Color Doppler allows the examiner to assess for aberrant vessels within the abscess cavity to avoid potential bleeding complications. Either simple aspiration for culture or placement of an indwelling catheter is possible depending on clinical circumstances. Follow-up of cavity resolution by ultrasound may obviate the need for repeated chest CT scans.

Percutaneous Dilational Tracheostomy

Tracheostomy is being performed with increasing frequency in the medical intensive care unit (MICU).[17] Most of these are performed in ICUs for prolonged respiratory failure. Given the safety of the procedure, percutaneous dilational tracheostomy (PDT) has been recommended as the procedure of choice in critically ill patients.[18,19] Although relatively safe, the known complications of tracheostomy include both acute and delayed bleeding. Ultrasonography offers several advantages to the IP. Ultrasound allows visualization of aberrant vasculature and other anatomic abnormalities (**Fig. 15**). Tracheal rings can be visualized, as well as the passing between the rings of instruments. Ultrasound can assist in patients with difficult anatomy, such as the large necks of the morbidly obese.

The superficial positioning of the proximal trachea, cricoid cartilage, cricothyroid membrane, thyroid gland, and thyroid cartilage allow for ultrasound imaging of these structures with a high-frequency linear transducer.[20] The tracheal rings

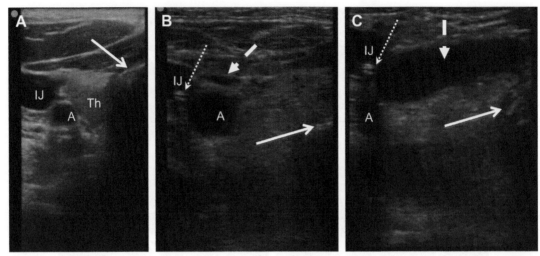

Fig. 15. High-riding brachiocephalic artery. (*A*) Normal neck anatomy obtained with high-frequency linear probe. The right common carotid artery (A) and the lateral lobe of the thyroid (Th) are visualized. Solid arrow marks the edge of the tracheal ring, and the internal jugular vein (IJ) can be seen on the edge of the image. (*B*) Candidate for PDT. The right common carotid artery (A) and right internal jugular vein (IJ) are visualized. Solid arrow marks the edge of the tracheal ring. The dashed arrow indicates an unidentified vascular structure. A central venous catheter can be seen within the IJ (*dotted arrow*). (*C*) Slight movement of the high-frequency linear probe caudally unveils a high-riding brachiocephalic artery (*dotted arrow*) overriding the tracheal ring. This patient should be referred for open tracheostomy.

appear as a series of hypoechoic ovoid structures in the sagittal or longitudinal plane (**Fig. 16**) and as a crescent-shaped structure backed by the reverberation artifact of the tracheal air column in the transverse scanning plane. The cricoid cartilage

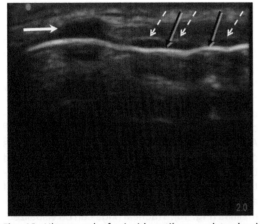

Fig. 16. Ultrasound of cricoid cartilage and tracheal rings using high-frequency linear probe in sagittal plane. Cephalad structures appear to the left. The cricoid cartilage is identified as a hypoechoic structure indicated by the solid arrow. The dashed arrows indicate the tracheal rings. The hyperechoic line running behind the cartilaginous structures is the tracheal air-tissue interface. The black vertical arrows identify possible needle puncture points for percutaneous tracheostomy.

is a larger hypoechoic structure cephalad to the tracheal rings. The cricothyroid membrane is recognized as the relatively hyperechoic structure linking the hypoechoic cricoid cartilage caudal to it with the hypoechoic thyroid cartilage cephalad. In addition to these structures, the vascular anatomy may be defined and aberrant vessels identified before needle insertion These include the internal and anterior jugular veins, the common carotid arteries, and thyroid vessels. The vasculature on ultrasound is identified by its strong hypoechoic properties. Venous and arterial vessels may be differentiated by the relative compressibility of the veins compared with the arteries and by their differing color and spectral Doppler properties. However, color and spectral Doppler are rarely needed to differentiate arteries from veins. Thyroid tissue, especially the isthmus, is identified during screening neck ultrasound (**Fig. 17**). The operator may unexpectedly observe either thyroid nodules/masses or a large thyroidal artery. Expert-level thyroid ultrasonography performed by trained personnel may be warranted.

Bleeding is a significant concern with PDT, with an incidence in one study of 5%.[21] However, life-threatening causes of bleeding are lacerations of aberrantly placed larger vessels of the neck (see **Fig. 15**). These include medial running carotid arteries and internal jugular veins, aberrant jugular systems, high-riding brachiocephalic vessels, and normal variants of the thyroid vasculature. The

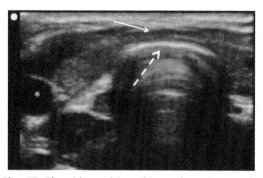

Fig. 17. Thyroid overlying the trachea. Image obtained using high-frequency linear probe. The right common carotid artery is visible on the left (*asterisk*). The thyroid isthmus (*arrow*) can be seen overlying the trachea (*dashed arrow*). Before PDT, this area should be evaluated for large thyroid vessels that may preclude puncture at that level.

thyroid and these more-prominent vascular anomalies are readily seen on ultrasound, allowing for avoidance of the vessels by meticulous placement of the tracheostomy or by transitioning to an open procedure.[22,23]

Placement of the tracheostomy during PDT is dependent on identification of the appropriate anatomic landmarks. Misidentification of the landmarks can lead to both inappropriately superior and inferior tracheostomy placements. In a small series, ultrasound guidance has been shown to eliminate the incidence of cranial placement.[24] In addition, ultrasound has been applied to allow for PDT in patients with landmarks that are difficult to palpate but are otherwise good candidates for PDT, as well as confirming patients who are not suited for PDT.[25] Ultrasound measurements of the skin-to-trachea distance may also assist in selection of the appropriate tracheostomy tube.[26]

Real-time ultrasound guidance of PDT has also been studied. One study performed 62 successful ultrasound-guided PDTs, using bronchoscopy only after the introduction cannula was inserted to confirm midline placement, avoiding risk to the bronchoscope.[27] Ultrasound guidance has also been used in a neurosurgical population without bronchoscopic guidance, with all subjects undergoing successful uncomplicated PDT, avoiding the transient increase in intracranial pressures commonly seen during bronchoscopy in this patient population.[28] Neither group reported posterior wall lacerations. Although promising, larger trials of ultrasound-guided PDT will need to be done before recommendations to eliminate bronchoscopy as a key component of the procedure can be considered.

Education

The ability to acquire, interpret, and act on ultrasound imaging requires additional training beyond what has traditionally been taught in ultrasound pulmonary fellowship training. There are different avenues to this training. Many courses on critical care ultrasound are commercially available and cover both the image-acquisition techniques and image interpretation necessary for IP applications, as the ultrasound scanning techniques remain constant. Some experts will also come to medical campuses and teach courses tailored to the learner's needs. Lacking in these courses, however, is the high-volume, longitudinal experience needed to master ultrasound techniques. The American College of Chest Physicians and the European Respiratory Society have issued a joint statement on the training requirements for critical care ultrasonography.[29]

A few courses are now starting to offer certificate programs in critical care ultrasonography. These courses typically entail a component similar to the commercial classes and then a period of image acquisition and interpretation at the learner's home institution. A faculty member then reviews the images, and once proficiency is demonstrated and both a video-based and cognitive-based examination passed, a certificate is awarded. These programs will likely continue to grow because of the need for credentialing documentation and longitudinal training.

Other learners obtain the longitudinal component at their home institutions through collaboration with radiologists, emergency medicine physicians, pulmonologists, and other physicians who have sufficient experience to mentor the learner in specific ultrasound techniques. However, given the need for the interventionalist to use ultrasound for diagnostic and procedural guidance, the ideal educational situation is with an IP who can teach both ultrasound and the procedures it is being used to guide. Although critical care physicians have a need for general critical care ultrasound training that encompasses goal-directed echocardiography, thoracic ultrasound, abdominal ultrasound, and vascular diagnostic and access, the IP must become proficient in pleural and lung ultrasound, as well as vascular imaging technique. This has practical considerations when considering time allocation for training.

Coding and Billing

The fee for ultrasonography is the sum of a professional component and technical component. The technical component is charged by the institution owning the equipment, whereas the physician who performs and interprets the examination charges the professional component. If the group performing the study also owns the machine, both components can be charged. The -26 modifier is used to indicate only the professional component is being charged. As billing codes are rules that are continuously changing, the IP practitioner is obligated to confirm codes are accurate and up to date.

Ultrasound codes currently of interest to IP include the following:

76604: Ultrasound, chest, real time with image documentation. This code is used for documenting ultrasound examinations of the chest, mediastinum, chest wall, or pleura for fluids or masses. A report and image documentation need to be placed in the chart.

76942: Ultrasonic guidance for needle placement. This is the ultrasound code for using ultrasound to guide needle placement for thoracentesis or chest tube placement. This code should be billed along with the appropriate procedure code for the corresponding procedure. This code may also be billed along with 76604 if a separate chest examination is performed; however, some private payers may bundle the ultrasound codes together. A report and image documentation need to be placed in the chart.

76536: Ultrasound examination, soft tissues, head and neck. This code would be appropriate for the diagnostic examination of the trachea, vasculature, and thyroid before PDT. As with the other codes, a report and image documentation need to be placed in the chart.

The amount reimbursed per code is dependent on location and payer. Given this, an economic evaluation of the feasibility of purchasing a machine for office use would need to include relevant local reimbursement rates and estimates of what examinations and how many examinations will be performed. The 76604-26 charge is approximately $30. 76942-26 reimburses in the range of $35 to $60. The professional component of 76536 is also in the $30 range. The technical components of all of these codes are significantly higher than the professional components.[30]

SUMMARY

Modern-day point-of-care ultrasonography is revolutionizing pulmonary and critical care practice. Ultrasound is a powerful tool in the hands of the IP, leading to increased patient safety,

enhanced decision making, and cost and time savings. With both reduced cost of portable ultrasound machines and the ease in acquiring competence, the IP will find ultrasound an integral part of daily practice as both a diagnostic tool and an adjunct to therapeutic remedies.

REFERENCES

1. Koenig SJ, Narasimhan M, Mayo PH. Thoracic ultrasonography for the pulmonary specialist. Chest 2011;140(5):1332–41.
2. Lichtenstein DA. Whole body ultrasonography in the critically ill. Berlin: Springer; 2010. p. 117–208.
3. Lichtenstein DA, Menu Y. A bedside ultrasound sign ruling out pneumothorax in the critically ill. Lung sliding. Chest 1995;108(5):1345–8.
4. Lichtenstein D, Mézière G, Biderman P, et al. The comet-tail artifact. An ultrasound sign of alveolar-interstitial syndrome. Am J Respir Crit Care Med 1997;156(5):1640–6.
5. Lichtenstein DA, Mezière GA, Lagoueyte JF, et al. A-lines and B-lines: lung ultrasound as a bedside tool for predicting pulmonary artery occlusion pressure in the critically ill. Chest 2009;136(4):1014–20.
6. Lichtenstein DA, Lascols N, Mezière G, et al. Ultrasound diagnosis of alveolar consolidation in the critically ill. Intensive Care Med 2004;30(2):276–81.
7. Lichtenstein D, Mezière G, Biderman P, et al. The "lung point": an ultrasound sign specific to pneumothorax. Intensive Care Med 2000;26(10):1434–40.
8. Lichtenstein D, Mezière G, Seitz J. The dynamic air bronchogram. A lung ultrasound sign of alveolar consolidation ruling out atelectasis. Chest 2009; 135(6):1421–5.
9. Diacon AH, Theron J, Schubert P, et al. Ultrasound-assisted transthoracic biopsy: fine-needle aspiration or cutting-needle biopsy? Eur Respir J 2007;29(2): 357–62.
10. Bandi V, Lunn W, Ernst A, et al. Ultrasound vs. CT in detecting chest wall invasion by tumor: a prospective study. Chest 2008;133(4):881–6.
11. Chen HJ, Tu CY, Ling SJ, et al. Sonographic appearances in transudative pleural effusions: not always an anechoic pattern. Ultrasound Med Biol 2008; 34(3):362–9.
12. Chian CF, Su WL, Soh LH, et al. Echogenic swirling pattern as a predictor of malignant pleural effusions in patients with malignancies. Chest 2004;126(1): 129–34.
13. Yang PC, Luh KT, Chang DB, et al. Value of sonography in determining the nature of pleural effusion: analysis of 320 cases. AJR Am J Roentgenol 1992; 159(1):29–33.
14. Diacon AH, Brutsche MH, Solèr M. Accuracy of pleural puncture sites: a prospective comparison

of clinical examination with ultrasound. Chest 2003; 123(2):436–41.

15. Yang PC. Ultrasound-guided transthoracic biopsy of the chest. Radiol Clin North Am 2000;38(2):323–43.

16. Yang PC, Luh KT, Lee YC, et al. Lung abscesses: US examination and US-guided transthoracic aspiration. Radiology 1991;180(1):171–5.

17. Cox CE, Carson SS, Holmes GM, et al. Increase in tracheostomy for prolonged mechanical ventilation in North Carolina, 1993-2002. Crit Care Med 2004; 32(11):2219–26.

18. Kornblith LZ, Burlew CC, Moore EE, et al. One thousand bedside percutaneous tracheostomies in the surgical intensive care unit: time to change the gold standard. J Am Coll Surg 2011;212:163–70.

19. Yarmus L, Pandian V, Gilbert C, et al. Safety and efficiency of interventional pulmonologists performing percutaneous tracheostomy. Respiration 2012; 84(2):123–7.

20. Kristensen MS. Ultrasound in the management of the airway. Acta Anaesthesiol Scand 2011;55:1155–73.

21. Muhammad JK, Major E, Wood A, et al. Percutaneous dilational tracheostomy: haemorrhagic complications and the vascular anatomy of the anterior neck. A review based on 497 cases. Int J Oral Maxillofac Surg 2000;29:217–22.

22. Guinot PG, Zogheib E, Petiot S, et al. Ultrasound-guided percutaneous tracheostomy in the critically ill obese patients. Crit Care 2012;16(2):R40.

23. Kollig E, Heydenreich U, Roetman B, et al. Ultrasound and bronchoscopic controlled percutaneous tracheostomy on trauma ICU. Injury 2000;31:663–8.

24. Sustić A, Kovac D, Zgaljardić Z, et al. Ultrasound-guided percutaneous dilational tracheostomy: a safe method to avoid cranial misplacement of the tracheostomy tube. Intensive Care Med 2000; 26(9):1379–81.

25. Muhammad JK, Patton DW, Evans RM, et al. Percutaneous dilational tracheostomy under ultrasound guidance. Br J Oral Maxillofac Surg 1999;37(4): 309–11.

26. Muhammad JK, Major E, Patton DW. Evaluating the neck for percutaneous dilational tracheostomy. J Craniomaxillofac Surg 2000;28(6):336–42.

27. Chacko J, Nikahat J, Gagan B, et al. Real-time ultrasound-guided percutaneous dilational tracheostomy. Intensive Care Med 2012;38(5):920–1.

28. Rajajee V, Fletcher JJ, Rochlen LR, et al. Real-time ultrasound-guided percutaneous dilatational tracheostomy: a feasibility study. Crit Care 2011;15(1):R67.

29. Mayo PH, Beaulieu Y, Doelken P, et al. American College of Chest Physicians/La Société de Réanimation de Langue Française statement on competence in critical care ultrasonography. Chest 2009;135(4): 1050–60.

30. AMA Coding Online. Available at: https://commerce.ama-assn.org/ocm/index.jsp. Accessed August 30, 2012.

Medical Pleuroscopy

Rahul Bhatnagar, MB ChB, MRCP, Nick A. Maskell, DM, FRCP*

KEYWORDS

- Pleuroscopy • Thoracoscopy • Pneumothorax • Empyema • Malignant pleural effusions

KEY POINTS

- There has been an exciting expansion in the practice of medical pleuroscopy in recent years.
- As technology has become more available and as confidence in the use of equipment has grown, medical thoracoscopy has become a core diagnostic and therapeutic tool in pleural disease care.
- Despite all of this, many areas of medical pleuroscopy practice remain conspicuously devoid of well-established evidence.
- More knowledge is needed in those areas where there is currently a degree of equipoise, such as whether thoracoscopic talc poudrage or talc slurry is a more effective method of pleurodesis.
- Similarly, many areas where pleuroscopy currently has a marginal role, such as the prevention of pneumothorax and the management of empyema, require high-quality randomized trials to be undertaken with a view to informing future practice and guidelines.

INTRODUCTION

Medical pleuroscopy recently celebrated its centenary as a recognized intervention[1] and has now firmly established itself as a valuable asset in the respiratory physician's toolbox. Known alternatively as medical thoracoscopy or local anesthetic thoracoscopy, the practice of medical pleuroscopy has seen great strides taken in the last 2 decades, energized by technological progress; improvements in sedation and local anesthetic techniques; and the growing recognition of the importance of pleural disease as a subspecialty of pulmonology.

The primary aim of medical pleuroscopy is to perform an endoscopic examination of the pleura in patients presenting with new undiagnosed pleural effusions, with a view to obtaining a definitive histologic diagnosis, in contrast to video-assisted thoracoscopic surgery (VATS), which was developed to allow surgeons to carry out operations in a minimally invasive fashion, which would otherwise require thoracotomy. Medical pleuroscopy, in the hands of most users, is performed under local anesthetic with amounts of sedation comparable to bronchoscopy, whereas VATS is typically undertaken with anesthetic support to provide single-lung ventilation. Interventions during medical pleuroscopy are therefore usually restricted to pleural fluid drainage, the breakdown of simple adhesions, parietal pleural biopsies, and the administration of pleurodesis agents. Although some practitioners do occasionally undertake some more invasive techniques, the role of the surgeon and the physician remains relatively well defined at this time.

This article aims to bring the reader up to date with the state of medical pleuroscopy, as well as examining the evidence behind current practices and recommendations in the context of its history and possible future directions.

Funding Sources: Dr Bhatnagar has received speaker fees from AstraZeneca and GlaxoSmithKline, and educational grants from Novartis and GlaxoSmithKline. Dr Maskell has received research funding from Novartis and CareFusion. He has also received honoraria from CareFusion for medical advisory board meetings.
Conflicts of Interest: The authors have no conflicts of interests to declare.
Academic Respiratory Unit, University of Bristol, Level 2, Learning and Research Building, Southmead Hospital, Southmead Road, Bristol BS10 5NB, UK
* Corresponding author.
E-mail address: Nick.Maskell@Bristol.ac.uk

Clin Chest Med 34 (2013) 487–500
http://dx.doi.org/10.1016/j.ccm.2013.04.001
0272-5231/13/$ – see front matter © 2013 Elsevier Inc. All rights reserved.

HISTORICAL PERSPECTIVE

Philipp Bozzini (1773–1809) is generally credited as the father of modern endoscopy.[2] Much of his life's work was devoted to perfecting his "light conductor," a device that may be seen as the ancestor of virtually all modern medical instruments which use an external light source to illuminate body cavities or passages. As early as 1807, far before technologies, or indeed attitudes, were able to adapt to his ideas, he predicted that being able to visualize the chest cavity could potentially have benefits in both the diagnosis and treatment of patients.[3]

By the 1840s, the specific term thoracoscopy, or derivatives of it, could be found in French dictionaries and encyclopedias,[4] although there is contention as to whether this constitutes evidence for pleuroscopy, as we would understand it, taking place during this time. Despite the term literally meaning "looking at the thorax," German dictionaries from this period indicate that "thorakoskopie" and "stethoskopie" were used interchangeably, and this may well have been the case across Europe.

There is precious little information to help establish when the practice of pleural endoscopy began to take hold, especially as there seems to have been no significant exchange of knowledge between those who might have been experimenting with it during the mid-nineteenth century. The first documented account of such an examination was, however, published by the Irish physician Samuel Gordon in 1866.[5] In a meticulously detailed paper, he recounts the 8 months of treatment given to an 11-year-old girl with a chronic empyema, which eventually required multiple drain insertions and resulted in the formation of a pleural fistula. Although the word "thoracoscopy" is not used, he tells of occasions when his urologist colleague, Francis Cruise, inserted an endoscope through the fistula opening to allow monitoring of disease progression and states that, to his knowledge, this was the first time such a procedure had been undertaken.

Although Cruise is now regarded as the first person to have performed such an examination, the invention of modern thoracoscopy is typically attributed to a Swedish physician named Hans Christian Jacobaeus (1879–1937). In 1910 he published a paper describing 2 thoracoscopies among a larger series of endoscopic examinations[6] and followed this up a year later with a report on a further 35 cases. He was able to perform his procedures under local anesthetic using an adapted cystoscope, detailing the ideal patient position, port site, and method for air insufflation, as well as describing the cauterization of fibrous bands in tuberculous effusions.[7] Indeed it

was in the management of tuberculosis that thoracoscopy found its first niche, regularly being used to help collapse infected lobes, which were tethered by adhesions, until the 1950s when medical therapy became established. Following this, its popularity declined except for in a few pockets of continental Europe.[1]

The modern resurgence in local anesthetic thoracoscopy began in the 1980s and was bolstered in the 1990s by rapid progress in both fiber optics and video technology. Although there is much overlap in technique, which can be traced back to their common origin, a division now exists between surgeon-led VATS and physician-led medical thoracoscopy, the former drawing heavily from open thoracotomy and laparoscopic practices. As progress continues in both fields, and as physicians' experience widens, it is likely that many techniques that are currently considered surgical will become available to the patients without the need for general anesthesia. For now, however, medical pleuroscopy remains a broadly diagnostic tool, with its surgical counterpart offering much more in terms of therapeutic options.

TECHNICAL AND TRAINING ASPECTS

The basic process involved in thoracoscopy has changed little since the time of Jacobaeus. Patients are placed in the lateral decubitus position, with the abnormal lung uppermost. A dissection is made down to the pleura following instillation of local anesthetic, and a port is placed to guide instruments. Additional ports can be created to allow procedures under direct vision, although the standard medical thoracoscopy tends to utilize a single port approach. Any fluid is drained away using a suction catheter before a camera, attached to a light source, is introduced in to the pleural cavity. This camera tends to be a rigid scope akin to that used during VATS and images are usually displayed on an adjacent monitor (**Fig. 1**). Following examination, biopsy, and/or talc poudrage, the port is replaced with a chest tube to allow the lung to re-expand, with patients typically remaining in the hospital for a few days afterward.[8,9]

Artificial Pneumothorax and Ultrasound

If a patient has a large pleural effusion, the chances of causing damage to the lung itself during the port and scope introduction are remote. However, without real-time ultrasound (US) imaging, it is almost impossible to discern whether portions of the lung may be abnormally adherent to the pleura, or how extensive diaphragmatic excursion may be. Many patients who require a medical

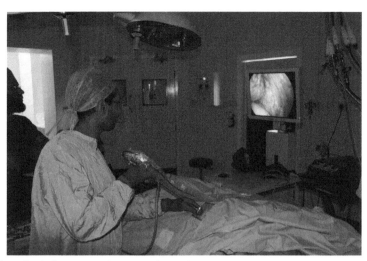

Fig. 1. A standard medical pleuroscopy being performed.

pleuroscopy do not have enough fluid to allow confident safe access to the safe triangle while in the lateral decubitus position, which means additional precautions must be taken. These precautions have historically involved the creation of a pneumothorax by the introduction of air through a blunt needle before the procedure,[10] but this process can be time-consuming.

Pleural intervention has been revolutionized by the widespread availability of bedside US, with national guidelines now recommending all such procedures be performed with US guidance.[11] Although the cost benefits of purchasing a machine purely for use during pleuroscopy could be argued against, most respiratory departments now have access to US machines intended for all pleural indications, allowing its use immediately before each procedure. A large series by Macha and colleagues[12] showed that 20 to 30 minutes could be saved from total pleuroscopy duration by using US to target port placement, and this is likely to be a conservative estimate. Another recent study was able to demonstrate a strong trend toward reducing access failure in those undergoing pleuroscopy as well as a reduction in the number of pneumothoraces needing to be induced.[13] There will undoubtedly be a continuing need to create an artificial pneumothorax in patients who have small volumes of pleural fluid (**Fig. 2**), but the routine use of US should be encouraged because it removes any uncertainty regarding access site in those with more significant collections. This US should be performed immediately before dissection begins and also in the outpatient setting (with the patient in the lateral decubitus position) during the process of deciding whether to perform the procedure.

Contraindications

The main concern when undertaking any form of pleural endoscopy is the potential to damage internal structures. For this reason, an operator should not attempt to insert a thoracoscope if a lung has been unable to collapse, which may occur because of obliteration of the pleural space by the underlying disease process. Beyond this, general contraindications to virtually any interventional procedure continue to apply in the case of medical pleuroscopy, including uncorrected bleeding diathesis, cardiovascular instability, pulmonary hypertension, and untreated hypoxemia. Patients should be able to tolerate the procedure by lying comfortably on their side, remembering that a significant proportion of any breathlessness will likely be improved by fluid drainage early on. With this in mind, guidelines suggest patients with a World Health Organization Performance Status of 2 or better (discounting fluid-related dyspnea) should be considered suitable for this procedure. However, it should also be mentioned that just because it is technically possible to undertake this procedure, it does not always mean this is the right way to manage a situation optimally. The questions should always be asked—"What is the added benefit of performing this invasive procedure to the patient?" and "Would a more conservative approach be more appropriate?"

Potential Complications

A reason for the on-going uptake in medical pleuroscopy is an acceptance that it is a safe and well-tolerated procedure. Nonetheless, patients should have consent taken with the knowledge that serious intraoperative or perioperative

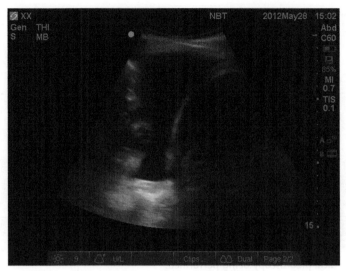

Fig. 2. An ultrasound image shows a small pleural effusion, taken in the lateral decubitus position. Some may choose to induce an artificial pneumothorax in the presence of a small-volume collection.

complications can occur. These complications include hemorrhage, port site tumor invasion, persistent air leak, pneumonia, and empyema, although all are rare. Pooled data from 51 studies, including 4956 patients (47 of which were analyzed by Rahman and colleagues[9] as part of a wide-ranging review),[8,14–16] showed a major complication rate of 2.1%. Mortality associated with pleuroscopy is extremely uncommon, with most deaths seemingly caused by pre-existing medical factors or as a result of reactions unrelated to the procedure itself.[17] In combined data from 5054 patients, the total number of deaths was 17 (0.34%).[8,9,14–16,18] The rates of both mortality and major complications for medical pleuroscopy are comparable to VATS.[19] Minor complications, such as transient hypoxemia or transient hypotension, and subcutaneous emphysema are less well reported. However, data assembled from 2411 patients in 31 studies have shown an expected overall rate of 7.3%,[9] most of which will not prolong hospital stay (see **Table 1**).[20]

There are also separate risks that result from the procedures associated with medical pleuroscopy, rather than the pleuroscopy itself. By adopting a local anesthetic approach, the risks of intubation, ventilation, and general anesthesia are removed. These risks tend to be replaced with the lower risk profile of short-acting sedatives, such as a benzodiazepine in combination with an opiate, but can vary considerably according to local expertise. This expertise can dramatically affect complication rates; a recent study that used titrated propofol noted hypotension in 64% of patients, 9% of them requiring corrective measures.[15] Other authors suggest the use of even sedation alone should warrant routine transcutaneous blood carbon dioxide measurement, alongside oxygen measurement, as patients have been found to hypoventilate significantly during thoracoscopy.[21]

Training and Competency

There is no international consensus on what constitutes adequate training in medical pleuroscopy. The American College of Chest Physicians recommend a minimum of 20 supervised procedures before operators are considered competent, with an additional minimum of 10 each year to maintain this,[22] although robust self-audit by practitioners will always be required to ensure standards are met locally. The British Thoracic Society outlines 3 levels of thoracoscopic competence, although the levels of training required for the levels I and II, into which basic and advanced medical pleuroscopy fall, have not yet been fully established.[9] The number of centers in the UK able to perform pleuroscopy tripled between 1999 and 2009,[9] despite many of these already having access to thoracic surgical expertise. Demand for services is likely to find a plateau, which means that the number of physicians who both need to be and can be trained will be limited.[23] For the time being, however, it is important that opportunities for exposure to pleuroscopy are maximized both locally, and through the provision of accredited training courses.

General Appearances

On entering the pleural space, an operator should be able to appreciate the collapsed lung, the mobile diaphragm, the visceral and parietal pleural surfaces, and the outline of ribs deep to the latter. The normal parietal pleural surface, seen under standard white light, is translucent and has a shiny appearance, allowing underlying structures such as ribs and muscles to be seen below. Erythematous or generally inflamed areas of pleura suggest abnormality and can represent a variety of pleural conditions including tuberculosis, which can also produce a widespread shallow nodularity. Such areas are likely biopsy targets (**Figs. 3** and **4**). Pleura that has been infiltrated by malignancy may also appear this way in its early stages, but as disease progresses often more pronounced pleural nodularity and thickening become apparent (**Figs. 5** and **6**). In patients with pneumothoraces, small discrete visceral pleural blebs may be appreciated on the lung surface. Exudative pleural effusions can cause fibrotic pleural deposition, appearing as an additional pleural layer that sloughs off easily during biopsy. More aggressive fibrotic processes such as empyema can also lead to adhesions or loculations forming, which appear as fixed bands traversing the pleural space with attachments to both the visceral and the parietal membranes (**Fig. 7**), sometimes tethering the lung to the diaphragm, limiting the movement of both. These membranes can often be divided by instrumentation, but this should be avoided if the adhesion looks to have a vascular component. Other commonly seen abnormalities include asbestos-related pleural plaques, appearing as discrete white patches that are rock hard to the touch (**Fig. 8**), and anthracosis, which appears as black spots in the lung parenchyma itself, visible

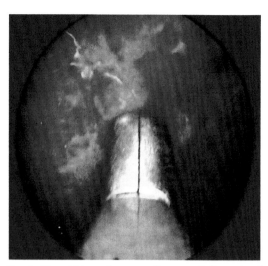

Fig. 4. Closed biopsy forceps adjacent to inflamed and nodular pleural surface.

through the visceral pleural layer. This latter abnormality may be associated with mineral dust exposure, or urban living, or as a result of smoking.

DIAGNOSTIC INDICATIONS

The identification and classification of pleural abnormalities have been at the heart of medical thoracoscopy since its inception, and this has remained true despite the increasing therapeutic possibilities afforded by technological advancements. The gold standard for pleural sampling remains open thoracotomy, which allows for complete hemi-thorax visualization, surgical field control, and effectively unlimited biopsy sample size. VATS has largely replaced thoracotomy as

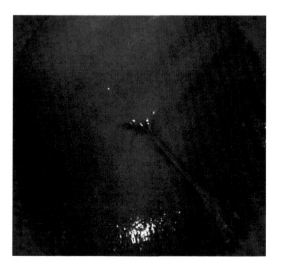

Fig. 3. Generalized inflammatory pleuritis, which may be seen in conditions such as tuberculosis. An adhesion is visible in the center of the image and stretches between the lung and the chest wall.

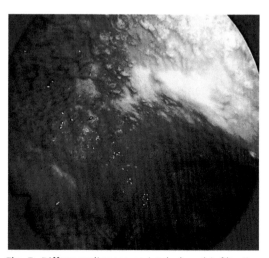

Fig. 5. Diffuse malignant parietal pleural infiltration with nodularity and erythema. The deflated lung is just visible at 7 o' clock.

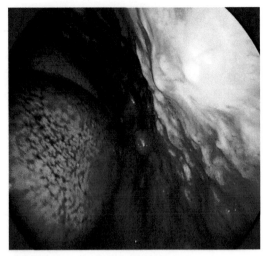

Fig. 6. Coarse nodular malignant infiltration of the parietal pleura. Note the anthracotic changes in the lung parenchyma.

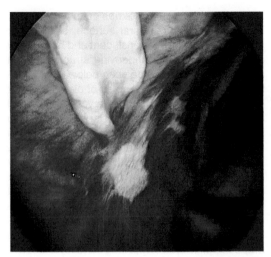

Figs. 8. 3 Asbestos-related pleural plaques can be appreciated, seen as a well-demarcated flat white area. The largest is just below the center of the camera's visual field. A large fatty deposit is also visible superiorly.

a routine procedure, but this still requires single-lung ventilation and general anesthesia, which many patients who present with pleural abnormalities, especially those who may have malignancy, may be unable to tolerate. However, by accessing the pleural space with conscious sedation and local anesthesia, the physician may be able to offer similar levels of diagnostic accuracy to a wider range of patients, but with diminished risk of mortality[19] and an associated reduction in the pressure on what are often limited surgical resources.

Undiagnosed Effusions and Pleural Malignancy

There are over 50 potential causes for a pleural effusion, with or without pleural thickening.[11] Many of these will be distinguishable through careful history and examination, or through basic tests performed following thoracentesis, and require little in terms of invasive investigation. However, around 20% of pleural effusions will remain undiagnosed,[24] even with percutaneous biopsy being used as a second-line investigation. The primary question in undiagnosed effusions is generally whether there is evidence of malignancy or not, and it is in answering this that pleuroscopy comes into its own.

For those patients in whom malignant pleural involvement is suspected, whether it be a primary or a metastatic process, the traditional and simplest methods of diagnosis can be disappointingly insensitive. Pleural fluid cytologic examination is unable to identify malignancy in any more than 60% of patients, even with multiple samples being taken,[25] and this figure is significantly lower in those with mesothelioma.[26] Blind pleural biopsy sampling has the ability to increase yields,[11] but is limited in its overall success rates because it is not uncommon for malignant disease to affect the pleura in a patchy manner, often with a predilection for relatively inaccessible paradiaphragmatic areas.[27] Progress has been made in image-guided biopsy techniques and, by using pleural-phase contrast computed tomography, radiologists are now increasingly able to aid in

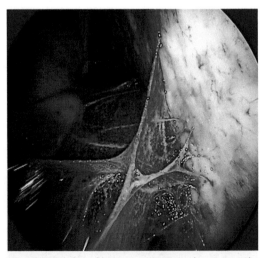

Fig. 7. Complex fibrous septations between the visceral and thickened parietal pleura as a result of pleural infection. Loculated fluid is appreciable below the fibrous layer, which would make complete drainage extremely difficult with standard tube drainage alone.

identifying cancerous pleural infiltration with accuracy far superior to blind methods and comparable to pleuroscopic biopsy.[28] Nonetheless, aside from the ever-present burden of service provision faced by imaging departments, image-guided biopsy is limited in the number of samples that may be taken at any one time, as opposed to pleuroscopy, during which an effectively unlimited number of pleural biopsy samples can be obtained, as long as hemostasis and patient comfort is maintained. Most practitioners recommend that a minimum of 8 to 12 biopsy samples are taken for histologic analysis, ideally over a rib, targeting areas of visual abnormality but avoiding the costophrenic recesses if possible. If no visible abnormality exists, samples are usually taken from areas of high lymphatic drainage. Pleuroscopy also has the advantage of allowing operators to perform therapeutic interventions such as immediate large volume thoracentesis, or preventative ones such as pleurodesis, as well as permitting direct visualization of pleural abnormalities.[27]

Several studies have reported on the diagnostic accuracy of thoracoscopy in malignancy (**Table 1**). Earlier series seemed to demonstrate significant variability, perhaps being limited by developing techniques, with overall values ranging from as low as 69% up to 100%.[29–32] Pooling results from all of these gives a combined diagnostic rate of 92.6%, based on a total sample of 1369 patients,[33] which is certainly comparable to rates achieved using VATS.[34] Some disparity in diagnostic values

also seems to exist when pleural mesothelioma is analyzed separately, with a series by Boutin and Rey[35] reporting a 98% success rate compared with 60% in another, marginally smaller, series.[30] Separate to diagnostic ability, however, is the appeal of the one-stop thoracoscopic approach, which is especially strong in mesothelioma given the extremely high rates of recurrent pleural effusion in this condition.[36]

Tuberculosis

Tissue culture is the ideal way to establish a diagnosis of tuberculosis (TB) because the disease has a strong tendency toward pleural infiltration. Blind pleural biopsy can identify TB in around 80% of cases,[41] which makes it a sensible first-line technique given that it is widely available and well-established around the world. Few studies have addressed the detection of TB pleurisy using pleuroscopy directly, but a prospective series by Diacon and colleagues[42] compared this method to both Abrams biopsy and standard fluid analysis. They showed that pleuroscopic biopsies were the most effective method for confirming TB, with an overall sensitivity of 100%. Current guidelines suggest that this method should be considered as an appropriate follow-on step in those patients in whom standard biopsy has failed to give a diagnosis.[9] Aside from this situation, pleuroscopy should also be considered if lung expansion is impeded by significant adhesions or if multidrug

Table 1
Complication rates and pick-up rates for malignancy from the current 10 largest series of diagnostic medical pleuroscopy

Study	Total Patients	Diagnostic Rate for Malignancy (%)	Mortality (%)	Major Complication Rate (%)	Minor Complication Rate (%)
Macha et al,[12] 1993	687	94	0	4/687 (0.6)	"Very few"
Boutin & Rey,[35] 1993	188	98	0	4/188 (2.1)	30/188 (6.9)
Hansen et al,[37] 1998	146	90.4	0	3/146 (2.1)	2/146 (1.4)
Sakuraba et al,[32] 2006	138	97.1	0	0/138 (0)	"Few"
Metintas et al,[28] 2010	124	94.1	0	3/124 (2.4)	22/124 (17.7)
Medford et al,[8] 2009	124	97.4	0.8	5/124 (4.0)	n/a
Kapsenberg,[38] 1981	115	95	0	0/115 (0)	0/115 (0)
Menzies & Charbonneau,[39] 1991	104	93.1	0	6/104 (5.8)	2/104 (1.9)
Wilsher & Veale,[40] 1998	58	85	0	4/58 (6.9)	n/a
Brims et al,[16] 2012	57	97.5	0	16/57 (28.1)	11/57 (19.3)

Major complications include pneumonia and empyema, significant hemorrhage, persistent air leak or pneumothorax, and port site metastasis. Minor complications include port site infection, transient hypotension, pyrexia, and minor bleeding.
Abbreviation: n/a, not applicable.

resistance is being considered, as this typically requires larger amounts of tissue to be taken for analysis.[43]

Parenchymal Lung Disease

Some centers, mainly European, advocate the use of pleuroscopy to aid the diagnosis of interstitial lung disease. Pleuroscopy usually takes place once bronchoscopic biopsy has proven inadequate and forms a bridge between this and open lung biopsy, allowing pinch samples to be taken. Such samples are of particular use in the diagnosis and classification of diffuse interstitial lung disease and pneumonitis in the immunocompromised.[44] A study by Vansteenkiste and colleagues[45] revealed an average biopsy sample size of 4 mm, which was good enough to provide a diagnosis in 75% of cases. Other studies suggest this figure can be improved on, but collating data reveals few patients have been formally analyzed in this way.[9,38] A lack of uptake in this area of thoracoscopy may mean that visceral biopsy represents the line over which most practitioners think only those with formal surgical training should cross; however, there is nothing to suggest that biopsies obtained this way are inherently more dangerous than open surgical biopsies, and indeed, some authors report thoracoscopic lung biopsies are better tolerated than bronchoscopic ones.[45] Nonetheless, a formal surgical lung biopsy currently remains the recommended definitive investigation for interstitial lung disease[46] in much of the world and is likely to remain so for the foreseeable future.

THERAPEUTIC INDICATIONS

One of the enduring appeals of pleural endoscopy is the ability to intervene in disease processes actively. Multiport procedures provide a high degree of flexibility and in appropriately trained hands can allow operations to be performed that would have historically needed a thoracotomy. Of course, the more complex a procedure, the higher the likelihood of complication, be that damage to viscera or other internal structures, or significant bleeding. This means that more advanced pleural intervention tends to be the domain of thoracic surgeons, who are often better equipped with the requisite skills to deal with difficulties as they arise, or to convert to thoracotomy if needed. Physician-led medical pleuroscopy typically relies on single-port access and this, along with a more limited level of technical expertise, tends to limit the type of intervention that can be achieved. Nonetheless, as pleuroscopy experience has grown in specialist centers around the world, more complex interventions such as sympathectomy or splanchnicolysis are now able to be managed with little or no surgical input whatsoever.[47,48]

Malignant Pleural Effusions and Pleurodesis

Debate continues to exist about the most appropriate way to manage malignant pleural effusions, with the role of medical pleuroscopy, and specifically talc poudrage, being at the heart of the issue.[49,50] Although every patient's case should be addressed individually and should take into account local provisions and policies, the options for dealing with such effusions can be broadly divided into 2 options: outpatient or inpatient. Outpatient management tends to revolve around the placement of an ambulatory indwelling pleural catheter (IPC) to allow repeated fluid drainage, whereas the inpatient approach involves administering a pleural sclerosant to try and induce pleurodesis and prevent future fluid recurrence. The use of an IPC effectively sacrifices an increased likelihood of pleurodesis (50% of patients at most will undergo spontaneous pleural adhesion with the drain in situ[51,52]) for the convenience of potentially avoiding all hospital admissions relating to fluid management. They are particularly useful in patients with trapped lung, in whom attempting pleurodesis is unlikely to be of benefit,[17] and some studies even suggest that IPCs can be cheaper than inpatient alternatives if they are used over a limited period of time.[53] It should also be remembered that although patients can have their IPC inserted and managed as an outpatient, health care contact may actually increase because community services may be called on to manage regular drainages.

For those patients requiring inpatient management of their malignant pleural effusion, the discussion revolves around what is the most effective way to perform a pleurodesis, essentially trying to limit the patient's hospital experience to a single definitive episode. Traditional management revolves around inserting a chest tube and following this with instillation of a chemical sclerosant, a process that typically takes around 1 week.[54] Various agents have historically been used, including bleomycin, doxycycline, tetracycline (which is no longer produced),[55] and bacterial protein derivatives such as OK-432.[56] The general consensus, however, is that sterile talc powder is the irritant with the best chance of success, and this has now become the standard in much of the world. For many years, the use of intrapleural talc was associated severe inflammatory response, including acute respiratory distress syndrome, but cases of such reactions have become very rare following the introduction of graded talc, in which smaller particles have been removed at source.[57,58]

When inserted via a chest drain, talc powder is first reconstituted as slurry, relying on adequate drainage having taken place to allow pleural apposition. Talc is then distributed over the pleural surfaces by respiratory motion. Studies that have looked to analyze pleurodesis with slurry have demonstrated variable percentage success rates, but on average, slurry pleurodesis with talc is quoted as successful 80% of the time.[59]

Intuitively, being able to distribute talc more evenly over the pleural surfaces should result in a more even inflammatory process, and therefore, a greater chance of meaningful pleurodesis. At the end of a thoracoscopy, with most of the pleural surface exposed, talc powder can be insufflated through the port site (poudrage), with visual inspection often confirming an even powder coating. Interestingly, however, computed tomography scans of patients who have undergone slurry treatment tend to have a typical "talc sandwich" appearance concentrated at the bases,[60] regardless of mode of application, implying a degree of redistribution occurs after poudrage.

The efficacy of talc poudrage for pleurodesis has been documented in several studies.[17,61–64] Published success rates tend to be slightly higher than those for slurry, although there is significant heterogeneity between study groups, which limits reliability. Direct comparison of talc slurry and talc poudrage was within the scope of the 2004 Cochrane review, which, along with suggesting talc was the most efficacious sclerosant, found talc poudrage at thoracoscopy to have an improved relative risk of non-recurrence (1.19) over talc slurry.[55] A subsequent large randomized trial by Dresler and colleagues[17] had some methodological flaws but did not show an overall significant difference between the talc slurry and poudrage. In post-hoc analysis, stratification by disease subtype revealed a clinically important 45% decrease in pleurodesis failure rate with thoracoscopy in good performance status patients with lung or breast cancer (thoracoscopy 18% failure vs tube 33%, $P = .02$). A further large, but nonrandomized, series showed talc poudrage also had fewer failures than talc slurry (12% vs 31%).[65] However, this study did not use the clinical outcome of repeat pleural drainage as an endpoint and had an unusually high proportion of patients with gastrointestinal malignancy.

Given the above evidence, a decision has not been reached on what is the best approach for managing malignant effusions, and thus what role pleuroscopy has to play beyond diagnosis. It is likely that some form of inpatient pleurodesis method will always be required for a proportion of patients. With this in mind, a large randomized controlled trial of talc poudrage versus slurry is currently being recruited to in the UK with results likely to be published in 24 months time.

For some authors, a merging of the outpatient approach, for patient convenience, and the inpatient approach, for a greater chance of pleurodesis success, has proven successful on a small scale. In a pilot study of 30 patients with recurrent malignant effusion, Reddy and colleagues[66] performed thoracoscopy and poudrage with simultaneous placement of an IPC under direct vision, which was then drained aggressively until output reduced. Patients had a median time in hospital of less than 2 days and had their IPC in place for a median of 7.5 days before removal. Both breathlessness and performance status improved and in the 26 patients who were alive at 6 months, 24 (92%) had remained free of fluid recurrence.

Although this was a small series, which undoubtedly represented a more costly approach in the initial stages, management pathways prioritizing outpatient techniques and minimal time in the hospital should certainly be the subject of larger randomized trials, the aim being to give patients with malignant effusions, in whom life expectancy is short, as high a quality of life as possible. Medical pleuroscopy clearly has a vital role in this because it is currently the method that allows the most rapid and complete application of talc for pleurodesis.

Pneumothorax

British and American management algorithms for primary spontaneous pneumothorax suggest definitive intervention (with a view to preventing recurrence) only needs to be taken in the event of a second ipsilateral primary pneumothorax, or a first contralateral episode.[67,68] Options for treatment include bleb or bullae removal, pleurectomy, and pleurodesis via either mechanical abrasion or talc poudrage. These treatments tend to be performed using VATS and general anesthetic as many feel treatment can be performed more effectively under single-lung ventilation, and because the application of talc to the normal pleural surface can be exquisitely painful to patients. Some would argue against this, especially as there is not necessarily a correlation between air leak and the location of visual abnormalities.[69]

European practice tends to favor a more aggressive initial approach, and in many centers medical thoracoscopy is a first-line treatment for primary spontaneous pneumothorax. Tschopp and colleagues[70] randomized 108 such patients to either thoracoscopy and poudrage, or chest drain and talc slurry, and were able to show a significantly reduced rate of recurrence at 5 years (5% vs 34%) in the thoracoscopy arm, suggesting this approach certainly has merit. Similar efficacy for poudrage at thoracoscopy has been demonstrated in patients with secondary pneumothoraces due to chronic obstructive pulmonary disease, albeit in a less robust manner,[71] with this group of patients potentially being of particular interest to medical thoracoscopy because they are more likely to be unfit for VATS interventions.

Pleural Infection

It is universally agreed on that complicated pleural space infection or empyema requires drainage, unless a late-stage fibrothorax has developed, in which case thoracic surgery is required. The timing and method by which drainage occurs remains a matter for debate. Although early trials with fibrinolytic therapy proved inconclusive overall, recent evidence suggests that complicated pleural effusions can be treated effectively with combination t-PA and DNase, with less than 5% of patients requiring surgical referral at 3 months.[72] Some practitioners, however, advocate the use of early medical pleuroscopy with the aim of breaking down adhesions, accurately placing chest tubes, and improving fluid outflow.[73] Although this is instinctively appealing, current practice relies heavily on expert opinion as there remain only 4 published studies in this area at the time of writing,[18,74–76] none of them randomized, which give a combined rate of 90% (172/191) for avoiding surgery. It should be noted that in the largest study among these,[76] which contributed 127 patients, 49% of patients had intrapleural fibrinolysis in association with their pleuroscopy, and that in the series by Ravaglia and colleagues,[18] only 50% of patients with evidence of intrapleural organization avoided surgery. These latter points suggest that if there is to be a more prominent role for medical pleuroscopy in the management of empyema, the ability to physically divide more difficult adhesions successfully is a key point, currently the remit of expert operators, but as experience grows, pleuroscopy, perhaps in combination with fibrinolytics, may become more widely used to ensure more patients avoid the need for surgery.

NOVEL TECHNIQUES AND FUTURE DIRECTIONS
Semi-rigid and Mini-Scopes

Although some consider it to be a harder skill than thoracoscopy,[10] the use of a flexible bronchoscope is perhaps more familiar to most respiratory physicians. Rigid thoracoscopes allow a large working channel to be maintained but reduce the area of the pleural cavity which is easily accessible, especially if a single entry port is used. Practitioners identified the potential for a more flexible scope early on, with studies experimenting with the introduction of a standard flexible bronchoscope into the pleural space instead of a rigid scope.[77,78] The conclusions were that that this adaptation could be made safely and easily but that more satisfactory biopsies were obtained using the standard instrument, perhaps because a lack of proximal rigidity reduces dexterity in the distal portion of the scope. Yokoyama and colleagues[79] looked to overcome this in a small series by directing the flexible bronchoscope through a 32-French chest tube, concluding that this technique may represent a cheap and accessible alternative to rigid thoracoscopy. A potentially more satisfactory alternative is an integrated device, which was first described in 1998.[80] Stiff at the site of chest entry but flexible distally, the semirigid thoracoscope has been shown to have a similar diagnostic sensitivity to its rigid alternative,[81,82] and, being autoclavable, can be reused rapidly. Biopsy samples tend to be smaller,[83] however, and so, although this hybrid device remains promising, further comparative studies are needed before rigid thoracoscopy can be displaced as the standard.

Minithoracoscopy uses smaller ports and instruments to perform pleural intervention in as minimally invasive a way as possible. Two access points are created: one for a scope, the other for interventional forceps, with both being less than 4 mm in diameter. This technique potentially allows safer access to smaller pleural spaces, or can be used in those with narrow intercostal spaces, with a sacrifice being made in the maximum possible biopsy size. The equipment is more fragile and takes longer to use, but patients are better able to tolerate the procedure and the smaller incision required necessitates smaller amounts of anesthesia postoperatively and also negates the need for sutures. Minithoracoscopy almost certainly has an ancillary role in the investigation of pleural disease, but as long as medical pleuroscopy is primarily applied to obtain diagnostic biopsies, it is unlikely to be used on anything other than a case-by-case basis.[84]

Autofluorescence Thoracoscopy

Standard endoscopic examination, whether that be bronchoscopic or thoracoscopic, uses white light to illuminate internal surfaces and structures.

This endoscopic examination allows visually abnormal areas to be targeted for intervention such as biopsy, or in the case of pneumothorax, bleb removal. The concept of using fluorescing chemicals to detect pleural abnormalities has been around for at least a decade, as Prosst and colleagues[85] instilled 5-ALA into rats who had been inoculated with tumor cells, showing promising results when later examined using VATS. In a more recent study, this same substance was administered orally to patients with undiagnosed pleural effusions before surgical thoracoscopy, the authors concluding that visualization of pleural malignancy was improved.[86] An alternative method is fluorescein-enhanced autofluorescence thoracoscopy (or "blue-light" thoracoscopy); this has been used in the medical setting. Nebulized fluorescein is inhaled before the procedure, with enough time left for it to permeate the outer portions of the lung. Following standard white-light examination, the scope is switched to blue-light mode, which allows any fluorescein on the visceral pleural surface to be seen. Noppen and colleagues[87] performed a small consecutive controlled series, which looked at fluorescein-enhanced autofluorescence thoracoscopy in primary spontaneous pneumothorax, and were able to demonstrate several important features. High levels of fluorescein leakage were only seen in patients with pneumothorax and typically occurred in zones that appeared normal on white-light examination. In addition, those areas that were abnormal using autofluorescence correlated poorly with the location of blebs and bullae seen on white light, all of which suggests that air leak may not be fully appreciable using traditional local anesthetic thoracoscopy methods.

Blue-light pleuroscopy remains in its infancy, with animal studies still being performed to clarify such factors as the optimum timing of fluorescein administration,[88] and pilot studies being performed to clarify its role in malignant pleural disease.[89] Nonetheless, with the contrast material readily available, and with autofluorescence equipment already familiar to many pulmonary physicians, it is possible that this technique may have a diagnostic role in the future.

SUMMARY

There has been an exciting expansion in the practice of medical pleuroscopy in recent years. As technology has become more available and as confidence in the use of equipment has grown, medical thoracoscopy has become a core diagnostic and therapeutic tool in pleural disease care. It now represents a de facto gold standard

in the management of undiagnosed effusions and perhaps offers the most effective way to manage malignant pleural effusions by affording the ability to apply talc while significantly reducing hospital attendance time. It is likely the boundaries of what is possible for physicians will continue to be pushed—there now being an ever-growing group of expert practitioners who are able to perform procedures and treat conditions under local anesthetic that were traditionally the domain of thoracic surgeons.

Despite all of this, many areas of medical pleuroscopy practice remain conspicuously devoid of well-established evidence. More knowledge is needed in those areas where there is currently a degree of equipoise, such as whether thoracoscopic talc poudrage or talc slurry is a more effective method of pleurodesis. Similarly, many areas where pleuroscopy currently has a marginal role, such as the prevention of pneumothorax and the management of empyema, require high-quality randomized trials to be undertaken with a view to informing future practice and guidelines.

REFERENCES

1. Marchetti GP, Pinelli V, Tassi GF. 100 Years of thoracoscopy: historical notes. Respiration 2011;82: 187–92.
2. Hoksch B, Birken-Bertsch H, Muller JM. Thoracoscopy before Jacobaeus. Ann Thorac Surg 2002; 74:1288–90.
3. Bozzini P. Der Lichtleiter Oder Die Beschreibung Einer Einfachen Vorrichtung Und Ihrer Anwendung Zur Erleuchtung Innerer Hohlen Und Zwischenraume des Lebenden Animalischen Korpers. Weimar (Germany): Verlag Des Landes Industrie Compoir; 1807.
4. Complement du Dictionnaire de l'Academie Francaise. Paris: Firmin Didot frères; 1842.
5. Gordon S. Clinical reports of rare cases, occurring in the Whitworth and Hardwicke hospitals: most extensive pleuritic effusion rapidly becoming purulent, paracentesis, introduction of a drainage tube, recovery, examination of interior of pleura by the endoscope. Dublin Quarterly Journal of Medical Science 1866;41:83–90.
6. Jacobaeus HC. Ueber Die Moglichkeit Die Zystoskopie Bei Untersuchung Seroser Hohlungen Anzuwenden. Munch Med Wochenschr 1910;57:2090–2.
7. Jacobaeus HC. Kurze Uebersicht Uber Meine Erfahrungen mit der Laparo-Thoracoscopie. Munch Med Wochenschr 1911;58:2017–9.
8. Medford AR, Agrawal S, Free CM, et al. A local anaesthetic video-assisted thoracoscopy service: prospective performance analysis in a UK tertiary respiratory centre. Lung Cancer 2009;66:355–8.

9. Rahman NM, Ali NJ, Brown G, et al. Local anaesthetic thoracoscopy: British Thoracic Society pleural disease guideline 2010. Thorax 2010;65(Suppl 2): ii54–60.

10. Loddenkemper R. Thoracoscopy–state of the art. Eur Respir J 1998;11:213–21.

11. Hooper C, Lee YC, Maskell N, et al. Investigation of a unilateral pleural effusion in adults: British Thoracic Society Pleural Disease Guideline 2010. Thorax 2010;65(Suppl 2):ii4–17.

12. Macha HN, Reichle G, Von Zwehl D, et al. The role of ultrasound assisted thoracoscopy in the diagnosis of pleural disease. Clinical experience in 687 cases. Eur J Cardiothorac Surg 1993;7:19–22.

13. Medford AR, Agrawal S, Bennett JA, et al. Thoracic ultrasound prior to medical thoracoscopy improves pleural access and predicts fibrous septation. Respirology 2010;15:804–8.

14. Agnoletti V, Gurioli C, Piraccini E, et al. Efficacy and safety of thoracic paravertebral block for medical thoracoscopy. Br J Anaesth 2011;106:916–7.

15. Tschopp JM, Purek L, Frey JG, et al. Titrated sedation with propofol for medical thoracoscopy: a feasibility and safety study. Respiration 2011;82: 451–7.

16. Brims FJ, Arif M, Chauhan AJ. Outcomes and complications following medical thoracoscopy. Clin Respir J 2012;6:144–9.

17. Dresler CM, Olak J, Herndon JE 2nd, et al. Phase III Intergroup Study of talc poudrage vs talc slurry sclerosis for malignant pleural effusion. Chest 2005;127:909–15.

18. Ravaglia C, Gurioli C, Tomassetti S, et al. Is medical thoracoscopy efficient in the management of multiloculated and organized thoracic empyema? Respiration 2012;84:219–24.

19. Imperatori A, Rotolo N, Gatti M, et al. Peri-operative complications of video-assisted thoracoscopic surgery (VATS). Int J Surg 2008;6(Suppl 1):S78–81.

20. Michaud G, Berkowitz DM, Ernst A. Pleuroscopy for diagnosis and therapy for pleural effusions. Chest 2010;138:1242–6.

21. Chhajed PN, Kaegi B, Rajasekaran R, et al. Detection of hypoventilation during thoracoscopy: combined cutaneous carbon dioxide tension and oximetry monitoring with a new digital sensor. Chest 2005;127:585–8.

22. Ernst A, Silvestri GA, Johnstone D, et al. Interventional pulmonary procedures: guidelines from the American College of Chest Physicians. Chest 2003;123:1693–717.

23. Medford AR, Bennett JA, Free CM, et al. Current status of medical pleuroscopy. Clin Chest Med 2010;31:165–72 Table of Contents.

24. Boutin C, Viallat JR, Cargnino P, et al. Thoracoscopy in malignant pleural effusions. Am Rev Respir Dis 1981;124:588–92.

25. Garcia LW, Ducatman BS, Wang HH. The value of multiple fluid specimens in the cytological diagnosis of malignancy. Mod Pathol 1994;7: 665–8.

26. Walters J, Maskell NA. Biopsy techniques for the diagnosis of mesothelioma. Recent Results Cancer Res 2011;189:45–55.

27. Canto A, Rivas J, Saumench J, et al. Points to consider when choosing a biopsy method in cases of pleurisy of unknown origin. Chest 1983; 84:176–9.

28. Metintas M, Ak G, Dundar E, et al. Medical thoracoscopy vs CT scan-guided Abrams pleural needle biopsy for diagnosis of patients with pleural effusions: a randomized, controlled trial. Chest 2010; 137:1362–8.

29. Enk B, Viskum K. Diagnostic thoracoscopy. Eur J Respir Dis 1981;62:344–51.

30. Page RD, Jeffrey RR, Donnelly RJ. Thoracoscopy: a review of 121 consecutive surgical procedures. Ann Thorac Surg 1989;48:66–8.

31. Weissberg D, Kaufmann M. Diagnostic and therapeutic pleuroscopy. Experience with 127 patients. Chest 1980;78:732–5.

32. Sakuraba M, Masuda K, Hebisawa A, et al. Diagnostic value of thoracoscopic pleural biopsy for pleurisy under local anaesthesia. ANZ J Surg 2006;76:722–4.

33. Davies HE, Nicholson JE, Rahman NM, et al. Outcome of patients with nonspecific pleuritis/ fibrosis on thoracoscopic pleural biopsies. Eur J Cardiothorac Surg 2010;38:472–7.

34. Harris RJ, Kavuru MS, Mehta AC, et al. The impact of thoracoscopy on the management of pleural disease. Chest 1995;107:845–52.

35. Boutin C, Rey F. Thoracoscopy in pleural malignant mesothelioma: a prospective study of 188 consecutive patients. Part 1: diagnosis. Cancer 1993;72: 389–93.

36. Robinson BW. Malignant mesothelioma. Chapter 41. In: Light RW, Gary Lee YC, editors. Textbook of pleural diseases. London, UK: Hodder Arnold; 2008. p. 507–15.

37. Hansen M, Faurschou P, Clementsen P. Medical thoracoscopy, results and complications in 146 patients: a retrospective study. Respir Med 1998;92: 228–32.

38. Kapsenberg PD. Thoracoscopic biopsy under visual control. Poumon Coeur 1981;37:313–6.

39. Menzies R, Charbonneau M. Thoracoscopy for the diagnosis of pleural disease. Ann Intern Med 1991; 114:271–6.

40. Wilsher ML, Veale AG. Medical thoracoscopy in the diagnosis of unexplained pleural effusion. Respirology 1998;3:77–80.

41. Loddenkemper R, Mai J, Scheffler N, et al. Prospective individual comparison of blind needle

biopsy and of thoracoscopy in the diagnosis and differential diagnosis of tuberculous pleurisy. Scand J Respir Dis Suppl 1978;102:196–8.

42. Diacon AH, Van De Wal BW, Wyser C, et al. Diagnostic tools in tuberculous pleurisy: a direct comparative study. Eur Respir J 2003;22:589–91.

43. Sheski FD. Indications for diagnostic thoracoscopy. 2012. Available at: www.uptodate.com/contents/indications-for-diagnostic-thoracoscopy. Accessed May 8, 2012.

44. Rodgers BM, Moazam F, Talbert JL. Thoracoscopy. Early diagnosis of interstitial pneumonitis in the immunologically suppressed child. Chest 1979; 75:126–30.

45. Vansteenkiste J, Verbeken E, Thomeer M, et al. Medical thoracoscopic lung biopsy in interstitial lung disease: a prospective study of biopsy quality. Eur Respir J 1999;14:585–90.

46. Bradley B, Branley HM, Egan JJ, et al. Interstitial lung disease guideline: the British Thoracic Society in collaboration with the Thoracic Society of Australia and New Zealand and the Irish Thoracic Society. Thorax 2008;63(Suppl 5):v1–58.

47. Elia S, Guggino G, Mineo D, et al. Awake one stage bilateral thoracoscopic sympathectomy for palmar hyperhidrosis: a safe outpatient procedure. Eur J Cardiothorac Surg 2005;28:312–7 [discussion: 17].

48. Noppen M, Meysman M, D'haese J, et al. Thoracoscopic splanchnicolysis for the relief of chronic pancreatitis pain: experience of a group of pneumologists. Chest 1998;113:528–31.

49. Lee P. Point: should thoracoscopic talc pleurodesis be the first choice management for malignant effusion? Yes. Chest 2012;142:15–7.

50. Light RW. Counterpoint: should thoracoscopic talc pleurodesis be the first choice management for malignant pleural effusion? No. Chest 2012;142:17–9.

51. Tremblay A, Michaud G. Single-center experience with 250 tunnelled pleural catheter insertions for malignant pleural effusion. Chest 2006;129:362–8.

52. Warren WH, Kalimi R, Khodadadian LM, et al. Management of malignant pleural effusions using the Pleur(X) catheter. Ann Thorac Surg 2008;85:1049–55.

53. Olden AM, Holloway R. Treatment of malignant pleural effusion: pleurx catheter or talc pleurodesis? A cost-effectiveness analysis. J Palliat Med 2010;13:59–65.

54. Antunes G, Neville E, Duffy J, et al. BTS guidelines for the management of malignant pleural effusions. Thorax 2003;58(Suppl 2):ii29–38.

55. Shaw P, Agarwal R. Pleurodesis for malignant pleural effusions. Cochrane Database Syst Rev 2004;(1):CD002916.

56. Kishi K, Homma S, Sakamoto S, et al. Efficacious pleurodesis with Ok-432 and doxorubicin against malignant pleural effusions. Eur Respir J 2004;24:263–6.

57. Maskell NA, Lee YC, Gleeson FV, et al. Randomized trials describing lung inflammation after pleurodesis with talc of varying particle size. Am J Respir Crit Care Med 2004;170:377–82.

58. Janssen JP, Collier G, Astoul P, et al. Safety of pleurodesis with talc poudrage in malignant pleural effusion: a prospective cohort study. Lancet 2007; 369:1535–9.

59. Roberts ME, Neville E, Berrisford RG, et al. Management of a malignant pleural effusion: British Thoracic Society pleural disease guideline 2010. Thorax 2010;65(Suppl 2):ii32–40.

60. Narayanaswamy S, Kamath S, Williams M. CT appearances of talc pleurodesis. Clin Radiol 2007; 62:233–7.

61. Debeljak A, Kecelj P, Triller N, et al. Talc pleurodesis: comparison of talc slurry instillation with thoracoscopic talc insufflation for malignant pleural effusions. J BUON 2006;11:463–7.

62. Diacon AH, Wyser C, Bolliger CT, et al. Prospective randomized comparison of thoracoscopic talc poudrage under local anesthesia versus bleomycin instillation for pleurodesis in malignant pleural effusions. Am J Respir Crit Care Med 2000;162:1445–9.

63. Danby CA, Adebonojo SA, Moritz DM. Video-assisted talc pleurodesis for malignant pleural effusions utilizing local anesthesia and I.V. sedation. Chest 1998;113:739–42.

64. Viallat JR, Rey F, Astoul P, et al. Thoracoscopic talc poudrage pleurodesis for malignant effusions. A review of 360 cases. Chest 1996;110:1387–93.

65. Stefani A, Natali P, Casali C, et al. Talc poudrage versus talc slurry in the treatment of malignant pleural effusion. A prospective comparative study. Eur J Cardiothorac Surg 2006;30:827–32.

66. Reddy C, Ernst A, Lamb C, et al. Rapid pleurodesis for malignant pleural effusions: a pilot study. Chest 2011;139:1419–23.

67. Baumann MH, Strange C, Heffner JE, et al. Management of spontaneous pneumothorax: an American College of Chest Physicians Delphi Consensus Statement. Chest 2001;119:590–602.

68. Macduff A, Arnold A, Harvey J, et al. Management of spontaneous pneumothorax: British Thoracic Society Pleural Disease Guideline 2010. Thorax 2010; 65(Suppl 2):ii18–31.

69. Tschopp JM, Frey JG. Treatment of primary spontaneous pneumothorax by simple talcage under medical thoracoscopy. Monaldi Arch Chest Dis 2002;57:88–92.

70. Tschopp JM, Boutin C, Astoul P, et al. Talcage by medical thoracoscopy for primary spontaneous pneumothorax is more cost-effective than drainage: a randomised study. Eur Respir J 2002;20:1003–9.

71. Lee P, Yap WS, Pek WY, et al. An audit of medical thoracoscopy and talc poudrage for pneumothorax prevention in advanced COPD. Chest 2004;125: 1315–20.

72. Rahman NM, Maskell NA, West A, et al. Intrapleural use of tissue plasminogen activator and dnase in pleural infection. N Engl J Med 2011;365:518–26.

73. Kern L, Robert J, Brutsche M. Management of parapneumonic effusion and empyema: medical thoracoscopy and surgical approach. Respiration 2011;82:193–6.

74. Colt HG. Thoracoscopy. A prospective study of safety and outcome. Chest 1995;108:324–9.

75. Soler M, Wyser C, Bolliger CT, et al. Treatment of early parapneumonic empyema by "medical" thoracoscopy. Schweiz Med Wochenschr 1997;127: 1748–53.

76. Brutsche MH, Tassi GF, Gyorik S, et al. Treatment of sonographically stratified multiloculated thoracic empyema by medical thoracoscopy. Chest 2005; 128:3303–9.

77. Gwin E, Pierce G, Boggan M, et al. Pleuroscopy and pleural biopsy with the flexible fiberoptic bronchoscope. Chest 1975;67:527–31.

78. Davidson AC, George RJ, Sheldon CD, et al. Thoracoscopy: assessment of a physician service and comparison of a flexible bronchoscope used as a thoracoscope with a rigid thoracoscope. Thorax 1988;43:327–32.

79. Yokoyama T, Toda R, Tomioka R, et al. Medical thoracoscopy performed using a flexible bronchoscope inserted through a chest tube under local anesthesia. Diagn Ther Endosc 2009;2009:394817.

80. Mclean AN, Bicknell SR, Mcalpine LG, et al. Investigation of pleural effusion: an evaluation of the new olympus ltf semiflexible thoracofiberscope and comparison with abram's needle biopsy. Chest 1998;114:150–3.

81. Wang Z, Tong ZH, Li HJ, et al. Semi-rigid thoracoscopy for undiagnosed exudative pleural effusions: a comparative study. Chin Med J (Engl) 2008;121: 1384–9.

82. Munavvar M, Khan MA, Edwards J, et al. The autoclavable semirigid thoracoscope: the way forward in pleural disease? Eur Respir J 2007;29:571–4.

83. Thangakunam B, Christopher DJ, James P, et al. Semi-rigid thoracoscopy: initial experience from a tertiary care hospital. Indian J Chest Dis Allied Sci 2010;52:25–7.

84. Tassi GF, Marchetti GP, Pinelli V. Minithoracoscopy: a complementary technique for medical thoracoscopy. Respiration 2011;82:204–6.

85. Prosst RL, Winkler S, Boehm E, et al. Thoracoscopic fluorescence diagnosis (TFD) of pleural malignancies: experimental studies. Thorax 2002;57: 1005–9.

86. Pikin O, Filonenko E, Mironenko D, et al. Fluorescence thoracoscopy in the detection of pleural malignancy. Eur J Cardiothorac Surg 2012;41: 649–52.

87. Noppen M, Dekeukeleire T, Hanon S, et al. Fluorescein-enhanced autofluorescence thoracoscopy in patients with primary spontaneous pneumothorax and normal subjects. Am J Respir Crit Care Med 2006;174:26–30.

88. Vandermeulen L, Makris D, Mordon S, et al. Thoracoscopic findings and pharmacokinetics of inhaled fluorescein in a pig model. Respiration 2010;80: 228–35.

89. Chrysanthidis MG, Janssen JP. Autofluorescence videothoracoscopy in exudative pleural effusions: preliminary results. Eur Respir J 2005;26:989–92.

Intracavitary Therapeutics for Pleural Malignancies

Andrew R. Haas, MD, PhD, Daniel H. Sterman, MD*

KEYWORDS

- Intracavitary therapeutics • Pleural • Malignancy • Tumors

KEY POINTS

- Pleural malignancies are ideal for novel therapeutic approaches, because they are invariable fatal with few treatment options.
- Intrapleural chemotherapy has only marginal benefit in pleural malignancies, but may prove efficacious with hyperthermic chemotherapy administered in combination with maximal tumor debulking.
- Intrapleural immunotherapies may be most effective in those patients with early-stage pleural malignancy, such as mesotheliomas limited to the parietal pleura, and may prove superior to standard pleurodesis methods in control of effusion and prolongation of survival.
- Gene therapy is a promising treatment of pleural malignancies, but awaits larger randomized clinical trials before it is available for routine clinical use.
- Mesothelioma is an ideal target for immunogene therapy, because there is no curative treatment and because the disease remains localized until the late stages.
- Although immunogene therapy may be unable to successfully treat bulky tumors on its own, greater success may be achieved with combination approaches that combine debulking surgery and chemotherapy with intrapleural genetic immunotherapy.

INTRODUCTION

Pleural malignancies are often refractory to standard treatment, including surgical resection, systemic chemotherapy, and external beam radiation therapy, but develop in a body cavity readily accessible for examination, biopsy, and repeated fluid sampling. Many pleural malignancies, in particular malignant mesothelioma (MM), cause morbidity and even mortality by local spread within the ipsilateral hemithorax. Novel therapeutics with intrapleural delivery can be readily analyzed for safety, efficacy, and induced immune and inflammatory responses with repeated pleural sampling.[1]

The concept of intrapleural (IP) therapy for thoracic malignancies arose from observations of improved survival in the setting of postoperative empyema status post surgical resection for non–small cell lung cancer.[2–4] In the early 1970s, the theory was posited that the inflammatory environment of the empyema engendered an antitumor immune response that improved disease control and patient survival, and that the pleural space was an ideal access point for the induction of a variety of antitumor responses against primary and metastatic pleural neoplasms.[5–7]

Several groups investigated the hypothesis that IP bacillus Calmette-Guérin (BCG) injection would initiate a nonspecific immune response that could generate similar antitumor immune effects as empyema, without the associated complications of severe pleural space infection. One small study randomized patients to a single dose of IP BCG versus saline instillation after lung cancer resection with the suggestion of improved survival in stage I disease,[8] but these results were not corroborated in several larger randomized trials.[9,10] However, these studies established that pleural space could

Section of Interventional Pulmonology and Thoracic Oncology, Division of Pulmonary, Allergy, and Critical Care, Department of Medicine, University of Pennsylvania Medical Center, Philadelphia, PA, USA
* Corresponding author. 833 West Gates Building, Philadelphia, PA 19104-4283.
E-mail address: daniel.sterman@uphs.upenn.edu

Clin Chest Med 34 (2013) 501–513
http://dx.doi.org/10.1016/j.ccm.2013.04.007
0272-5231/13/$ – see front matter © 2013 Elsevier Inc. All rights reserved.

be an ideal site for safe delivery of novel therapeutics. These investigations have been pursued in 3 major areas: IP cytotoxic chemotherapy, IP immunotherapy, and IP gene therapy.

IP CHEMOTHERAPY

Pleural malignancies such as mesothelioma are characterized by predominantly locoregional spread of disease for which surgical resection can be attempted, but with the certainty of residual microscopic disease. Therefore, there is a rationale for attempted local control of pleural malignancies by IP instillation of cytotoxic chemotherapeutic agents. For example, Refaely and colleagues[11] in 2002 reported their experience with intraoperative IP hyperthermic cisplatin chemotherapy in 15 patients with metastatic thymic carcinoma or thymoma after surgical resection. The hyperthermia was used to break down tight intracellular junctions and increase tumor cell access to cytotoxic chemotherapy. One patient with thymic carcinoma was alive at 54 months and 8 patients with thymoma were alive without evidence of recurrence at 9 to 70 months. Although two patients had significant post-operative bleeding, no other major toxicities from IP chemotherapy were reported.

Given the poor response rates to therapies for pleural malignancies, some investigators have developed multimodality treatment approaches involving both IP and systemic chemotherapy. For example, Pinto and colleagues[12] treated 22 patients with MM with IP mitoxantrone in combination with intravenous methotrexate and mitomycin. Although the overall median survival time of patients enrolled was equivalent to historical median survival with standard chemotherapy (13.5 months), responders to IP chemotherapy achieved a median survival of 18 months compared with 8 months for nonresponders. Furthermore, treatment with IP chemotherapy resulted in significant reductions in dyspnea and pain.

Some groups have taken an aggressive approach to the management of pleural malignancies such as MM by combining maximal tumor debulking with extrapleural pneumonectomy (EPP) followed by IP chemotherapy to control microscopic residual disease. The Thoracic Surgical group at the Brigham[13] and Women's Hospital reported several clinical trials combining EPP with intraoperative hyperthermic chemotherapy with cisplatin or gemcitabine. These studies showed that hyperthermic intraoperative intracavitary chemotherapy perfusion following EPP can be performed with acceptable morbidity and mortality, and may enhance local control in the chest.[14]

Although MM and thymic tumors are rare malignancies, metastatic disease to the pleura from other primary sites (eg, lung) is a common clinical scenario associated with significant morbidity and mortality. Many groups have consequently investigated whether IP chemotherapy could be a modality to control malignant pleural effusions (MPEs), particularly those caused by lung cancer given its high incidence of pleural dissemination, as well as to improve overall survival.

For example, Tohda and colleagues[15] treated 68 patients with malignant effusions caused by lung cancer with IP cisplatin and etoposide with acceptable toxicity, an overall response rate (control of effusion) of 46.2%, and a median survival time of 8 months. Shoji and colleagues[16] studied biweekly IP instillation of 5-flourouracil and cisplatin via an indwelling pleural catheter in 22 patients with MPE, with reasonable safety and a median survival period of 13 months.

Su and colleagues[17] reported a more extensive combination therapy approach wherein 27 patients with lung cancer–related malignant effusions received IP cisplatin followed by intravenous gemcitabine and docetaxel, and thoracic irradiation. The overall response rate was 55% with 7% complete response (CR), and only 2 of 27 patients had recurrence of the malignant effusion. Matsuzaki and colleagues[18] studied 11 consecutive patients with lung cancer associated with pleural dissemination who underwent resection of the primary tumor followed by treatment with IP cisplatin. The median survival time for patients receiving IP chemotherapy was 20 months, and 6 months for the control group.

More recent studies of IP chemotherapy have been conducted with modern chemotherapeutic agents that have greater efficacy in malignant effusions, particularly those related to lung cancer. Jones and colleagues[19] from the University of Virginia conducted a phase I dose escalation trial with the primary aim of determining the maximally tolerated dose of IP docetaxel in 15 patients with MPE. Subjects received escalating single doses of IP docetaxel after drainage of the effusion and insertion of a tunneled pleural catheter. All patients tolerated the therapy well and most had a complete radiographic response. Pleural exposure to docetaxel was 1000 times higher than systemic exposure, which accounted for the minimal systemic toxicities seen.[19]

IP IMMUNOTHERAPY

Among the malignancies of the pleural space, MM has been thought to be resistant to immunotherapy compared with more classically immunogenic tumors such as melanoma or renal cell carcinoma. In these diseases, exogenous cytokines, monoclonal antibodies, and tumor vaccines have contributed to antitumor responses. Immunotherapy has been attempted in MM, despite observations of a significant immunosuppressive tumor microenvironment.[20–22] In addition to the tumor's innate mechanisms of immune evasion, patients with MM have impaired immune systems: abnormal humoral and cell-mediated immunity, abnormal cell-mediated antibody-dependent cellular toxicity, and defective macrophage and natural killer (NK) cell function.[22–25] However, high local levels of certain proinflammatory cytokines may be able to overcome the innate immune resistance of MM. For this reason, human clinical trials of IP or systemic infusion of various cytokines, including interleukin (IL)-2,[26] interferon (IFN)-α,[27] and IFN-γ have been conducted, showing varying degrees of tumor regression.[28,29]

One of the most promising studies was a phase I/II clinical trial conducted by Boutin and colleagues[28,29] in Marseille assessing the activity of IP gamma-interferon twice weekly for 8 weeks on an outpatient basis in 22 patients with MM. Toxicity was minimal with no dose-limiting side effects. CRs (confirmed by repeat thoracoscopy) were seen in 4 of 9 patients with stage IA disease (tumor limited to the parietal and diaphragmatic pleurae), all of whom had pleural nodules less than 5 mm in diameter at the time of baseline thoracoscopy.

Based on these encouraging results in early-stage patients with MM, Boutin and colleagues[28] conducted a prospective, multi-institutional phase II study of IP IFN-γ. Eighty-nine patients with stage I to III disease and both epithelial and mixed histologies were enrolled in the study. There were 8 histologically confirmed CRs and 9 partial response (PRs), with an overall response rate of 20% and a response rate of 45% in patients with stage I disease. In general, IP IFN-γ was safe, with the most serious complication being empyema in 7 of 89 patients, 6 of whom required removal of the pleural catheter. In an adjunctive study, the pharmacokinetics of IP IFN-γ in pleural fluid and blood were measured in 6 patients, and clearly showed that significantly higher levels of immunostimulatory cytokines can be achieved in the pleural space by direct instillation as opposed to intravenous administration, with the likelihood of decreased systemic toxicity of cytokine therapy.

A shortage of IFN-γ for clinical use in Europe limited further study, but a pilot study of IP IFN-γ for MPE secondary to lung carcinoma was subsequently conducted in Japan.[30] Six patients with MPE underwent 1 to 3 weekly instillations of IFN-γ via a pleural catheter; 2 of the 6 patients had complete clearance of malignant cells from their pleural fluid. An additional patient had a partial radiographic response after 2 IP instillations of IFN-γ. No significant toxicities were noted. However, IFN-γ infusions did not induce effective pleurodesis.[30]

There have been additional cytokines studied for their potential role in IP immunotherapy for pleural malignancies. Phase I to II clinical trials of IP IL-2 administered by continuous infusion via an indwelling pleural catheter showed a 19% PR rate with significant dose-related toxicity, most notably pleural space infections.[31] Researchers at the University of Turin (Italy) conducted a clinical trial involving combined systemic and IP IL-2, achieving an estimated a response rate of 22.5%, and significant reductions in pleural effusion volume in 90% of patients. Toxicities were minimal; primarily fever and eosinophilia.[31]

In a prospective, randomized trial comparing IP chemotherapy with IP immunotherapy, Sartori and colleagues[32] studied IP bleomycin versus IP IFN-α2b in patients with recurrent MPE. Although there was no significant difference in median survival (96 days, bleomycin; 85 days, IFN-α2b), 30-day response was 84.3% in the bleomycin arm and 62.3% in IFN-α2b arm ($P = .002$), and median time to progression was 93 days in bleomycin group and 59 days in the IFN-α2b group ($P<.001$).[32] This study suggested that, for control of MPE, IP chemotherapy with bleomycin was superior to IP immunotherapy with IFN-α2b. However, there was no survival advantage, but a palliative advantage in terms of MPE control, which may be attributable to the effect of IP bleomycin to induce pleurodesis rather than cytotoxicity to pleural tumor.

In addition to the specific immunotherapeutic agents, other investigators have attempted to generate an antitumor immune response within the pleural space using nonspecific immunostimulatory agents to treat pleural malignancy. These immune-activating agents included inactivated bacterial superantigens from Streptococcus (OK-432) or Staphylococcus. Yamaguchi and colleagues[33] studied combinations of IP OK-432 with IP IL-2 in 16 patients with MPE from colorectal cancer. There was a cytologic response and decrease in effusion volume in 9 of 11 (82%) patients treated with OK-432 alone and in all 5 patients treated with OK-432 plus IL-2. Ikehara and colleagues[34] treated 15 patients with MPE in a phase II study with IP OK-432 followed by standard systemic chemotherapy with cisplatin and gemcitabine. Of the 15 patients, 1 achieved PR, 13 had stable disease, and 1 progressive disease, with an overall response rate of 6.7%. The median survival time was 13.5 months and the 1-year survival rate was 60.0%.

Ren and colleagues[35] instilled staphylococcal superantigen (SSAg) once or twice weekly into the pleural space of 14 consecutive patients with stage IVa non–small cell lung cancer with poor performance status (Eastern Cooperative Oncology Group performance status ≥2). Eleven patients had a CR and 3 patients had a PR (CR was defined as complete resolution of MPE). In 12 patients, the response endured for longer than 90 days, with a median time to recurrence of 5 months (range, 3–23 months). Median survival of the 14 SSAg-treated cases and 13 control talc-poudrage–treated patients with comparable pretreatment performance status was 7.9 months and 2.0 months, respectively (P = .0023). Nine of 14 patients treated with SSAg survived for longer than 6 months, whereas 1 of the 13 talc-treated patients survived for longer than 6 month.[35] These findings suggest that IP delivery of nonspecific immunostimulatory agents can have significant effects on recurrence of MPE, as well as on overall survival.

IP GENE THERAPY

Advances in molecular genetics and gene transfer technology facilitated the development of gene therapy: the modification of the genetic makeup of cells for therapeutic purposes. The concept of gene therapy now encompasses the treatment of any pathophysiologic state based on the transfer of genetic material, including complementary DNA (cDNA), full-length genes, small-interfering RNA (si-RNA), or oligonucleotides. This definition also includes approaches involving delivery of genetically altered cells such as bone marrow–derived stem cells.

Gene therapy involving the pleural space offers several potential advantages. The pleural space has a large surface area lined by a thin layer of mesothelium, an ideal configuration for efficient gene transfer by liquids or cell suspensions injected into the pleural space In addition, access to the pleural space is easy and safe (**Fig. 1**). Unlike the peritoneal cavity, where adhesions and inflammation can cause severe complications, fusion of the pleural space is benign, and, in the case of MPEs, may even be desirable.

The most likely role for pleural gene therapy is in the treatment of pleural malignancies. Pleural malignancies have several characteristics that make them attractive targets for gene therapy, including (1) absence of curative therapy; (2) accessibility in the pleural space for biopsy, vector delivery, and analysis of treatment effects; and (3) benefit from only transient gene expression. MM is an especially attractive target because local extension of disease, rather than distant metastases, is responsible for much of its morbidity and mortality.[1]

VECTORS USED IN PLEURAL GENE THERAPY

The first requirement for successful gene therapy is efficient gene delivery and a variety of viral and nonviral gene transfer vectors have been developed.[36,37] As summarized in **Table 1**, each of these vectors has certain advantages with regard to DNA carrying capacity, types of cells targeted, in vivo gene transfer efficiency, duration of expression, and induction of inflammation.

Retroviruses

The principal advantages of this vector derive from its availability to accomplish efficient gene transfer in vitro in a broad range of targeted cells, with the capacity to achieve integration into the host genome and long-term expression. Retroviruses have been used to transduce mesothelial or tumor cells in vitro for subsequent reinjection (discussed later).[38] However, successful use of retroviruses for in vivo transduction of therapeutic genes into the pleural and peritoneal space has been limited.[39] The usefulness of retroviral gene delivery in pleural malignancies may be limited by IP chondroitin sulfate proteoglycans/glycosaminoglycans that inhibit successful gene transfer.[40]

Adeno-associated Virus

Another viral vector that has generated significant interest is the adeno-associated virus (AAV), a defective parvovirus with a single-strand DNA genome and a naked protein coat.[41] AAV has not been associated with any known human disease state, suggesting a significant safety margin for this vector. In addition, after wild-type AAV entry to the host cell, there is a site-specific DNA integration step. To date, there have been no published reports of AAV-mediated gene therapy in human pleural diseases.

Adenoviruses

The most widely used vector in human clinical trials of IP gene therapy has been recombinant adenovirus with deleted viral gene regions replaced with therapeutic genes under the control of general or tumor-specific promoters.[42] This vector system offers several advantages including high-efficiency transduction of target cells (including nondividing cells) and high expression levels of the delivered transgene.[43] The two

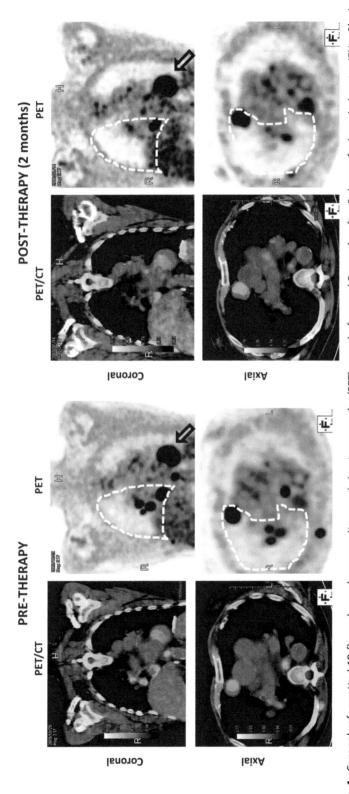

Fig. 1. Coronal reformatted 18-fluorodeoxyglucose positron emission tomography (PET) scans before and 2 months after 2 doses of adenoviral vector IFN-α-2b via surgically implanted right pleural catheter in patient with progressive mesothelioma status post prior right radical pleurectomy, intraoperative photodynamic therapy, and adjuvant pemetrexed-based combination chemotherapy. Follow-up PET scan at 2 months showed decrease in hypermetabolic foci in right hemithorax, as well as in right hilar and mediastinal nodes. Repeat PET computed tomography scan at 6 months showed a near-CR (anatomic and metabolic) in right hemithorax and mediastinum (data not shown). Arrows delineate normal FDG uptake in left ventricle.

Table 1
Gene therapy vectors used for IP delivery

Vector	Advantages	Disadvantages	Use in Clinical Trials in the Pleura
Retrovirus	Efficient entry into dividing cells Stable integration into host genome	Difficult to produce in sufficient titers for human trials Insertional oncogenesis	Used ex vivo for transfection of allogeneic tumor cells
Ad	Entry into dividing and nondividing cells High level gene expression No integration into host genome	Viral genes must be in vector Induces immune responses that can limit repeat dosing	Most commonly used vector for IP gene therapy trials in humans
AAV	Chromosomal integration at defined site Minimal immune response	Small insert size Difficult to produce in sufficient titers for human trials Inconsistent tumor cell delivery	No trials of direct IP instillation in humans
Liposomes	Easy to produce in large amounts Minimal immune responses that do not inhibit repeat dosing	Variable entry into target cells	Single human trial with E1A gene delivery
Allogeneic tumor cells	Homing to tumor cells in pleura High transgene expression	Induces immune responses Often requires bystander effect	Single human trial with PA1-STK delivery in MPM

Abbreviations: AAV, adeno-associated virus; Ad, adenovirus.

primary disadvantages of adenoviruses in traditional gene therapy are transient gene expression and induction of local and systemic inflammatory responses may be advantageous for cancer gene therapy.[44]

Mesothelial and mesothelioma cells (as well as other tumor cell lines) are readily transduced by adenoviral vectors in vitro and in vivo.[45–48] Our group has injected adenoviral vectors into the pleural space of patients with MM and confirmed intratumoral gene transfer of tumor by detection of transgene DNA, RNA, and protein at 3 days after vector instillation (discussed later).[49]

Nonviral Vectors

A variety of nonviral vectors have also been developed for in vivo and in vitro gene delivery, with liposomes being the most common nonviral vector used in animal models and human clinical trials. Liposomes are artificial lipid bilayers designed to translocate drugs or nucleic acids into the cell cytosol via a cell-membrane fusion event or endocytosis. Liposomal/DNA complexes are less efficient than viral vectors and they produce only transitory transgene expression, but they offer simplicity of construction, enhanced DNA packaging capacity, and greater safety.[50]

Liposomes have been used for IP gene transfer in both animal models of metastatic pleural disease and in human clinical trials.[51] Hortobagyi and colleagues[52] conducted a phase 1 trial examining the weekly injection of liposomes containing the adenoviral E1A gene (DCC-E1A) into the thoracic or peritoneal cavities of 18 patients with metastatic breast or ovarian cancer. E1A gene expression in tumor cells was detected by immunohistochemical staining and reverse transcriptase–polymerase chain reaction (RT-PCR), and accompanied by HER-2/neu downregulation and tumor cell apoptosis. The most common treatment-related toxicities were fever, nausea, and injection site discomfort.[52]

Several different cancer gene therapy approaches are currently being explored for malignant pleural tumors including use of suicide genes, tumor suppressor genes, and immunomodulatory genes (**Table 2**).

Suicide gene therapy

Suicide gene therapy involves delivery of a cDNA encoding for an enzyme capable of converting a prodrug to a toxic metabolite. The enzyme used most commonly in human clinical trials and in animal models is the herpes simplex virus-1

Table 2
IP gene therapy trials for pleural malignancy

Study	Phase	Histology	Total No. Evaluable	Agent	Delivery	Best Clinical Response	Additional Outcome Measures
Sterman et al,[49] 1998	I	MM	21	Ad.HSVtk	IP (single dose)	Gene transfer confirmed in 11 of 20 patients	Antiadenoviral immune responses, including high titers of Nabs and T-cell proliferation to Ad antigens
Sterman et al,[66] 2000	I	MM	8	Ad.HSVtk + corticosteroids	IP (single dose)	Two long-term survivors (>6 y after)	Safety and toxicity without difference but with decreased febrile response
Hortobagyi et al,[52] 2001	I	MPE (Breast, ovary)	18	DCC-E1A	IP Intraperitoneal (weekly injection)	E1A expression detected by IHC and RT-PCR	HER-2/neu downregulation, increased tumor cell apoptosis, and reduced tumor proliferation
Sterman et al,[73] 2007	I	MM MPE	10	Ad.IFN-β	IP (single dose)	1 CR, 2 PR, 4 SD	IFN-β gene transfer, induction of humoral/innate immune response
Dong et al,[79] 2008	I	MM MPE	27	Ad.wt-p53	IP Intraperitoneal (weekly injection)	Effusion control rates for the treatment group 63.0%	Safety and toxicity
Zhao et al,[80] 2009	I	Stage IVA NSCLC (MPE)	17	Ad.wt-p53	IP (weekly × 4)	Effusion control rates for the treatment group 82.35%	Safety and toxicity
Sterman et al,[74] 2010	I	MM MPE	17	Ad.IFN-β	IP (2 doses)	3 PR/MR; 11 SD	IFN-α gene transfer after first dose only, induction of Nabs
Sterman et al,[75] 2011	I	MM	9	Ad.IFN-α-2b (SCH721015)	IP (2 doses)	2 PR, 4 SD	Increased and persistent IFN-α induction in pleural fluid
Schwarzenberger et al,[59] 2011	I	MM	15	PA1-STK Cells	Multiple IP infusion (every 4 wk × 3)	SD (9) and (3) at 3 and 6 mo	Median survival from the time of treatment 7.7 mo
Haas and Sterman,[81] 2013	I/IIA	MM	25 (ongoing accrual)	Ad.IFN-α-2b (SCH721015)	IP (2 doses) 1. Pemetrexed + Platin 2. Gemcitabine ± Platin	Ongoing	Gene transfer, immune response, safety, and toxicity

Abbreviations: Ad.wt-p53, adenovirus wild-type p53 gene construct; DCC-E1A, liposomal E1A gene conjugate; IHC, immunohistochemical staining; MR, mixed response; Nabs, antiadenoviral neutralizing antibodies; PD, progressive disease; SD, stable disease.

thymidine kinase (HSV*tk*) gene, which renders malignant cells sensitive to the nucleoside analogues ganciclovir (GCV) and valcyclovir.[53] Therapeutic efficacy is enhanced because transgene expression in every cell is not required for complete tumor regression,[54,55] and can induce antitumor immune responses capable of killing tumor cells not expressing HSV*tk*.[56]

Tumor cells transduced ex vivo with HSV*tk* and injected into the peritoneal or pleural cavity in combination with GCV resulted in the death of the transduced cells and the subsequent release of immunostimulatory cytokines that engendered killing of nontransduced cells.[57] This approach showed marked increase in survival in mouse models of MM involving injection of an HSVtk-transduced ovarian cancer cell line (PA1) followed by GCV.[58]

Schwarzenberger and colleagues[59] conducted a phase I clinical trial involving direct IP infusion of escalating doses of HSVtk suicide gene–modified PA1-STK cells in 15 patients with MM followed by 7 days of intravenous GCV. The first 2 cohorts received a single IP dose via an indwelling pleural catheter; cohorts 3 to 5 received 3 weekly doses. The investigators showed that PA1-STK cells home to MM deposits in patients after IP instillation. The treatment was well tolerated without any grade 3 or 4 toxicity. Significant inductions of both Th1 and Th2 cytokines up to 20-fold more than baseline were observed.[60]

Adenovirus is the most extensively studied vector for suicide gene delivery. Replication-deficient adenoviral HSV*tk* vectors (Ad.HSV*tk*) efficiently transduced and killed mesothelioma cells both in tissue culture and in animal models in combination with GCV.[61,62] Ad.HSV*tk* gene transfer subsequently successfully treated established tumors in immunodeficient murine and rat models of MM and lung cancer.[47,63,64]

Based on success in animal models, Sterman and colleagues[49] conducted a phase 1 clinical trial of IP Ad.HSV*tk* and systemic GCV in 21 patients with MM.[65] Side effects were minimal, and dose-dependent gene transfer was confirmed in 11 of 20 evaluable patients. Antiadenoviral humoral and cellular immune responses were generated.[49] A second trial involving peri–gene transfer treatment with systemic corticosteroids showed decreased IP and systemic inflammatory responses, but no inhibition of the generation of anti-Ad antibodies or Ad-induced peripheral blood mononuclear cell activation.[66] Despite the early nature of these trials, some clinical responses were seen: PRs were observed in several of the patients at the higher dose levels, and 2 patients remained tumor free 3 years after treatment.[49,65]

An additional 8 patients with MM were treated with an Ad.HSV*tk* virus (E1/E4 deleted) modified for a lower incidence of recombination to form wild-type virus. Of these 8 patients, 2 were long-term survivors both treated at the higher dose level of 5.0×10^{13} viral particles (vp). Both of these patients had radiographically stable disease without other antitumor therapy for more than 6 years after treatment.[66]

Cytokine gene therapy

There has been significant interest in the delivery of genes encoding cytokines in patients with pleural malignancies. Expression of cytokine genes by tumor cells generates a high level of intratumoral cytokines in an autocrine and paracrine fashion, inducing tumor cell apoptosis and inhibition of tumor angiogenesis and generating humoral and cellular antitumor immune responses. Cytokine gene delivery activates tumor-infiltrating dendritic cells (DCs), which can migrate to regional lymph nodes, stimulating proliferation of tumor-specific CD8 and CD4 T lymphocytes, facilitating antitumor cytotoxicity at distant sites. In addition, increases in intratumoral proinflammatory cytokines such as IL-2 and IL-12 can overcome tolerance signals to produce tumor-specific cytotoxic T lymphocytes and also activate NK cells.[67,68]

The first human clinical trial of direct intratumoral delivery of cytokine genes in pleural malignancy was conducted by investigators at Queen Elizabeth II Hospital in Perth, Australia, using a recombinant vaccinia virus (VV) expressing the human IL-2 gene. The VV–IL-2 vector was serially injected into palpable chest wall lesions of 6 patients with advanced MM. Toxicities were minimal, and there was no clinical or serologic evidence of spread of VV to patient contacts. VV–IL-2 mRNA was detected by RT-PCR in serial tumor biopsies for up to 6 days after injection, but declined to low levels by day 8. No significant tumor regression was seen, and only modest intratumoral T-cell infiltration was detected on tumor biopsies.[69]

As discussed earlier, several clinical trials in the early 1990s showed safety and efficacy of IP recombinant IFN proteins in patients with early-stage MM.[28,29,70,71] IP IFN-β protein administration for metastatic pleural effusions also showed clinical promise with a reasonable safety profile, but was hampered by the same issues that limited application of recombinant IFN-γ in mesothelioma, including short in vivo half-life and lack of sustained tissue levels of the recombinant proteins. To overcome these problems, our group conducted preclinical studies of IFN-β gene transfer in syngeneic murine models of MM.[72]

The success of these in vivo experiments led to the publication in 2007 of the first human trial of IP IFN gene therapy for MM and MPE.[73] The study evaluated the safety and feasibility of single-dose IP IFN-β gene transfer using an adenoviral vector IFN-β (Ad.IFN-β) administered in escalating doses via an indwelling pleural catheter in heavily pre-treated patients. IP Ad.IFN-β was well tolerated, with transient lymphopenia as the most common side effect. Gene transfer was documented in 7 of the 10 patients by demonstration of IFN-β mRNA or protein in pleural fluid. Antitumor immune responses were shown in 7 of 10 patients. Four of 10 patients showed clinically meaningful radio-graphic responses defined as disease stability and/or regression on positron emission tomography (PET) and computed tomography (CT) scans at day 60 after vector instillation.[73]

Our group subsequently conducted a second phase I trial to determine the safety and efficacy of repeated dosing of Ad.IFN-β vector via an indwelling pleural catheter in 10 patients with MM and MPE.[74] Repeated doses were generally well tolerated, with the most common side effects being lymphopenia, hypoalbuminemia, hypoten-sion, anemia, hypocalcemia, and mild cytokine release syndrome (CRS). One patient developed pericardial tamponade, which was successfully treated by therapeutic pericardiocentesis; pericar-dial fluid analysis did not reveal malignant cells or the presence of adenoviral vector.[74] High levels of IFN-β protein were detected in pleural fluid after the first dose, but were undetectable after the sec-ond, correlating with the rapid induction of neutral-izing Ad antibodies (Nabs). Antibody responses against tumor antigens were induced in most pa-tients. At 2-month follow-up imaging, 1 patient had a PR, 2 had stable disease (SD), and 9 had progressive disease (PD). There were 7 patients with survival times longer than 18 months.[74]

Based on these results, we designed a new phase I trial to evaluate a shortened dosing interval of 3 days after the first dose, before the expected Nabs peak. For this trial, we used a recombinant adenovirus vector expressing the human IFN-α2b gene (Ad.IFN-α2b) obtained from Schering-Plough/Merck (SCH721015).[75] IP Ad.IFN-α2b was instilled on study days 1 and 4 via an indwelling pleural catheter at a starting vector of 1×10^{12} vp, thereafter reduced to 3×10^{11} vp after the first 3 en-rollees developed significant CRS symptoms after the initial vector dose. In general, Ad.IFN-α2b vec-tor instillation was well tolerated, although most pa-tients developed some CRS symptoms after the initial dose. Increased and sustained serum IFN-α levels were sometimes associated with protracted flulike symptoms lasting 7 to 10 days. Pleural catheter-related infections occurred in 2 patients; however, both were treated successfully with anti-biotics and catheter removal.[75] Significant IP IFN-α levels were shown even in patients treated at the lower vector dose. In addition, the second Ad.IFN-α2b dose at the shortened time interval re-sulted in successful gene transfer. All patients had marked increases in Nabs 1 week after Ad.IFN-α2b administration. Posttreatment humoral and cellular immunologic responses were noted in 7 of 8 evaluable patients, including antibodies against allogeneic tumor-associated antigens, as well as activation of circulating NK cells.[75]

At the time of first radiographic assessment us-ing modified RECIST (Response Evaluation Criteria in Solid Tumors) (60 days), 3 subjects had PD, 4 had SD, and 2 had objective PRs. Two patients were subsequently able to undergo radical pleurectomy, with no signs of postopera-tive recurrence at 12 and 24 months. One patient, status post prior radical pleurectomy, intraopera-tive photodynamic therapy, and adjuvant chemo-therapy with multifocal recurrence, had a dramatic radiographic tumor response on 6-month follow-up PET/CT (see **Fig. 1**). PET/CT after Ad.IFN-α2b was characterized by near-complete resolution of all sites of metabolic tumor activity, including foci distant from vector instillation.[75]

IFN gene therapy trials have mostly documented safety, successful gene transfer, and induction of antitumor humoral and cellular immune responses, but have shown only limited efficacy. Given the complex nature of pathogenesis of many malig-nancies, the future may lie in combination gene therapy approaches, concomitant use of other im-munostimulatory cytokines, or tumor vaccines.[76] Multimodality cancer treatment (ie, surgical de-bulking, chemotherapy, and/or radiotherapy) in conjunction with IFN gene transfer may provide improved long-term outcomes in MM and other pleural malignancies. Based on promising preclin-ical data, our group has initiated a phase I/II clinical trial of repeated-dose IP Ad.IFN-α2b in combina-tion with standard chemotherapy and high-dose celecoxib for patients with MM.[77]

IP DELIVERY OF TUMOR SUPPRESSOR GENES

One of the primary approaches to cancer gene therapy has been mutation compensation: the replacement of absent or mutated tumor suppres-sor genes responsible, in part, for the malignant phenotype of the cancer cell. Intratumoral delivery of the wild-type p53 (wt-p53) gene, for example, has been used in human gene therapy trials for lung cancer and other solid tumors. Despite most mesotheliomas having wt-p53, p53 function may be abnormal in mesothelioma cells secondary to p53 binding by inhibitor proteins such as SV40 large T antigen. There is therefore a rationale for gene therapy for mesothelioma via overexpression of wt-p53 even in the absence of mutations. Giuliano and colleagues[78] transfected human mesothelioma cells with a replication-deficient adenoviral vector carrying the wt-p53 gene (Ad.wt-p53), and showed inhibition of tumor cell growth in vitro associated with induction of apoptosis. In addition, they showed inhibition of tumor growth and prolonged survival with both ex vivo and in vivo wt-p53 gene in immunodeficient murine models of MM.

IP p53 gene therapy clinical trials have been conducted in China for the treatment of malignant effusions secondary to mesothelioma and pleural metastases.[79,80] Recombinant adenoviral vectors carrying wt-p53 have been approved in China for intratumoral injection in head and neck cancer, and have been used clinically with intratumoral injection in lung cancer. Dong and colleagues[79] evaluated the efficacy of adenovirus wt-p53 (rAd-p53) injection combined with IP (or intraperitoneal) cisplatin for the treatment of malignant pleural or peritoneal effusion. After thoracentesis or paracentesis, patients received intracavitary administration of rAd-p53 once weekly for 4 successive weeks. At 48 hours after rAd-p53, patients were given intracavitary administration of cisplatin. The total effective rates (evaluated by control of the malignant effusion) for the treatment group (63.0%) were significantly higher than for the control group (42.9%).[79] Zhao and colleagues[80] evaluated the clinical efficacy and toxicity of rAd-p53 combined with cisplatin in 35 patients with MPE related to lung cancer. Both treatment and control groups were administered intracavitary cisplatin with or without rAd-p53 once weekly for 4 weeks. The total effective rates (based on control of MPE) in the treatment and control groups were 82.35% and 50.00% ($P<.05$), respectively. The principal toxicity in the treatment group was self-limited fever ($P<.05$).

Both studies noted superior control of pleural (and peritoneal) effusion in patients who received the Ad.p53-based combination therapy, but both studies were limited by the lack of data on tumor response rates or survival.[79,80] Therefore, it is possible that this approach may have only been useful in achieving pleurodesis as a result of an inflammatory reaction to repeated IP administration of the adenoviral vector.

SUMMARY

Pleural malignancies are ideal for novel therapeutic approaches, because they are invariably fatal, with few treatment options. In addition, research efforts into the efficacy of novel therapies are aided by the ease of access of the pleural space for thoracoscopic examination and/or pleural fluid sampling. IP chemotherapy has only marginal benefit in pleural malignancies, but may prove efficacious with hyperthermic chemotherapy administered in combination with maximal tumor debulking. IP immunotherapies may be most effective in those patients with early-stage pleural malignancy, such as mesotheliomas limited to the parietal pleura, and may prove superior to standard pleurodesis methods in control of effusion and prolongation of survival. Gene therapy is a promising treatment of pleural malignancies, but awaits larger randomized clinical trials before it is available for routine clinical use. Clinical trials of IP wt-p53 gene delivery have shown excellent control of pleural effusions in patients with stage IVa lung cancer, but have not yet shown evidence of objective tumor responses. Recent clinical trials involving adenoviral vectors encoding for human IFN genes revealed induction of humoral and cellular antitumor immune responses and objective tumor reductions in heavily pretreated patients with pleural malignancies. Mesothelioma is an ideal target for immunogene therapy because there is no curative treatment and because the disease remains localized until the late stages. Although immunogene therapy may be unable to successfully treat bulky tumors on its own, greater success may be achieved with combination approaches that combine debulking surgery and chemotherapy with IP genetic immunotherapy.

REFERENCES

1. Sterman DH, Albelda SM. Advances in the diagnosis, evaluation and management of malignant pleural mesothelioma. Respirology 2005;10: 266–83.
2. Bone G. Postoperative empyema and survival in lung cancer. Br Med J 1973;2(5859):178.
3. Ruckdeschel JC, Codish SD, Stranahan A, et al. Postoperative empyema improves survival in lung cancer. Documentation and analysis of a natural experiment. N Engl J Med 1972;287(20):1013–7.
4. Vaisrub S. Empyema in lung cancer–the cloud with a silver lining. JAMA 1973;224(12):1644.
5. Minasian H, Lewis CT, Evans SJ. Influence of postoperative empyema on survival after pulmonary resection for bronchogenic carcinoma. Br Med J 1978;2(6148):1329–31.
6. Lawaetz O, Halkier E. The relationship between postoperative empyema and long-term survival after pneumonectomy. Results of surgical treatment of bronchogenic carcinoma. Scand J Thorac Cardiovasc Surg 1980;14(1):113–7.

7. Pastorino U, Valente M, Piva L, et al. Empyema following lung cancer resection: risk factors and prognostic value on survival. Ann Thorac Surg 1982;33(4):320–3.

8. McKneally MF, Maver C, Lininger L, et al. Four-year follow-up on the Albany experience with intrapleural BCG in lung cancer. J Thorac Cardiovasc Surg 1981;81(4):485–92.

9. Bakker W, Nijhuis-Heddes JM, Wever AM, et al. Postoperative intrapleural BCG in lung cancer: lack of efficacy and possible enhancement of tumour growth. Thorax 1981;36(11):870–4.

10. Bakker W, Nijhuis-Heddes JM, van der Velde EA. Post-operative intrapleural BCG in lung cancer: a 5-year follow-up report. Cancer Immunol Immunother 1986;22(2):155–9.

11. Refaely Y, Simansky DA, Paley M, et al. Resection and perfusion thermochemotherapy: a new approach for the treatment of thymic malignancies with pleural spread. Ann Thorac Surg 2001;72(2): 366–70.

12. Pinto C, Marino A, Guaraldi M, et al. Combination chemotherapy with mitoxantrone, methotrexate, and mitomycin (MMM regimen) in malignant pleural mesothelioma: a phase II study. Am J Clin Oncol 2001;24(2):143–7.

13. Chang MY, Sugarbaker DJ. Innovative therapies: intraoperative intracavitary chemotherapy. Thorac Surg Clin 2004;14(4):549–56.

14. Tilleman TR, Richards WG, Zellos L, et al. Extrapleural pneumonectomy followed by intracavitary intraoperative hyperthermic cisplatin with pharmacologic cytoprotection for treatment of malignant pleural mesothelioma: a phase II prospective study. J Thorac Cardiovasc Surg 2009; 138(2):405–11.

15. Tohda Y, Iwanaga T, Takada M, et al. Intrapleural administration of cisplatin and etoposide to treat malignant pleural effusions in patients with non-small cell lung cancer. Chemotherapy 1999;45(3): 197–204.

16. Shoji T, Tanaka F, Yanagihara K, et al. Phase II study of repeated intrapleural chemotherapy using implantable access system for management of malignant pleural effusion. Chest 2002;121(3):821–4.

17. Su WC, Kitagawa M, Xue N, et al. Combined intrapleural and intravenous chemotherapy, and pulmonary irradiation, for treatment of patients with lung cancer presenting with malignant pleural effusion. A pilot study. Oncology 2003;64(1):18–24.

18. Matsuzaki Y, Edagawa M, Shimizu T, et al. Intrapleural hyperthermic perfusion with chemotherapy increases apoptosis in malignant pleuritis. Ann Thorac Surg 2004;78(5):1769–72 [discussion: 1772–3].

19. Jones DR, Taylor MD, Petroni GR, et al. Phase I trial of intrapleural docetaxel administered through an implantable catheter in subjects with a malignant pleural effusion. J Thorac Oncol 2010;5(1):75–81.

20. Fitzpatrick DR, Peroni DJ, Bielefeldt-Ohmann H. The role of growth factors and cytokines in the tumorigenesis and immunobiology of malignant mesothelioma. Am J Respir Cell Mol Biol 1995; 12(5):455–60.

21. Fitzpatrick DR, Bielefeldt-Ohmann H, Himbeck RP, et al. Transforming growth factor-beta: antisense RNA-mediated inhibition affects anchorage-independent growth, tumorigenicity and tumor-infiltrating T-cells in malignant mesothelioma. Growth Factors 1994;11(1):29–44.

22. Jarnicki AG, Musk AW, Robinson BW, et al. Altered CD3 chain and cytokine gene expression in tumor infiltrating T lymphocytes during the development of mesothelioma. Cancer Lett 1996;103(1):1–9.

23. Lew F, Tsang P, Holland JF, et al. High frequency of immune dysfunctions in asbestos workers and in patients with malignant mesothelioma. J Clin Immunol 1986;6(3):225–33.

24. Kagan E. The alveolar macrophage: immune derangement and asbestos-related malignancy. Semin Oncol 1981;8(3):258–67.

25. Henderson DW, Attwood HD, Constance TJ, et al. Lymphohistiocytoid mesothelioma: a rare lymphomatoid variant of predominantly sarcomatoid mesothelioma. Ultrastruct Pathol 1988;12(4):367–84.

26. Astoul P, Viallat JR, Laurent JC, et al. Intrapleural recombinant IL-2 in passive immunotherapy for malignant pleural effusion. Chest 1993;103(1): 209–13.

27. Christmas TI, Manning LS, Garlepp MJ, et al. Effect of interferon-alpha 2a on malignant mesothelioma. J Interferon Res 1993;13(1):9–12.

28. Boutin C, Nussbaum E, Monnet I, et al. Intrapleural treatment with recombinant gamma-interferon in early stage malignant pleural mesothelioma. Cancer 1994;74(9):2460–7.

29. Boutin C, Viallat JR, Van Zandwijk N, et al. Activity of intrapleural recombinant gamma-interferon in malignant mesothelioma. Cancer 1991;67(8): 2033–7.

30. Yanagawa H, Haku T, Hiramatsu K, et al. Intrapleural instillation of interferon gamma in patients with malignant pleurisy due to lung cancer. Cancer Immunol Immunother 1997;45(2):93–9.

31. Goey SH, Eggermont AM, Punt CJ, et al. Intrapleural administration of interleukin 2 in pleural mesothelioma: a phase I-II study. Br J Cancer 1995; 72(5):1283–8.

32. Sartori S, Tombesi P, Tassinari D, et al. Prospective randomized trial of intrapleural bleomycin versus interferon alfa-2b via ultrasound-guided small-bore chest tube in the palliative treatment of malignant pleural effusions. J Clin Oncol 2004;22(7): 1228–33.

33. Yamaguchi Y, Ohshita A, Kawabuchi Y, et al. Locoregional immunotherapy of malignant effusion from colorectal cancer using the streptococcal preparation OK-432 plus interleukin-2: induction of autologous tumor-reactive CD4+ Th1 killer lymphocytes. Br J Cancer 2003;89(10):1876–84.

34. Ikehara M, Oshita F, Suzuki R, et al. Phase II study of OK-432 intrapleural administration followed by systemic cisplatin and gemcitabine for non-small cell lung cancer with pleuritis carcinomatosa. J Exp Ther Oncol 2004;4(1):79–83.

35. Ren S, Terman DS, Bohach G, et al. Intrapleural staphylococcal superantigen induces resolution of malignant pleural effusions and a survival benefit in non-small cell lung cancer. Chest 2004;126(5):1529–39.

36. Wivel NA, Wilson JM. Methods of gene delivery. Hematol Oncol Clin North Am 1998;12(3):483–501.

37. Curiel DT, Pilewski JM, Albelda SM. Gene therapy approaches for inherited and acquired lung diseases. Am J Respir Cell Mol Biol 1996;14(1):1–18.

38. Nagy JA, Shockley TR, Masse EM, et al. Systemic delivery of a recombinant protein by genetically modified mesothelial cells reseeded on the parietal peritoneal surface. Gene Ther 1995;2(6):402–10.

39. Yang L, Hwang R, Pandit L, et al. Gene therapy of metastatic pancreas cancer with intraperitoneal injections of concentrated retroviral herpes simplex thymidine kinase vector supernatant and ganciclovir. Ann Surg 1996;224(3):405–14 [discussion: 414–7].

40. Batra RK, Dubinett SM, Henkle BW, et al. Retroviral gene transfer is inhibited by chondroitin sulfate proteoglycans/glycosaminoglycans in malignant pleural effusions. J Biol Chem 1997;272(18):11736–43.

41. Monahan PE, Samulski RJ. AAV vectors: is clinical success on the horizon? Gene Ther 2000;7(1):24–30.

42. Zhang WW. Development and application of adenoviral vectors for gene therapy of cancer. Cancer Gene Ther 1999;6(2):113–38.

43. Yeh P, Perricaudet M. Advances in adenoviral vectors: from genetic engineering to their biology. FASEB J 1997;11(8):615–23.

44. Wold WS, Doronin K, Toth K, et al. Immune responses to adenoviruses: viral evasion mechanisms and their implications for the clinic. Curr Opin Immunol 1999;11(4):380–6.

45. Smythe WR, Hwang HC, Amin KM, et al. Use of recombinant adenovirus to transfer the herpes simplex virus thymidine kinase (HSVtk) gene to thoracic neoplasms: an effective in vitro drug sensitization system. Cancer Res 1994;54(8):2055–9.

46. Brody SL, Jaffe HA, Han SK, et al. Direct in vivo gene transfer and expression in malignant cells using adenovirus vectors. Hum Gene Ther 1994;5(4):437–47.

47. Esandi MC, van Someren GD, Vincent AJ, et al. Gene therapy of experimental malignant mesothelioma using adenovirus vectors encoding the HSVtk gene. Gene Ther 1997;4(4):280–7.

48. Batra RK, Dubinett SM, Henkle BW, et al. Adenoviral gene transfer is inhibited by soluble factors in malignant pleural effusions. Am J Respir Cell Mol Biol 2000;22(5):613–9.

49. Sterman DH, Treat J, Litzky LA, et al. Adenovirus-mediated herpes simplex virus thymidine kinase/ganciclovir gene therapy in patients with localized malignancy: results of a phase I clinical trial in malignant mesothelioma. Hum Gene Ther 1998;9(7):1083–92.

50. Chesnoy S, Huang L. Structure and function of lipid-DNA complexes for gene delivery. Annu Rev Biophys Biomol Struct 2000;29:27–47.

51. Nagamachi Y, Tani M, Shimizu K, et al. Suicidal gene therapy for pleural metastasis of lung cancer by liposome-mediated transfer of herpes simplex virus thymidine kinase gene. Cancer Gene Ther 1999;6(6):546–53.

52. Hortobagyi GN, Ueno NT, Xia W, et al. Cationic liposome-mediated E1A gene transfer to human breast and ovarian cancer cells and its biologic effects: a phase I clinical trial. J Clin Oncol 2001;19(14):3422–33.

53. Tiberghien P. Use of suicide genes in gene therapy. J Leukoc Biol 1994;56(2):203–9.

54. Mesnil M, Yamasaki H. Bystander effect in herpes simplex virus-thymidine kinase/ganciclovir cancer gene therapy: role of gap-junctional intercellular communication. Cancer Res 2000;60(15):3989–99.

55. Elshami AA, Saavedra A, Zhang H, et al. Gap junctions play a role in the 'bystander effect' of the herpes simplex virus thymidine kinase/ganciclovir system in vitro. Gene Ther 1996;3(1):85–92.

56. Pope IM, Poston GJ, Kinsella AR. The role of the bystander effect in suicide gene therapy. Eur J Cancer 1997;33(7):1005–16.

57. Kolls J, Freeman S, Ramesh R, et al. The treatment of malignant pleural mesothelioma with gene modified cancer cells: a phase I study. Am J Respir Crit Care Med 1998;157:A563.

58. Schwarzenberger P, Harrison L, Weinacker A, et al. Gene therapy for malignant mesothelioma: a novel approach for an incurable cancer with increased incidence in Louisiana. J La State Med Soc 1998;150(4):168–74.

59. Schwarzenberger P, Byrne P, Gaumer R, et al. Treatment of mesothelioma with gene-modified PA1STK cells and ganciclovir: a phase I study. Cancer Gene Ther 2011;18(12):906–12.

60. Harrison LH Jr, Schwarzenberger PO, Byrne PS, et al. Gene-modified PA1-STK cells home to tumor

sites in patients with malignant pleural mesothelioma. Ann Thorac Surg 2000;70(2):407–11.

61. Smythe WR, Hwang HC, Elshami AA, et al. Treatment of experimental human mesothelioma using adenovirus transfer of the herpes simplex thymidine kinase gene. Ann Surg 1995;222(1):78–86.

62. Smythe WR, Kaiser LR, Hwang HC, et al. Successful adenovirus-mediated gene transfer in an in vivo model of human malignant mesothelioma. Ann Thorac Surg 1994;57(6):1395–401.

63. Hwang HC, Smythe WR, Elshami AA, et al. Gene therapy using adenovirus carrying the herpes simplex-thymidine kinase gene to treat in vivo models of human malignant mesothelioma and lung cancer. Am J Respir Cell Mol Biol 1995; 13(1):7–16.

64. Elshami AA, Kucharczuk JC, Zhang HB, et al. Treatment of pleural mesothelioma in an immunocompetent rat model utilizing adenoviral transfer of the herpes simplex virus thymidine kinase gene. Hum Gene Ther 1996;7(2):141–8.

65. Molnar-Kimber KL, Sterman DH, Chang M, et al. Impact of preexisting and induced humoral and cellular immune responses in an adenovirus-based gene therapy phase I clinical trial for localized mesothelioma. Hum Gene Ther 1998;9(14): 2121–33.

66. Sterman DH, Molnar-Kimber K, Iyengar T, et al. A pilot study of systemic corticosteroid administration in conjunction with intrapleural adenoviral vector administration in patients with malignant pleural mesothelioma. Cancer Gene Ther 2000;7(12): 1511–8.

67. Leong CC, Marley JV, Loh S, et al. The induction of immune responses to murine malignant mesothelioma by IL-2 gene transfer. Immunol Cell Biol 1997; 75(4):356–9.

68. Addison CL, Braciak T, Ralston R, et al. Intratumoral injection of an adenovirus expressing interleukin 2 induces regression and immunity in a murine breast cancer model. Proc Natl Acad Sci U S A 1995; 92(18):8522–6.

69. Mukherjee S, Haenel T, Himbeck R, et al. Replication-restricted vaccinia as a cytokine gene therapy vector in cancer: persistent transgene expression despite antibody generation. Cancer Gene Ther 2000;7(5):663–70.

70. Rosso R, Rimoldi R, Salvati F, et al. Intrapleural natural beta interferon in the treatment of malignant pleural effusions. Oncology 1988; 45(3):253–6.

71. Cascinu S, Isidori PP, Fedeli A, et al. Experience with intrapleural natural beta interferon in the treatment of malignant pleural effusions. Tumori 1991; 77(3):237–8.

72. Odaka M, Sterman DH, Wiewrodt R, et al. Eradication of intraperitoneal and distant tumor by adenovirus-mediated interferon-beta gene therapy is attributable to induction of systemic immunity. Cancer Res 2001;61(16):6201–12.

73. Sterman DH, Recio A, Carroll RG, et al. A phase I clinical trial of single-dose intrapleural IFN-beta gene transfer for malignant pleural mesothelioma and metastatic pleural effusions: high rate of anti-tumor immune responses. Clin Cancer Res 2007; 13(15 Pt 1):4456–66.

74. Sterman DH, Recio A, Haas AR, et al. A phase I trial of repeated intrapleural adenoviral-mediated interferon-beta gene transfer for mesothelioma and metastatic pleural effusions. Mol Ther 2010; 18(4):852–60.

75. Sterman DH, Haas A, Moon E, et al. A trial of intrapleural adenoviral-mediated interferon-α2b gene transfer for malignant pleural mesothelioma. Am J Respir Crit Care Med 2011;184(12):1395–9.

76. Selvaraj P, Yerra A, Tien L, et al. Custom designing therapeutic cancer vaccines: delivery of immunostimulatory molecule adjuvants by protein transfer. Hum Vaccin 2008;4(5):384–8.

77. Vachani A, Moon E, Wakeam E, et al. Gene therapy for mesothelioma and lung cancer. Am J Respir Cell Mol Biol 2010;42(4):385–93.

78. Giuliano M, Catalano A, Strizzi L, et al. Adenovirus-mediated wild-type p53 overexpression reverts tumourigenicity of human mesothelioma cells. Int J Mol Med 2000;5(6):591–6.

79. Dong M, Li X, Hong LJ, et al. Advanced malignant pleural or peritoneal effusion in patients treated with recombinant adenovirus p53 injection plus cisplatin. J Int Med Res 2008;36(6):1273–8.

80. Zhao WZ, Wang JK, Li W, et al. Clinical research on recombinant human Ad-p53 injection combined with cisplatin in treatment of malignant pleural effusion induced by lung cancer. Ai Zheng 2009; 28(12):1324–7.

81. Haas AR, Sterman DH. Malignant pleural mesothelioma: Update on treatment options with a focus on novel therapies. Clin Chest Med 2013;34(1):99–111.

Percutaneous Dilational Tracheostomy

David W. Hsia, MD[a],*, Uzair K. Ghori, MD[b],
Ali I. Musani, MD[c]

KEYWORDS

- Percutaneous dilational tracheostomy • Chronic respiratory failure • Flexible bronchoscopy
- Critical illness

KEY POINTS

- There are numerous indications for PDT placement in the management of chronic respiratory failure.
- PDT has been safely performed by surgical and medical physicians, including critical care intensivists and interventional pulmonologists.
- There are multiple methods of performing the procedure and the single dilator variant of the Ciaglia method is currently the most widely used.
- PDT compares favorably with surgical tracheostomy in regards to procedure time, complications, and cost.
- Flexible bronchoscopy is commonly used as a procedural adjunct and has been shown to decrease complications.
- Because of its advantages, PDT has become one of the most common procedures performed in the modern ICU.

INTRODUCTION

Tracheostomy is one of the oldest surgical procedures and has been performed for several thousand years. There are many indications for tracheostomy placement, such as the need for prolonged mechanical ventilator support, improved clearance of secretions, protection from aspiration, and maintenance of the airway because of sequelae from upper airway obstructions or trauma. In addition, tracheostomy has additional potential benefits over endotracheal tube (ETT) intubation because it decreases the work of breathing,[1] reduces ventilator-associated pneumonia,[2] provides a more secure airway, and permits patient phonation and swallowing. Tracheostomy plays a prominent role in the treatment of prolonged respiratory failure

and more than 50% of all tracheostomies are placed in critically ill patients.[3]

The modern operative procedure remains largely unchanged from the methodology described by Chevalier Jackson in the early 1900s.[4] Jackson's approach involved a long incision, good exposure of the anatomic structures, and division of the thyroid isthmus. His guidelines on the procedure were instrumental in improving procedural safety and outcomes. Subsequent refinements to the procedure and improvements in equipment have resulted in decreased procedure-related morbidity and mortality.[5] In 1957, Sheldon and Pudenz[6] described a Seldinger method of percutaneous tracheostomy placement. The procedure became more widely used after the introduction of the percutaneous dilational method by Ciaglia in

Sources of Support: The authors have no financial disclosures.
[a] Department of Medicine, Harbor-UCLA Medical Center, 1000 West Carson Street, Box #405, Torrance, CA 90509, USA; [b] Department of Medicine, Military Hospital Rawalpindi, Main Peshawar Road, 46000 Rawalpindi, Pakistan; [c] National Jewish Health, 1400 Jackson Street, J225, Molly Blank Building, Denver, CO 80206, USA
* Corresponding author.
E-mail address: dhsia@labiomed.org

Clin Chest Med 34 (2013) 515–526
http://dx.doi.org/10.1016/j.ccm.2013.04.002

chestmed.theclinics.com

1985.[7] Percutaneous tracheostomy is now recognized as a cost-effective procedure that can be performed easily and safely at the bedside by interventional pulmonologists, critical care physicians, and surgeons in the intensive care unit (ICU).

PERCUTANEOUS DILATIONAL TRACHEOSTOMY TECHNIQUES

Percutaneous dilational tracheostomy (PDT) uses the insertion of a tracheal cannula by a modified Seldinger approach. A guidewire is inserted through the anterior tracheal wall; dilation is then performed until the tracheal stoma is large enough to permit insertion of the tracheal cannula. Cannula insertion is generally performed between the second and third tracheal rings, with a suggestion of decreased risk of bleeding when placed above the fourth tracheal ring.[8] Several variations of the procedure have been developed and are in use today.

The Ciaglia method[7] is currently the most commonly used PDT technique; it was originally described using serial dilation with progressively larger hydrophilic coated dilators and is now adapted in commercially available kits to use a single conical dilator (Ciaglia Blue Rhino Tracheostomy Introducer Kit, Cook Critical Care, Bloomington, IN; Per-Fit Kit, SIMS Portex, Keene, NH) (**Fig. 1**). Before the procedure, the distal tip of the ETT is repositioned within the subglottic space proximal to the intended tracheostomy dilation site. A midline incision is made over the anterior trachea and the pretracheal soft tissue is bluntly dissected with mosquito clamps. The underlying trachea is then identified using a needle and introducer sheath. Flexible bronchoscopic visualization is commonly used to provide endoscopic guidance from within the trachea (**Fig. 2**). Removal of the needle allows an introduction of a J-shaped guidewire through the introducer sheath into the trachea and directed caudally into the distal airways. The introducer sheath is then removed and dilation of the trachea and soft tissue is performed initially with a short dilator followed by a curved, conical dilator. Special precautions must be taken to ensure proper midline puncture of the anterior trachea wall and introduction of the guidewire and subsequent dilation through the anterior wall while avoiding puncture of the posterior membranous portion of the trachea. A trachestomy tube is loaded onto an introducer dilator and inserted into the trachea over the guidewire through the dilated stoma and secured in place. The use of the single dilator method is theorized to decrease the risk of injury to the posterior tracheal wall and prevent the risk of oxygen desaturation or

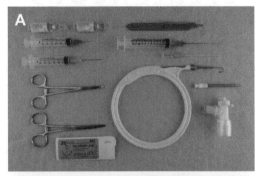

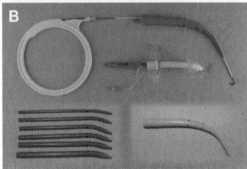

Fig. 1. Single and multiple dilator methods based on the Ciaglia technique. (*A*) Example of equipment found in commercially available PDT kits. (*B*) Multiple and single dilator systems. The guidewire and guide catheter are shown inserted through a single conical-shaped Blue Rhino dilator. A tracheostomy cannula is loaded onto a specialized introducer. Inset shows a set of multiple dilators with sizes ranging from 18F to 36F catheter compared with a single dilator.

inadequate ventilation by minimizing the period of time needed to dilate the tracheostomy stoma and insert the tracheostomy cannula. Another modification of the Ciaglia method (Ciaglia Blue Dolphin Tracheostomy Introducer Kit; Cook Critical Care) using a balloon dilator has also been developed (**Fig. 3**).[9] PDT using single dilation has been shown to decrease procedure time compared with the multiple and balloon dilation methods.[10–12]

Numerous kits using other PDT dilation methods are also commercially available. The Griggs' dilational forceps technique (Portex PDT Kit; Portex, Hyathe, Kent, UK) uses curved Howard-Kelly forceps with a special groove that permits passage of the guidewire through the forceps.[13] The guidewire directs the path of the forceps, which are used to dilate the soft tissue and trachea. The translaryngeal tracheostomy method (Translaryngeal Tracheostomy Kit; Mallinckrodt, Courtaboeuf, France) directs the guidewire caudally either within or external to the ETT. The ETT is removed and the patient is reintubated with a

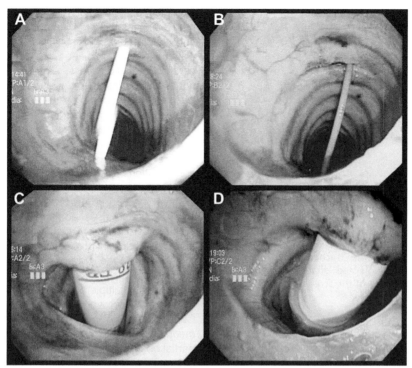

Fig. 2. Bronchoscopic guidance of PDT using a single dilator. Endotracheal images of PDT insertion visualized by a bronchoscope positioned within the ETT. The distal tip of the ETT can be seen at the bottom of each image. (*A*) Insertion of the guide catheter through the anterior tracheal wall. (*B*) Insertion of the guidewire, which is then directed distally in the trachea. (*C*) Blunt dilation with a single conical-shaped Blue Rhino dilator over the guide-wire by modified Seldinger technique. (*D*) Insertion of the tracheostomy cannula through the dilated tracheostomy tract.

special 5-mm ETT. The guidewire is directed retrograde through the anterior tracheal wall until the tip exits the mouth. A conical tracheal cannula is attached to the cranial end of the dilator and pulled back into the trachea where it is used to dilate the

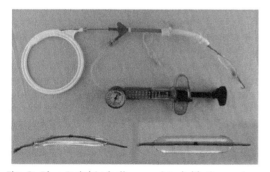

Fig. 3. Blue Dolphin balloon-assisted dilation system. The Blue Dolphin saline-filled inflation dilator is shown with guidewire and inflation syringe. The tracheostomy cannula is loaded directly onto the device and deployed after performing balloon dilation. Inset shows a close-up of the distal tip with the balloon deflated and inflated.

trachea and pretracheal soft tissue from within the tracheal lumen. When the cannula protrudes from the soft tissue of the neck, the external tip is cut off and attached to the mechanical ventilator while the tracheal portion of the cannula is directed toward the carina by an obturator. One potential benefit of the translaryngeal tracheostomy method is that it avoids anterior compression of the trachea, which may be useful in younger patients with highly elastic tracheas.[14] A single-step screw-like dilator (PercuTwist; Rüsch, Kernen, Germany) has also been developed that uses rotation to advance the dilator to avoid complications associated with direct compression of the trachea (**Fig. 4**).[15] Additional methods include use of a specialized speculum-like tracheostome,[16] a cutting bougie device,[17] and Rapitrac tracheostome (SurgiTech Medical, Sydney, Australia).[18]

Although PDT has gained in popularity, not all of these commercial kits are universally available. Recent surveys of ICU directors suggest that the Ciaglia single dilator has become the most popular tracheostomy placement technique and is the method of choice in up to 69% of ICUs.[19,20] As with any procedure, however, the experience of

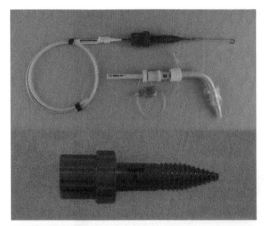

Fig. 4. "PercuTwist" screw-like dilation system. The "PercuTwist" dilator is shown with guidewire and introducer catheter. The tracheostomy cannula is introduced after single-step dilation is performed. Inset shows a close-up of the screw-like dilator.

the physician with the procedural method is of paramount importance.

PROCEDURAL ADJUNCTS

Flexible bronchoscopy is commonly used to provide endoscopic procedural guidance and is routinely used in 83% to 97.7% of ICUs.[19,20] Bronchoscopy provides real-time visual guidance from within the tracheal lumen. This includes confirmation of appropriate ETT positioning, midline placement of the introducer needle and catheter within the tracheal lumen, direction of the guidewire, proper placement of the tracheal cannula, and helps prevent injury to the posterior tracheal wall by visually guiding stoma dilation. Composite evaluation of 1385 patients (15 studies) undergoing PDT without endoscopic guidance demonstrated a complication rate of 16.8% compared with 8.7% in 1351 patients (nine studies) with endoscopic guidance.[21] PDT performed with bronchoscopy was also associated with lower rates of accidental extubation, false passage, pneumomediastinum and pneumothorax, and other technical difficulties. However, it is difficult to control for variations in patient populations, PDT technique, and operator experience across studies. Few trials have directly examined the impact of bronchoscopy on PDT complications. A prospective study by Berrouschot and colleagues[22] demonstrated a similar perioperative complication rate while prospectively evaluating PDT with and without bronchoscopy (7% vs 6%), but had more severe complications in the group without bronchoscopy. Jackson and colleagues[23] reported no difference in complications, including bleeding and late

complications. Use of bronchoscopy with PDT has been associated with transient hypercarbia and respiratory acidosis[24–26]; this may lead to an elevation in intracranial pressure and decrease in cerebral perfusion pressure.[27] These findings are not surprising because transient increases in positive end-expiratory pressure (PEEP) and partial pressure of carbon dioxide are known to occur during flexible bronchoscopy on mechanically ventilated patients because of partial occlusion of the ETT by the bronchoscope.[28] Nevertheless, complications resulting from these physiologic changes are rare and bronchoscopy remains a routinely performed procedure in the ICU. Bronchoscopy also uses additional equipment and personnel resources, affects procedural costs, and may result in procedure-related damage to the bronchoscope. Nevertheless, given the benefits of endoscopic visual guidance compared with its low risk, multiple authors have recommended its use to improve procedural safety.[13,21,29–32] Care should be taken to monitor and adjust mechanical ventilator settings to account for the partial obstruction of the ETT by the flexible bronchoscope and the resulting physiologic and ventilatory effects.

Ultrasonography is another adjunct method used to ensure accurate placement of the introducer needle into the trachea, estimate the distance from the skin to the trachea, identify anomalous vascular anatomy, and prevent damage to vascular and adjacent structures (**Fig. 5**).[33] Ultrasound evaluation of the anterior neck has been shown to change the intended tracheostomy site in up to 24% of cases to avoid subcutaneous vasculature.[34] Ultrasonography can also provide real-time procedural guidance for introduction of the introducer needle and guide catheter into the tracheal lumen[35,36] and ETT positioning.[37] Bedside ultrasound machines are readily available in the ICU setting and are a familiar imaging modality to interventional pulmonologists and intensivists. Performing ultrasonography is inexpensive and has essentially no procedure-related drawbacks. However, further studies are required to evaluate its impact on procedural performance and safety.

Inadvertent extubation of the ETT and puncture of the ETT cuff are potential complications that may lead to catastrophic hypoxia or loss of the airway. The laryngeal mask airway (LMA) has been considered as an alternative method of airway management during PDT. The position of the LMA external to the trachea prevents it from interfering with the PDT procedure. There are concerns that this method of ventilation is not adequately secure in critically ill patients who may require significant mechanical ventilator

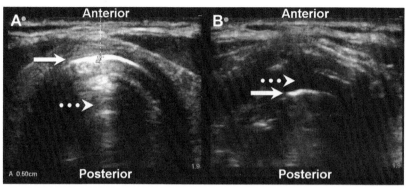

Fig. 5. Ultrasonography for PDT. Demonstration of ultrasound images of the neck and trachea. (*A*) Normal trachea imaged above a tracheal ring. Tracheal cartilage (*solid arrow*) creates a shadow artifact (*dotted arrow*). Image depth of 1.9 cm is indicated in the lower right corner. The *dotted line* measures the distance between the skin and anterior trachea to be 0.50 cm, as indicated in the lower left corner. (*B*) Intubated trachea imaged between tracheal rings. The ETT (*solid arrow*) and associated shadow artifact is visualized within the tracheal lumen (*dotted arrow*).

support with high airway pressures, levels of oxygen supplementation, or PEEP. Several trials comparing PDT with bronchoscopic guidance through an LMA versus ETT have been performed with varying results. Dosemeci and colleagues[38] demonstrated a greater incidence of hypercarbia along with higher associated rise in partial pressure of carbon dioxide ($Paco_2$) with ETT (56.7% of patients; 6.8 ± 3.5 mm Hg) compared with LMA (38.5% of patients; 4.5 ± 2.4 mm Hg). Visualization of tracheal structures during PDT has also been found to be improved with the use of an LMA.[39,40] However, in a randomized comparison of 60 patients undergoing PDT, 6.6% of patients using ETT had cuff puncture and 3.3% had accidental extubation; in comparison, 33% performed with LMA had potentially catastrophic airway-related complications, including loss of the airway, significant hypoxia, and aspiration of gastric contents.[41] Therefore, although the use of an LMA with PDT has been shown to be feasible, its safety has not been convincingly demonstrated.

PROCEDURE-RELATED COMPLICATIONS

PDT is a safe procedure when performed in the properly selected patient, in an appropriate setting, and with trained physicians and staff. Overall complication rates of 5.6% to 54% have been reported, most of which were considered minor.[21,42–45] Periprocedural and early postprocedural complications include bleeding; hemodynamic instability; cardiac arrhythmias; airway obstruction or loss of the airway (eg, accidental extubation or decannulation); hypoxia; tracheal ring fracture; underdilation or overdilation of the trachea; damage to mediastinal structures (eg, damage to the tracheal wall, creation of a false

passage, development of subcutaneous emphysema, pneumomediastinum, or pneumothorax); wound infection; technical difficulties requiring conversion to a surgical approach; and death. Procedure-related mortality is low, with reported rates of 0% to 0.7%.[21,42–45]

Procedural or postprocedural bleeding is usually rare, with reported incidence of 0.4% to 8%.[21,42–45] As a result, PDT does not require routine use of electrocautery to control hemostasis. Bleeding may be reduced because of the creation of a tight tracheostomy stoma with blunt dilation, which shifts and compresses vascular structures that may be perforated with sharp surgical dissection techniques. Most bleeding results from soft tissue oozing because the procedure is performed in the midline to avoid vascular structures. Given the tight nature of the PDT tract, hemostasis is usually obtained from tamponade by the tracheostomy cannula. Bleeding may be decreased with the use of stay sutures securing the flanges of the tracheostomy tube.[46] Occasionally, digital compression or a suture may be required to control superficial bleeding.[47]

Head-to-head trials involving different PDT methods are rare, which makes the comparison of complication rates difficult and problematic. **Table 1** highlights findings from prospective, randomized PDT comparison trials.[10–12,24,25,48–51] The single dilator Ciaglia technique has been associated with greater rates of tracheal ring fracture compared with the multiple dilator Ciaglia and the Griggs' dilational forceps methods.[11,49] The translaryngeal tracheostomy technique has been associated with loss of the airway and technical difficulties requiring physicians to switch to an alternate tracheostomy method.[25] Other conclusions regarding complications rates are conflicting

Table 1
PDT complications from prospective, randomized direct comparison trials

Study	Number of Subjects	Dilaton Methods	Significant Findings
Johnson et al,[10] 2001	50	Multiple vs single	No significant difference in complication rates
Byhahn et al,[11] 2000	50	Multiple vs single	Decreased tracheal ring fracture with multiple dilator (8% vs 36%)
Cianchi et al,[12] 2010	70	Single vs balloon	Decreased resistance to cannula insertion (5.7% vs 28.6%) with single dilator
Nates et al,[48] 2000	100	Multiple vs forceps	Decreased surgical complications (1.9% vs 24%) and bleeding (1.9% vs 15%) with multiple dilator
Kaiser et al,[24] 2006	100	Single vs forceps	Decreased major complications (0% vs 12.5%), minor bleeding (12% vs 35%), and hypoxemia (0% vs 10%) with forceps dilator
Ambesh et al,[49] 2002	60	Single vs forceps	Decreased overdilation or underdilation (7% vs 53%) and bleeding (3% vs 17%) with single dilator. Decreased change in P_{Peak} (+5 vs +16.5 cm H_2O) and tracheal ring fracture (0% vs 30%) with forceps dilator
Anon et al,[50] 2004	53	Single vs forceps	Nonsignificant trend toward decreased procedural complications with single dilator (7.4% vs 26.9%; $P = .07$)
Montcriol et al,[51] 2011	90	Forceps vs rotational	No significant difference in complication rates
Cantais et al,[25] 2002	100	Forceps vs translaryngeal	Decreased need to convert to alternate method (0% vs 23%), loss of airway (0% vs 15%), and bleeding (4% vs 23%) with forceps dilator

Abbreviation: P_{Peak}, peak airway pressure.
Data from Refs.[10–12,24,25,48–51]

or limited given the relative paucity of data available. It is therefore difficult to determine which technique is superior.

Comparison of long-term complications, such as tracheal stenosis, delayed stoma closure, airway symptoms (eg, dyspnea, cough, phonetic impairment), and scarring/cosmesis is difficult to evaluate given the low occurrence rate; analysis of these complications requires long-term follow-up of a large study population.

PERCUTANEOUS VERSUS SURGICAL TECHNIQUES

Surgical tracheostomy involves dissection through the pretracheal soft tissue until the trachea is identified. The trachea is then cannulated under direct visualization. It is typically performed in the operating room, in contrast to PDT, which is usually performed in the ICU. Meta-analysis of 15 randomized, controlled trials involving 973 patients has demonstrated several important clinical outcome differences between PDT and surgical tracheostomy.[52] Most PDTs included in this analysis were performed using the multiple dilator method placed in the ICU setting. PDT was associated with a significant decrease in unfavorable scarring (odds ratio [OR], 0.44; 95% confidence interval [CI], 0.23–0.83) and wound infections (OR, 0.31; 95% CI, 0.22–0.62). Decreased wound infection is likely related to the minimal trauma and tissue manipulation associated with PDT and is consistent with the decrease in surgical site infections associated with other minimally invasive surgical procedures.[53] There was no significant difference in minor or major hemorrhage, development of subglottic stenosis, creation of a false passage, or death. However, PDT had a higher risk of complications associated with decannulation and mucous obstruction (OR, 2.79; 95% CI, 1.29–6.03), which may be related to the use of smaller tracheostomy tracts and cannulas with PDT.

By performing PDT at the bedside, morbidity associated with patient transport can also be avoided. Intrahospital transportation of critically ill patients has been shown to adversely impact patients physiologically and psychologically.[54] In addition, the numerous intravascular lines, endoluminal tubes, monitoring devices, and other hardware associated with the care of critically ill patients may become displaced during transport. Significant adverse events have been shown to occur in up to 8.9% of intrahospital transports of critically ill patients.[55,56] It is therefore beneficial when diagnostic or therapeutic interventions can be safely performed at the bedside without transport of the critically ill patient away from the ICU.

Performing procedures in the operating room setting uses a limited hospital resource and is associated with higher associated costs. PDT has been shown to reduce procedural costs by $851 to $1645 largely because of cost savings related to operating room and anesthesiologist charges.[57–60] Compared with surgical tracheostomy, mean PDT procedure length is shorter by approximately 4.6 minutes.[52] In some institutions, bedside PDT may also decrease the length of time between the point when a tracheostomy is deemed necessary and the time when the procedure occurs.[61,62] Logistic limitations of performing surgical tracheostomy in the operating room may play a role in the procedural delay associated with surgical tracheostomy. PDT reduces the amount of time before a permanent airway is secured and potentially decreases ICU and hospital length of stay in select patient populations[62]; benefits in logistic efficiency and length of stay, however, are not consistent in all institutions.[60]

SPECIAL CIRCUMSTANCES

It is estimated that 11% to 35% of patients with cervical spine injuries may require a tracheostomy for long-term airway management.[63] Cervical spine injury limits the amount of neck extension permissible when positioning a patient for PDT. In addition, patients undergoing anterior cervical spine fixation are at higher risk for infection given the close proximity of the wound to the tracheostomy site, concomitant use of high-dose steroids, and relative immunosuppression resulting from severe injury.[63] Several small case series involving PDT in patients with cervical spine fixation reported only rare procedural bleeding and wound infection without any worsening in neurologic status.[63,64] Retrospective comparison of PDT and surgical tracheostomy in this population demonstrated comparable procedure-related complication rates with 5.9% bleeding, 10% tracheal stenosis, and 15% stomal cellulitis.[65] In a small prospective randomized trial, PDT procedure time was significantly shorter than surgical tracheostomy (8 ± 6 vs 21 ± 7 minutes) without significant difference in periprocedure or postprocedure complications.[66] Furthermore, PDT in trauma patients clinically or radiographically cleared of cervical spine injury may not have worse outcomes compared with patients who have neck injuries or are unable to be cleared of neck injury.[67]

The critically ill obese population has greater perioperative and postprocedural complications with surgical tracheostomies and is considered another relative contraindication to PDT.[50,68] Neck landmarks may be harder to identify given the abundance of soft tissue, especially in patients with short neck length. Greater neck diameter may play a role in the formation of a false passage or inadvertent decannulation. Obesity may also compromise mechanical ventilation and oxygenation. A trial using multiple PDT techniques demonstrated a 2.7-fold increased risk for perioperative complications (43.8% vs 18.2%) and 4.9-fold increased risk for serious complications (9.6% vs 0.7%) in obese patients[69]; the complication rates in this study, however, were higher than in many comparable studies and interpretation of the results may be hindered by the use of multiple PDT methods. In contrast, several trials using a single dilator technique found no significant difference in complication rates between obese and nonobese populations.[36,70,71] Although these studies categorized obesity based on body mass index, this index may not accurately reflect the impact of obesity on the soft tissue of the neck. Tabaee and colleagues[72] stratified patients based on the cricosternal distance in the neutral and extended positions and did not find correlation between neck length and PDT outcomes. Finally, a retrospective comparison between 89 PDT and 53 surgical tracheostomies in morbidly obese patients showed no difference in serious adverse outcomes (6.5% vs 6.5%).[73] These data suggest that PDT can be safely performed by skilled operators in this potentially high-risk population.

During the PDT procedure, the ETT cuff is deflated to reposition the ETT. Cuff deflation affects PEEP generated by the mechanical ventilator and may result in derecruitment of alveoli.[74] PDT may therefore adversely affect patients with severe hypoxic respiratory failure and high PEEP requirements. Beiderlinden and colleagues[75] investigated bronchoscopic-guided PDT in patients with hypoxic respiratory failure and did not demonstrate any significant decrease in arterial oxygen levels. This included patients with PEEP greater than 10 cm H_2O (mean, 16.7 $\pm$ 4 cm H_2O) whose peripheral oxygen saturation (Spo_2) did not decrease during the procedure. Furthermore, arterial oxygen to fraction of inhaled oxygen ratios (Pao_2/Fio_2) remained unchanged before the procedure compared with 1 hour and 24 hours postprocedure (243 $\pm$ 90 vs 223 $\pm$ 83 vs 260 $\pm$ 86 mm Hg) suggesting that derecruitment did not occur. It is possible, however, that the use of bronchoscopic guidance may have minimized the potential loss of PEEP during PDT because of the effect of the bronchoscope on PEEP. Recruitment maneuvers before PDT may also help prevent potential derecruitment as demonstrated in a small trial with sustained improvement in oxygenation during the procedure and postprocedure.[76] PDT has also been performed in patients undergoing high-frequency oscillatory ventilation.[77] Despite these data, it is preferable to perform PDT when hypoxic respiratory failure and PEEP requirements have improved.

Unfortunately, ICU patients often have underlying coagulopathy or thrombocytopenia related to their comorbid conditions. Critically ill patients may also require treatment of medical issues with aspirin and clopidigrel or venous thromboembolic prophylaxis with heparin products. As a result, they are often at higher risk for procedure-related bleeding. There is wide variability in physician practices regarding periprocedural holding of anticoagulation,[78] but prophylactic anticoagulation may not adversely affect bleeding risk.[78,79] Prothrombin time,[80] activated partial thromboplastin time,[79] and thrombocytopenia[79,80] are associated with increased PDT procedural bleeding risk. These data are contradicted, however, by a small prospective, randomized trial demonstrating no difference in bleeding when coagulopathy or thrombocytopenia was corrected with fresh frozen plasma or platelet transfusion.[81] PDT has also been successfully performed in patients with refractory coagulopathy from severe liver disease[82] and organ transplant.[83] Although PDT has been successfully performed in these high-risk populations, further studies to evaluate the risk of bleeding from coagulopathy and thrombocytopenia are needed.

Part of the appeal of PDT is the relative simplicity of the procedure, which allows it to be adapted to potentially difficult situations. PDT has been safely performed in several situations where the patient may be at higher risk for complications. Additional circumstances where PDT has been successfully used include establishment of an emergent airway,[84] prior tracheostomy,[80,85,86] thyromegaly,[86] difficult airway,[87] and extreme age.[88] However, it is important to recognize that the physician's experience is crucial when evaluating if PDT can be safely performed; demonstration of the ability to perform PDT in a few select cases does not imply that PDT is the method of choice in all cases involving these patient populations.

PROCEDURAL TRAINING AND GUIDELINES

PDT can be safely performed by a variety of physician specialists, including interventional pulmonologists, medical critical care intensivists, neurointensivists, surgeons, and anesthesiologists.[47,89–92] Specific training is required to perform PDT with most guidelines using expert opinion to determine a recommended number of procedures to be used as a surrogate marker for the establishment of procedural competency. Although procedure volume is not the only determinant of competency, procedural outcomes in other specialties have been demonstrated to be directly related to outcomes.[93] Procedural simulation has also been used for PDT training.[94] The American College of Chest Physicians recommends a minimum of 20 procedures, whereas the American Thoracic Society and European Respiratory Society recommend 5 to 10 procedures before performing PDT independently with a minimum of 10 procedures per year to maintain proficiency.[95,96] In addition, it is recommended that physicians performing PDT have extensive experience in airway management and the treatment of critically ill patients.[96]

SUMMARY

There are numerous indications for PDT placement in the management of chronic respiratory failure. PDT has been safely performed by surgical and medical physicians, including critical care intensivists and interventional pulmonologists. There are multiple methods of performing the procedure and the single dilator variant of the Ciaglia method is currently the most widely used. PDT compares favorably with surgical tracheostomy in regards to procedure time, complications, and cost. Flexible bronchoscopy is commonly used as a procedural adjunct and has been shown to decrease complications. Because of its advantages, PDT has become one of the most common procedures performed in the modern ICU.

REFERENCES

1. Diehl JL, El Atrous S, Touchard D, et al. Changes in the work of breathing induced by tracheotomy in ventilator-dependent patients. Am J Respir Crit Care Med 1999;159:383–8.
2. Nseir S, Di Pompeo C, Jozefowicz E, et al. Relationship between tracheotomy and ventilator-associated pneumonia: a case control study. Eur Respir J 2007; 30:314–20.
3. Zeitouni A, Kost K. Tracheostomy: a retrospective review of 281 patients. J Otolaryngol 1994;23:61–6.
4. Jackson C. Tracheotomy. Laryngoscope 1909;19: 285–90.
5. Dulguerov P, Gysin C, Perneger TV, et al. Percutaneous or surgical tracheostomy: a meta-analysis. Crit Care Med 1999;27:1617–25.
6. Sheldon C, Pudenz R. Percutaneous tracheotomy. JAMA 1957;165:2068–70.
7. Ciaglia P, Firsching R, Syniec C. Elective percutaneous dilational tracheostomy; a new simple bedside procedure; preliminary report. Chest 1985;87: 715–9.
8. Muhammad JK, Major E, Wood A, et al. Percutaneous dilational tracheostomy: haemorrhagic complications and the vascular anatomy of the anterior neck. A review based on 497 cases. Int J Oral Maxillofac Surg 2000;29:217–22.
9. Gromann TW, Birkelbach O, Hetzer R. Balloon dilational tracheostomy. Technique and first clinical experience with the Ciaglia Blue Dolphin method. Chirurg 2009;80:622–7 [in German].
10. Johnson JL, Cheatham ML, Sagraves SG, et al. Percutaneous dilational tracheostomy: a comparison of single versus multiple-dilator techniques. Crit Care Med 2001;29:1251–4.
11. Byhahn C, Wilke HJ, Halbig S, et al. Percutaneous tracheostomy: ciaglia Blue Rhino versus the basic Ciaglia technique of percutaneous dilational tracheostomy. Anesth Analg 2000;91:882–6.
12. Cianchi G, Zagli G, Bonizzoli M, et al. Comparison between single-step and balloon dilational tracheostomy in intensive care unit: a single-centre, randomized controlled study. Br J Anaesth 2010;104: 728–32.
13. Griggs WM, Worthley LI, Gilligan JE, et al. A simple percutaneous tracheostomy technique [letter reply]. Surg Gynecol Obstet 1990;170:543–5, 512–3.
14. Fantoni A, Ripamonti D. A non-derivative, non-surgical tracheostomy: the translaryngeal method. Intensive Care Med 1997;23:386–92.
15. Frova G, Quintel M. A new simple method for percutaneous tracheostomy: controlled rotating dilation. A preliminary report. Intensive Care Med 2002;28:299–303.
16. Shelden CH, Pudenz RH, Freshwater DB, et al. A new method for tracheostomy. J Neurosurg 1955;12:428–31.
17. Toye FJ, Weinstein JD. A percutaneous tracheostomy device. Surgery 1969;65:384–9.
18. Schachner A, Ovil Y, Sidi J, et al. Percutaneous tracheostomy: a new method. Crit Care Med 1989;17: 1052–6.
19. Kluge S, Baumann HJ, Maier C, et al. Tracheostomy in the intensive care unit: a nationwide survey. Anesth Analg 2008;107:1639–43.
20. Krishnan K, Elliot SC, Mallick A. The current practice of tracheostomy in the United Kingdom: a postal survey. Anaesthesia 2005;60:360–4.
21. Kost KM. Endoscopic percutaneous dilational tracheotomy: a prospective evaluation of 500 cases. Laryngoscope 2005;115:1–30.
22. Berrouschot J, Oeken J, Steiniger L, et al. Perioperative complications of percutaneous dilational tracheostomy. Laryngoscope 1997;107:1538–44.
23. Jackson LS, Davis JW, Kaups KL, et al. Percutaneous tracheostomy: to bronch or not to bronch – that is the question. J Trauma 2011;71:1553–6.
24. Kaiser E, Cantais E, Goutorbe P, et al. Prospective randomized comparison of progressive dilational vs forceps dilational percutaneous tracheostomy. Anaesth Intensive Care 2006;34:51–4.
25. Cantais E, Kaiser E, Le-Goff Y, et al. Percutaneous tracheostomy: prospective comparison of the translaryngeal technique versus the forceps-dilational technique in 100 critically ill adults. Crit Care Med 2002;30:815–9.
26. Reilly PM, Sing RF, Giberson FA, et al. Hypercarbia during tracheostomy: a comparison of percutaneous endoscopic, percutaneous Doppler, and standard surgical tracheostomy. Intensive Care Med 1997;23:859–64.
27. Reilly PM, Anderson HL III, Sing RF, et al. Occult hypercarbia: an unrecognized phenomenon during percutaneous endoscopic tracheostomy. Chest 1995;107:1760–3.
28. Lindholm CE, Ollman B, Snyder JV, et al. Cardiorespiratory effects of flexible fiberoptic bronchoscopy in critically ill patients. Chest 1978;74:362–8.
29. Marelli D, Paul A, Manolidis S, et al. Endoscopic guided percutaneous tracheostomy: early results of a consecutive trial. J Trauma 1990;30:433–5.
30. Kost KM. The optimal technique of percutaneous tracheostomy. Int J Intens Care 2001;8:82–8.
31. Trottier SJ, Hazard PB, Sakabu SA, et al. Posterior tracheal wall perforation during percutaneous dilational tracheostomy: an investigation into its mechanism and prevention. Chest 1999;115:1383–9.

32. Polderman KH, Spijkstra JJ, De Bree R, et al. Percutaneous tracheostomy in the intensive care unit: which safety precautions? [letter]. Crit Care Med 2001;29:221–2.

33. Muhammad JK, Patton DW, Evans RM, et al. Percutaneous dilational trachesotomy under ultrasound guidance. Br J Oral Maxillofac Surg 1999;37:309–11.

34. Kollig E, Heydenreich U, Roetman B, et al. Ultrasound and bronchoscopic controlled percutaneous tracheostomy on trauma ICU. Injury 2000; 31:663–8.

35. Rajajee V, Fletcher JJ, Rochlen LR, et al. Real-time ultrasound-guided percutaneous dilatational tracheostomy: a feasibility study. Crit Care 2011;15:R67.

36. Guinot PG, Zogheib E, Petiot S, et al. Ultrasound-guided percutaneous tracheostomy in critically ill obese patients. Crit Care 2012;16(2):R40.

37. Werner SL, Smith CE, Goldstein JR, et al. Pilot study to evaluate the accuracy of ultrasonography in confirming endotracheal tube placement. Ann Emerg Med 2007;49:75–80.

38. Dosemeci L, Yilmaz M, Gurpinar F, et al. The use of the laryngeal mask airway as an alternative to the endotracheal tube during percutaneous dilatational tracheostomy. Intensive Care Med 2002; 28:63–7.

39. Cattano D, Abramson S, Buzzigoli S, et al. The use of the laryngeal mask airway during guidewire dilating forceps tracheostomy. Anesth Analg 2006; 103:453–7.

40. Linstedt U, Zenz M, Krull K, et al. Laryngeal mask airway or endotracheal tube for percutaneous dilatational tracheostomy: a comparison of visibility of intratracheal structures. Anesth Analg 2010;110: 1076–82.

41. Ambesh SP, Sinha PK, Tripathi M, et al. Laryngeal mask airway vs endotracheal tube to facilitate bedside percutaneous tracheostomy in critically ill patients: a prospective comparative study. J Postgrad Med 2002;48:11–5.

42. Moe KS, Stoeckli SJ, Schmid S, et al. Percutaneous tracheostomy: a comprehensive evaluation. Ann Otol Rhinol Laryngol 1999;108:384–91.

43. Fernandez L, Norwood S, Roettger R, et al. Bedside percutaneous tracheostomy with bronchoscopic guidance in critically ill patients. Arch Surg 1996;131:129–32.

44. Marx WH, Ciaglia P, Graniero KD. Some important details in the technique of percutaneous dilational tracheostomy via the modified Seldinger technique. Chest 1996;110:763–6.

45. Hill BB, Zweng TN, Maley RH, et al. Percutaneous dilational tracheostomy: report of 356 cases. J Trauma 1996;40:238–43.

46. Halum SL, Ting JY, Plowman EK, et al. A multi-institutional analysis of tracheotomy complications. Laryngoscope 2012;122:38–45.

47. Susarla SM, Peacock ZP, Alam HB. Percutaneous dilational tracheostomy: review of technique and evidence for its use. J Oral Maxillofac Surg 2012; 70:74–82.

48. Nates JL, Cooper DJ, Myles PS, et al. Percutaneous tracheostomy in critically ill patients: a prospective, randomized comparison of two techniques. Crit Care Med 2000;28:3734–9.

49. Ambesh SP, Pandey CK, Srivastava S, et al. Percutaneous tracheostomy with single dilatation technique: a prospective, randomized comparison of Ciaglia Blue Rhino versus Griggs' guidewire dilating forceps. Anesth Analg 2002;95:1739–45.

50. Anon JM, Escuela MP, Gomez V, et al. Percutaneous tracheostomy: ciaglia blue rhino versus griggs' guide wire dilating forceps. A prospective randomized trial. Acta Anaesthesiol Scand 2004; 48:451–6.

51. Montcriol A, Bordes J, Asencio Y, et al. Bedside percutaneous tracheostomy: a prospective randomised comparison of PercuTwist versus Griggs' forceps dilational tracheostomy. Anaesth Intensive Care 2011;39:209–16.

52. Higgins KM, Punthakee X. Meta-analysis comparison of open versus percutaneous tracheostomy. Laryngoscope 2007;117:447–54.

53. Targarona EM, Balague C, Knook MM, et al. Laparoscopic surgery and surgical infection. Br J Surg 2000;87:536–44.

54. Fanara B, Manzon C, Barbot O, et al. Recommendations for the intra-hospital transport of critically ill patients. Crit Care 2010;14:R87.

55. Szem JW, Hydo JL, Fischer E, et al. High-risk intrahospital transport of critically ill patients: safety and outcome of the necessary "road trip." Crit Care Med 1995;23(10):1660–6.

56. Papson JP, Russell KL, Taylor DM. Unexpected events during the intrahospital transport of critically ill patients. Acad Emerg Med 2007;14:574–7.

57. Van Natta TL, Morris JA Jr, Eddy VA, et al. Elective bedside surgery in critically injured patients is safe and cost-effective. Ann Surg 1998;227(5):618–24.

58. Bowen CP, Whitney LR, Truwit JD, et al. Comparison of safety and cost of percutaneous versus surgical tracheostomy. Am Surg 2001;67(1):54–60.

59. Cobean R, Beals M, Moss C, et al. Percutaneous dilational tracheostomy. A safe, cost-effective bedside procedure. Arch Surg 1996;131(3):265–71.

60. Freeman BD, Isabella K, Cobb JP, et al. A prospective, randomized study comparing percutaneous with surgical tracheostomy in critically ill patients. Crit Care Med 2001;29:926–30.

61. Friedman Y, Fildes J, Mizock B, et al. Comparison of percutaneous and surgical tracheostomies. Chest 1996;110:480–5.

62. Mirski MA, Pandian V, Bhatti N, et al. Safety, efficiency, and cost-effectiveness of a multidisciplinary

percutaneous tracheostomy program. Crit Care Med 2012;40:1827–34.

63. O'Keeffe T, Goldman RK, Mayberry JC, et al. Tracheostomy after anterior cervical spine fixation. J Trauma 2004;57:855–60.

64. Ben Nun A, Orlovsky M, Best LA. Percutaneous tracheostomy in patients with cervical spine fractures: feasible and safe. Interact Cardiovasc Thorac Surg 2006;5:427–9.

65. Ganuza JR, Forcada AG, Gambarrutta C, et al. Effect of technique and timing of tracheostomy in patients with acute traumatic spinal cord injury undergoing mechanical ventilation. J Spinal Cord Med 2011;34(1):76–84.

66. Sustic A, Krstulovic B, Eskinja N, et al. Surgical tracheostomy versus percutaneous dilational tracheostomy in patients with anterior cervical spine fixation: preliminary report. Spine 2002;27:1942–5.

67. Mayberry JC, Wu IC, Goldman RK, et al. Cervical spine clearance and neck extension during percutaneous tracheostomy in trauma patients. Crit Care Med 2000;28:3436–40.

68. El Solh AA, Jaafar W. A comparative study of the complications of surgical tracheostomy in morbidly obese critically ill patients. Crit Care 2007;11(1):R3.

69. Byhahn C, Lischke V, Meininger D, et al. Peri-operative complications during percutaneous tracheostomy in obese patients. Anaesthesia 2005;60:12–5.

70. Romero CM, Cornejo RA, Ruiz MH, et al. Fiberoptic bronchoscopy-assisted percutaneous tracheostomy is safe in obese critically ill patients: a prospective and comparative study. J Crit Care 2009;24(4):494–500.

71. McCague A, Aljanabi H, Wong DT. Safety analysis of percutaneous dilational tracheostomies with bronchoscopy in the obese patient. Laryngoscope 2012;122:1031–4.

72. Tabaee A, Geng E, Lin J, et al. Impact of neck length on the safety of percutaneous and surgical tracheotomy: a prospective, randomized study. Laryngoscope 2005;115:1685–90.

73. Heyrosa MG, Melniczek DM, Rovito P, et al. Percutaneous tracheostomy: a safe procedure in the morbidly obese. J Am Coll Surg 2006;202: 618–22.

74. Sydow M, Burchardi H, Ephraim E, et al. Long-term effects of two different ventilatory modes on oxygenation in acute lung injury. Comparison of airway pressure release ventilation and volume-controlled inverse ratio ventilation. Am J Respir Crit Care Med 1994;149:1550–6.

75. Beiderlinden M, Groeben H, Peters J. Safety of percutaneous dilational tracheostomy in patients ventilated with high positive end-expiratory pressure (PEEP). Intensive Care Med 2003;29:944–8.

76. Franchi F, Cubattoli L, Faltoni A, et al. Recruitment maneuver in prevention of hypoxia during percutaneous dilational tracheostomy: randomised trial. Respir Care 2012;57(11):1850–6.

77. Shah S, Morgan P. Percutaneous dilation tracheostomy during high-frequency oscillatory ventilation. Crit Care Med 2002;30:1762–4.

78. Barton CA, McMillian WD, Osler T, et al. Anticoagulation management around percutaneous bedside procedures: is adjustment required? J Trauma 2012;72:815–20.

79. Beiderlinden M, Eikermann M, Lehmann N, et al. Risk factors associated with bleeding during and after percutaneous dilational tracheostomy. Anaesthesia 2007;62:342–6.

80. Rosseland LA, Laake JH, Stubhaug A. Percutaneous dilatational tracheostomy in intensive care unit patients with increased bleeding risk or obesity. A prospective analysis of 1000 procedures. Acta Anaesthesiol Scand 2011;55:835–41.

81. Veelo DP, Vlaar AP, Dongelmans DA, et al. Correction of subclinical coagulation disorders before percutaneous dilatational tracheotomy. A randomised controlled trial. Blood Transfus 2012;10: 213–20.

82. Auzinger C, O'Callaghan GP, Bernal W, et al. Percutaneous tracheostomy in patients with severe liver disease and a high incidence of refractory coagulopathy: a prospective trial. Crit Care 2007;11(5): R110.

83. Waller EA, Aduen JF, Kramer DJ, et al. Safety of percutaneous dilatational tracheostomy with direct bronchoscopic guidance for solid organ allograft recipients. Mayo Clin Proc 2007;82:1502–8.

84. Ben-Nun A, Altman E, Best LA. Emergency percutaneous tracheostomy in trauma patients: an early experience. Ann Thorac Surg 2004;77:1045–7.

85. Meyer M, Critchlow J, Mansharamani N, et al. Repeat bedside percutaneous dilational tracheostomy is a safe procedure. Crit Care Med 2002;30: 986–8.

86. Ben Nun A, Altman E, Best LA. Extended indications for percutaneous tracheostomy. Ann Thorac Surg 2005;80:1276–9.

87. Gerig HJ, Schnider T, Heidegger T. Prophylactic percutaneous transtracheal catheterization in the management of patients with anticipated difficult airways: a case series. Anaesthesia 2005;60: 801–5.

88. Drendel M, Primov-Fever A, Talmi YP, et al. Outcome of tracheostomy in patients over 85 years old (oldest-old patients). Otolaryngol Head Neck Surg 2009;140:395–7.

89. Yarmus Y, Pandian V, Gilbert C, et al. Safety and efficiency of interventional pulmonologists performing percutaneous tracheostomy. Respiration 2012; 84(2):123–7.

90. Hsia D, Musani AI. Interventional pulmonology. Med Clin North Am 2011;95:1095–114.

91. Klein M, Agassi R, Shapira AR, et al. Can intensive care physicians safely perform percutaneous dilational tracheostomy? A analysis of 207 cases. Isr Med Assoc J 2007;9:717–9.

92. Seder DB, Lee K, Rahman C, et al. Safety and feasibility of percutaneous tracheostomy performed by neurointensivists. Neurocrit Care 2009; 10:264–8.

93. Lamb CR, Feller-Kopman D, Ernst A, et al. An approach to interventional pulmonary fellowship training. Chest 2010;137:195–9.

94. Gardiner Q, White PS, Carson D, et al. Technique training: endoscopic percutaneous tracheostomy. Br J Anaesth 1998;81:401–3.

95. Ernst A, Silvestri GA, Johnstone D, American College of Chest Physicians. Interventional pulmonary procedures: guidelines from the American College of Chest Physicians. Chest 2003;123:1693–717.

96. Bolliger CT, Mathur PN, Beamis JF, et al, European Respiratory Society/American Thoracic Society. ERS/ATS statement on interventional pulmonology. Eur Respir J 2002;19:356–73.

Tracheobronchomalacia and Excessive Dynamic Airway Collapse

Septimiu Murgu, MD[a],*, Henri Colt, MD[b]

KEYWORDS

- Tracheobronchomalacia • Excessive dynamic airway collapse • Airway stents • Tracheoplasty
- Noninvasive positive pressure ventilation • Airflow dynamics • Choke points
- Functional bronchoscopy

KEY POINTS

- Tracheobronchomalacia is characterized as weakened or destroyed cartilage in the central airways resulting in expiratory flow limitation.
- Excessive dynamic airway collapse is characterized by excessive bulging of the posterior membrane inside the central airway lumen.
- A careful physiologic assessment of the impact of expiratory central airway collapse on airflow and functional status is warranted before treatment.
- Identification of the flow-limiting airway segments can be obtained by performing functional bronchoscopy before invasive interventions.
- Even when the central airway collapse is identified as responsible for symptoms, we suggest a conservative approach with medical treatment and noninvasive positive pressure ventilation before committing patients to potentially harmful effects resulting from airway stents or open surgical procedures.

DEFINITIONS AND CLASSIFICATIONS

Unambiguous definitions and clinically useful classifications provide a common language for health care providers managing expiratory central airway collapse (ECAC). By applying accepted terminology in their practices, clinicians and scientists can stratify patients according to predefined objective criteria and analyze data. Consensual frameworks offered by classification systems allow comparison of data within populations over time and between populations at the same point in time, thus facilitating meaningful research.[1,2]

In this regard, the collapse of the intrathoracic trachea and mainstem bronchi in adult patients has been described using a variety of terms, including tracheobronchomalacia (TBM), tracheobronchial collapse, expiratory tracheobronchial collapse, expiratory tracheobronchial stenosis, tracheobronchial dyskinesia, dynamic airway collapse (AC), and ECAC.[3] However, these terms do not distinguish between collapse of the pars membranosa and collapse of the cartilaginous wall. ECAC is an accepted term to describe the narrowing of the central airways during expiration; it is a

Disclosure: The authors have no relationship with any commercial company that has a direct financial interest in the subject matter or materials discussed in this article or with any company making a competing product.
[a] Department of Medicine, University of Chicago Pritzker School of Medicine, 5841 South Maryland Avenue, Chicago, IL 60637, USA; [b] Department of Medicine, University of California Irvine, 101 The City Drive South, 400 City Tower, Orange, CA 92868, USA
* Corresponding author.
E-mail address: tim.murgu@gmail.com

Clin Chest Med 34 (2013) 527–555
http://dx.doi.org/10.1016/j.ccm.2013.05.003
0272-5231/13/$ – see front matter © 2013 Elsevier Inc. All rights reserved.

chestmed.theclinics.com

syndrome comprising 2 different pathophysiologic entities: TBM, characterized by weakness of the tracheobronchial cartilaginous structures, and excessive dynamic AC (EDAC), defined as excessive bulging of the posterior membrane into the airway lumen during expiration without cartilage collapse.[2–6]

A major controversy in the published literature and among experts managing these patients is represented by the amount of collapse labeled as excessive. The frontier between normal and abnormal narrowing of the central airways during exhalation has not been clarified, and investigators propose various cutoff values.[6–12] There is variability among studies in regards to anatomic location and respiratory maneuver used to measure narrowing of the expiratory airway (**Table 1**).[10–15] These facts may be the main source of inconsistency in reported prevalence of these disorders. The anatomic site used for measuring the collapse needs to be standardized, because physiologic airway narrowing is more pronounced in the bronchus intermedius and main carina than at the aortic arch or cricoid level.[12]

Results of dynamic computed tomography (CT) studies show that 70% to 80% of normal individuals meet the 50% criteria used for abnormal collapse.[6,12,16] Healthy volunteers with normal lung function have shown mean levels of expiratory collapse of 54% in the trachea, 67% in the right main bronchus (RMB), 61% in the left main bronchus (LMB), and even total collapse in the bronchus intermedius.[12] A different study showed that the mean % collapse of normal volunteers was 66.9% in the RMB and 61.4% in the LMB, with 73% of participants exceeding the currently accepted cutoff value of 50% threshold for defining bronchomalacia.[17] Even in a disease process such as chronic obstructive pulmonary disease (COPD), in which the central AC is more pronounced, the degree of narrowing may be independent of disease severity and does not correlate significantly with physiologic parameters.[6,11] Excessive expiratory tracheal collapse defined as more than 80% expiratory reduction in tracheal luminal cross-sectional during dynamic CT was shown to not significantly correlate with the pulmonary function tests (PFTs) or quality-of-life (QOL) measures.[6,11]

To reduce false-positive diagnoses and avoid unwarranted treatments, EDAC may be defined only if clinically relevant excessive collapse is noted during tidal breathing (**Fig. 1**). The degree of pathologic expiratory collapse has not yet been established on physiologic basis because work of breathing and symptoms depend not only on the degree of airway narrowing but also

on its geometry and flow velocity.[18] Therefore, the accurate assessment of the reduction in airway lumen cross-sectional area becomes relevant for the purpose of having a common language when evaluating patients and communicating about TBM and EDAC, and not necessarily only to decide on need for therapeutic interventions.

The degree of narrowing is only 1 factor involved in flow limitation; it is only 1 criterion included in classifications for this syndrome. Most systems are limited by inconsistent definitions or by criteria addressing only the extent, severity, or cause but not the 2 separate morphologic types of TBM and EDAC or the patient's functional impairment (**Table 2**).[10,13–15,19] A classification based on objective quantifiable criteria has been developed and can be applied before and after therapeutic interventions to objectively document not only the changes in the extent and severity of AC but also the impact of these changes on functional class (**Table 3**).[2] The criteria of this system can be grouped in 2 sets: the descriptive factors including morphology and etiology, and stratification factors that can be scored objectively. The morphology criterion describes the shape of the airway lumen, which is reduced during expiration as assessed by bronchoscopy or radiologic studies. ECAC has 5 morphologic types (**Fig. 2**). Origin (etiology) describes the underlying mechanism responsible for the abnormality: idiopathic or secondary to other disorders (**Table 4**). To describe functional class, this system used the World Health Organization functional impairment scale, because of its easy clinical applicability and because it does not address just dyspnea but the overall impact of symptoms on patient's functional status. The extent criterion describes the location and distribution of the abnormal airway segment as assessed by bronchoscopy or radiographic studies. The severity criterion describes the degree of the AC during expiration as assessed by bronchoscopy or radiographic studies. Since its introduction in 2005, the terminology proposed in this system has been applied in clinical research of these disorders.[5,6,20–24] This classification allows monitoring of the progression or improvement of the disease process and the outcome and durability of different treatment strategies on airway lumen patency and patient symptoms. Five domains are addressed: functional class (F), extent (E), morphology (M), origin (O), and severity of AC (S). The F, E, and S parts of the system have an ordinal scale of 1 to 4 (see **Table 3**). Outcomes are documented as subscripts, for example $F_2 E_2 S_4$, and should not be combined to form a single number. This information can be tabulated or plotted to provide a visual temporal treatment

Table 1
Studies using different cutoff values to define excessive central AC

Reference	Cutoff Value to Define Abnormal, Excessive AC During Expiration	Comments
Aquino et al,[7] 2001	>28% expiratory reduction in sagittal diameter >18% expiratory reduction in CSA in the upper trachea >28% expiratory reduction in CSA in the middle trachea	Only for tracheal collapse Used paired inspiratory–static end-expiratory CT
Stern et al,[8] 1993	35% expiratory reduction in CSA in normal individuals	Only for tracheal collapse Used paired inspiratory–dynamic-expiratory CT
Nuutinen,[9] 1977	>50% expiratory reduction in sagittal diameter	For tracheal and bronchial collapse Used bronchoscopic estimations
Zhang et al,[75] 2003	>50% expiratory reduction in CSA	Only for tracheal collapse Low-dose CT (40–80 mA) was just as accurate as the standard dose (240–280 mA) Used paired inspiratory–dynamic-expiratory CT
Gilkeson et al,[130] 2001	>50% expiratory reduction in CSA	For tracheal and bronchial collapse Paired inspiratory–dynamic-expiratory CT
Hein et al,[66] 2000	>50% expiratory reduction in CSA	Only for tracheal collapse Used paired inspiratory–dynamic-expiratory electron beam tomography
Boiselle et al,[12] 2009	>50% expiratory reduction in CSA	Only for tracheal collapse in healthy volunteers Used low-dose paired inspiratory–dynamic-expiratory CT 80% of healthy study participants met the criteria for abnormal collapse
Litmanovich et al,[17] 2010	>50% expiratory reduction in CSA	Only for bronchial collapse Used low-dose paired inspiratory–dynamic-expiratory CT 73% of healthy participants exceeded the diagnostic threshold level for abnormal bronchial collapse
Masaoka et al,[10] 1996	>80% expiratory narrowing	For tracheal and bronchial collapse Used bronchoscopic estimations and frontal and lateral radiograph films to estimate the narrowing Narrowing is not clearly defined as reduction of CSA or reduction in diameter
Boiselle et al,[6] 2012	>80% expiratory reduction in CSA	Only for tracheal collapse in patients with COPD Used low-dose paired inspiratory–dynamic-expiratory CT

Abbreviations: COPD, chronic obstructive pulmonary disease; CSA, cross-sectional area; CT, computed tomography.

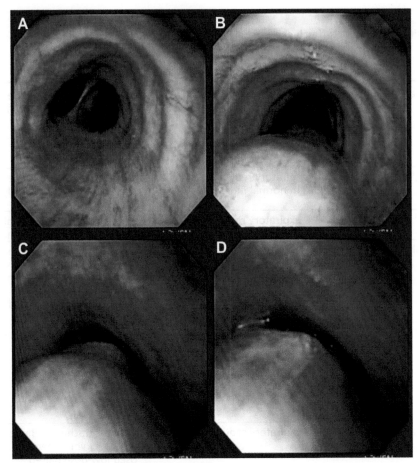

Fig. 1. Impact of respiratory maneuver and effort on degree of airway narrowing. Images A–D are obtained from the same patient undergoing flexible bronchoscopy for an unrelated reason (ie, right lower lobe atelectasis). The tracheal cartilaginous wall is intact during all respiratory maneuvers. Normal tracheal lumen during inspiration (*A*). Physiologic, dynamic airway compression during tidal expiration (*B*). EDAC during forced expiration (*C*) and coughing (*D*).

map, charting patient progress through treatment. In this article, a description is given of how this system can be used in 2 clinical scenarios: TBM and EDAC.

Clinical Application: TBM

A patient with a history of extensive mediastinal lymph node calcifications and bilateral upper lobe fibrosis was unable to clear secretions, had progressive dyspnea on exertion, and cough limiting normal physical activities. The patient was treated for asthma with inhaled and systemic steroids for more than a year before a bronchoscopy, which revealed collapse of the anterior wall of the lower trachea. During tidal expiration, this collapse reached a 100% closure of the lumen (**Fig. 3**). This morphology was characteristic of

crescent-type malacia and was considered to be caused by secondary tracheobronchomegaly (caused by bilateral upper lobe fibrosis). Because of the patient's lack of discomfort at rest, but presence of increased symptoms with normal physical activity, his functional class was labeled as F_2. The process was limited to the lower trachea, therefore the extent was labeled E_2, and because the 2 walls of the trachea were touching each other during expiration (100% closure), severity of airway narrowing was labeled as S_4. Rigid bronchoscopy was performed and a straight silicone stent inserted in to the lower trachea. After intervention, the patient was tapered off the steroids for his presumed asthma and symptoms improved to normal (F_1). Bronchoscopy showed no residual malacia (E_1) and normal expiratory airway lumen (S_1) (see **Fig. 3**).

Clinical Application: EDAC

A patient with COPD and obesity presented with worsening dyspnea. She had a history of severe oxygen and corticosteroid-dependent COPD limiting her daily activities. The main finding on bronchoscopy was bulging of the posterior membrane in the lower trachea during tidal breathing, with narrowing of the airway lumen by 100% at the level of main carina. This finding was consistent with EDAC morphology. The findings extended in the lower tracheal and mainstem bronchi, and the extent was labeled E_4; the severity was S_4 (100% closure during exhalation), and given her symptoms with minimal activity, functional class was F_3. The patient underwent a Y silicone stent insertion, and after this procedure, she was classified as F_2 E_1 S_1 (see **Fig. 3**). The lack of complete symptomatic response to stent insertion was explained by confounding disorders (COPD and obesity) and by the choke point migration seen just distal to the stent (see **Fig. 3**).

Definitions and classifications: key points

1. TBM is characterized by weakness or destruction of the airway cartilaginous wall.

2. EDAC is characterized by bulging of the pars membranosa inside the airway lumen.

3. The 50% reduction in airway cross-sectional area (CSA) during forced expiration is inadequate to define abnormal collapse.

4. Multidimensional classification systems for ECAC include an assessment of the patient's functional status, craniocaudal extent, morphology of the airway during expiration, cause, and degree of AC.

PATHOPHYSIOLOGY

TBM and EDAC have different morphology on imaging studies and bronchoscopy. The 2 processes are also distinct in terms of impact on flow dynamics. Physiologic studies addressing the collapse of the central airways suggest that EDAC is likely a consequence of peripheral airway obstruction from emphysema, chronic bronchitis, or asthma or resulting from the restrictive physiology and positive pleural pressures in morbid obesity.[25–29] TBM, on the other hand, is a true central airway cartilaginous disease resulting in AC and flow limitation. Theories and mathematical models have been proposed and tested to explain expiratory flow limitation in health and obstructive ventilatory disorders and are relevant to understanding flow limitation in EDAC and TBM.[30,31]

Flow-Limitation Theories

Equal pressure point theory: dynamic compression and determinants of maximal expiratory flow

There is a region within the intrathoracic airway where intraluminal and extraluminal pressures become equal once expiratory flow becomes limited at a given lung volume.[30] The point within the airway at which this situation occurs is called the equal pressure point (EPP) (**Fig. 4**). This concept is based on the following facts: alveolar pressure is the driving pressure that causes gas to flow through airways during expiration. This pressure (Palv) is determined by the recoil pressure of the lungs (Pst) and the pleural pressure (Ppl):

$$Palv = Ppl + Pst \qquad (1)$$

A pressure decrease is required to accelerate air as it moves from an upstream (toward the alveoli) region of low velocity to a downstream (toward the mouth) region of high velocity. Because of this pressure decrease, the intraluminal pressure (P_L) eventually becomes equal to pleural pressure (Ppl). The point in the airway at which this process occurs, the EPP, divides the airways into upstream segments (alveolarward from the EPP), at which transmural pressure (P_L–Ppl) is positive, and downstream segments (mouthward from the EPP), at which the transmural pressure is positive within the extrathoracic airways and negative within the intrathoracic airways. For a given lung volume, driving pressure upstream from the EPP would be equal to lung elastic recoil (driving pressure = Palv–P_L, but at EPP, P_L = Ppl and based on Equation 1, driving pressure = Pst and becomes effort independent); downstream from the EPP, airways are compressed during expiration (see **Fig. 4**). This region of airway compression is referred to as a flow-limiting segment (FLS). This compressed airway segment develops close to the EPP where Ppl exceeds P_L and where there is absence or inadequate cartilaginous support or traction provided by neighboring alveoli. This situation explains collapse of the trachea and mainstem bronchi at the weakest point in the airway wall, namely the pars membranosa, which is not supported by airway cartilage.

As lung volume decreases during expiration, elastic and alveolar pressures are reduced with respect to pleural pressure, and EPP moves toward the alveoli. This situation results in a lengthening of the increasingly narrow downstream segment. This lengthening can be seen on bronchoscopy or dynamic CT as EDAC (see **Fig. 4**). Thus, the FLS have tracheal location at high lung

Table 2
Classification systems used for ECAC

Reference	Criteria Included in the System	Comments
Rayl,[13] 1965	Extent: proximal (type I), mediastinal (type II), and intrapulmonary (type III) airways	Tracheobronchial collapse was assessed during cough on cine-bronchography
Johnson et al,[14] 1973	Severity: 4° of airway narrowing	TM: >50% collapse during coughing on fluoroscopy
Feist et al,[15] 1975	Cause: congenital and acquired	TM: >50% collapse during coughing on fluoroscopy
Jokinen et al,[19] 1977	Severity: mild (<50%), moderate (50%–75%), severe (100%) Extent: TM, TBM, BM	TBM: expiratory reduction of 50% or more in the anteroposterior diameter of the airways First classification based on bronchoscopic findings
Mair et al,[131] 1992	Cause: congenital (type 1), extrinsic compression (type 2), acquired (type 3) Severity: mild (<70%), moderate (70%–90%), severe (>90%) collapse	Described for pediatric TBM Empirical severity score
Masaoka et al,[10] 1996	Cause and extent criteria Pediatric, adult, and secondary	TBM: >80% collapse during expiration Based on bronchoscopic estimations and frontal and lateral radiograph films to estimate the narrowing

Abbreviations: BM, bronchomalacia; TM, tracheomalacia.

Table 3
Stratification factors from FEMOS classification system for ECAC

Definition	Criterion Grade			
	1	2	3	4
Functional status Refers to degree of functional impairment as defined by World Health Organization	Asymptomatic	Symptomatic on exertion	Symptomatic with daily activity	Symptomatic at rest
Extent Defines the length of the tracheobronchial wall affected and the location of the abnormal airway segment	No abnormal AC	1 main, lobar, or segmental bronchus or 1 tracheal region (upper, mid, or lower)	In 2 contiguous or ≥2 noncontiguous regions	In >2 contiguous regions
Severity Describes the degree of the AC during expiration as documented by bronchoscopic or radiologic studies	Expiratory AC of 0%–50%	Expiratory AC of 50%–75%	Expiratory AC of 75%–100%	Expiratory AC of 100%; the airway walls make contact

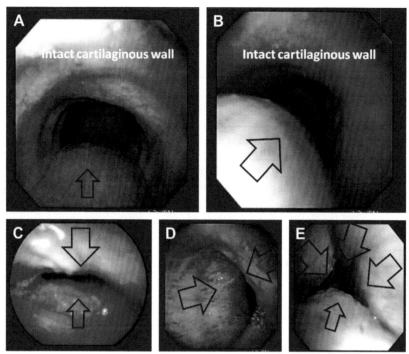

Fig. 2. Morphologic types of ECAC based on the shape of the airway lumen during expiration. (*A*) Normal dynamic airway compression during exhalation with the posterior membrane slightly bulging within the airway lumen (*arrow*). This compression usually narrows the airway lumen by less than 50%. (*B*) In EDAC, the posterior membrane bulges in (*arrow*) and excessively narrows the airway lumen by 50% or more. This process occurs without cartilaginous wall weakness. (*C*) In crescent-type TBM, the anterior cartilaginous wall is weakened and collapses inside the lumen (*large arrow*). (*D*) In saber-sheath TBM, the lateral walls are collapsing inside the lumen (*arrows*). (*E*) In circumferential-type TBM, typically seen in relapsing polychondritis, the anterior and lateral cartilaginous walls are collapsing inside the lumen (*large arrows*) and there is diffuse airway edema and hyperemia. The small arrows denote normal expected physiologic dynamic compression, whereas the large arrows denote abnormal airway wall collapse.

volumes (ie, total lung capacity [TLC]), but as lung volume decreases during exhalation, FLS move peripherally but still stay in the central airways (in the lobar, segmental, and at the most subsegmental bronchi), as shown in previous experimental and human studies. Even at residual volume (RV), the FLS were found in the central airways, fixed and in parallel in the right middle lobe, left upper lobe, and left lower lobe bronchi. These lobar and segmental locations of FLS were shown in normal individuals and individuals with obstructive ventilatory impairment over considerable ranges of lung volume.[32–34] Based on the EPP theory, if the FLS are located in the lobar or segmental airways, then the downstream resistance should not affect flow. Intraluminal pressure monitoring with airway catheters shows the lack of decrease in pressure in airways between the mouth and the FLS.[34] Therefore, tracheal and mainstem bronchial collapsibility observed on dynamic bronchoscopy or dynamic CT in the form of EDAC should not impede flow.[35]

The EPP theory explains how lung compliance and airway resistance affect airflow limitation and how changes in these 2 factors result in increased compression of the airway downstream from the FLS responsible for the bronchoscopic or radiographic EDAC. For instance, a decrease in elastic recoil of the lungs (either because of low lung volume as seen in morbid obesity or because of emphysema) reduces the airway pressure relative to pleural pressure, resulting in greater dynamic compression. A decrease in elastic recoil of the lungs results in less traction on the adjacent airways and therefore greater dynamic compression. As for airway resistance, the greater the pressure decrease along the airway from the alveoli to the EPP (along the upstream segment), the sooner the development of an EPP and the greater the dynamic compression. The EPP theory, therefore, sustains the theory that central airway compression downstream from EPP (bronchoscopic/radiographic EDAC) is not pathologic from a flow dynamic standpoint.

Table 4
Secondary causes of ECAC

Morphologic Type of ECAC	Associated Disease or Process	Potential Mechanism
BM	After lung transplantation	Impaired blood supply and necrosis
TM	History of ETT or tracheostomy tube	Pressure necrosis, impaired blood supply, and chondritis
TM	Chest trauma	Cartilage fracture
TBM	Relapsing polychondritis	Cartilage inflammation
TBM	Chronic recurrent airway infections	Cartilage inflammation
TBM	Chronic indwelling ETT or tracheostomy tube	Chronic inflammation of the airway walls
TM, BM	Cancer (lung, thyroid, esophageal, or metastasis from extrathoracic malignancies)	Direct tumor invasion of the cartilaginous wall
TM, BM	Radiation therapy	Cartilage necrosis
	Bronchoscopic electrocautery and laser	Thermal energy destruction of the cartilaginous wall
TM, BM, TBM	After thyroidectomy, postpneumonectomy syndrome, severe scoliosis	Mechanical factors
TM, BM	Mediastinal goiter Tumors (carcinoma, teratoma, lymphoma, neuroblastoma) Vascular anomalies (innominate artery, aortic arch ring, pulmonary artery sling, aberrant right subclavian) Cysts (thymic cyst, bronchogenic cyst, lymphatic malformation) Cardiac (enlarged left atrium, enlarged pulmonary arteries or veins)	Chronic extrinsic compression and secondary weakness of the cartilage
EDAC	COPD	Decreased elastic recoil[a] Small airway inflammation[a] Atrophy of elastic fibers
EDAC	Asthma, bronchiectasis, bronchiolitis	Small airway inflammation[a]
EDAC	Obesity	Decreased elastic recoil[a] Positive pleural pressures[a]
EDAC	Healthy individuals during forced exhalation and coughing	Increased pleural pressures[a]
EDAC	Mounier-Kuhn syndrome	Congenital atrophy of elastic fibers

Abbreviations: BM, bronchomalacia; ETT, endotracheal tube; TM, tracheomalacia.
[a] For explanations on how decreased elastic recoil, small airway inflammation, and increased pleural pressures cause EDAC, please refer to the section on flow-limitation theories.

Wave speed theory: airway compliance and impact on choke point physiology

A different approach to explain expiratory flow limitation is offered by the wave speed theory, which states that flow limitation in elastic tubes occurs at the speed at which the fluid (eg, air) in the tube (eg, airways) propagates pressure waves.[31] These waves develop from the interaction of recoil force of the elastic airway wall and the axial inertial force of the flowing gas. The wave speed is the speed at which a small disturbance travels in a fluid-filled compliant tube. Thus, expiratory flow limitation occurs when flow velocity equals the speed of propagation of pressure pulse waves at some point within the tubes; this point, called the choke point or FLS, tends to be at a region of minimum CSA and minimum intraluminal airway pressure when maximal flow has been reached:

$$\dot{V}\,ws = A[A/(\rho \times Caw)]^{0.5} \qquad (2)$$

This wave-speed flow ($\dot{V}$ ws) depends on the CSA (A), airway compliance ($Caw = dA/dPtm$),

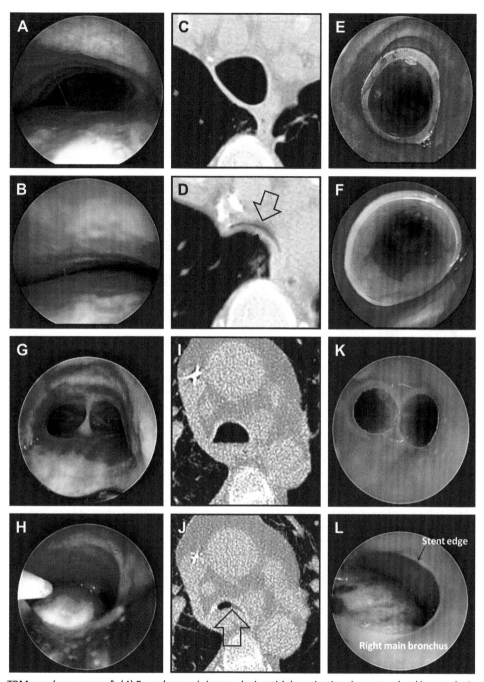

Fig. 3. TBM case (*upper panel*): (*A*) Bronchoscopic image during tidal respiration: lower tracheal lumen during inspiration; (*B*) lower tracheal lumen during expiration showing 100% closure resulting in severity grade S4; (*C*) paired inspiratory–dynamic-expiratory CT showing lower tracheal lumen during inspiration; (*D*) lower tracheal lumen during expiration shows that in addition to the normal dynamic airway compression (*small arrow*), there is flattening of the anterior wall of the lower trachea (*large arrow*), consistent with focal (E_2) crescent-type tracheomalacia; (*E*) rigid bronchoscopic image after stent insertion during inspiration; (*F*) bronchoscopic image during tidal expiration shows patent airway with no residual malacia (E_1) and normal airway caliber (S_1). EDAC case (*lower panel*): (*G*) lower tracheal lumen during inspiration; (*H*) during tidal expiration, the collapse of the posterior membrane closes the airway completely, resulting in severity grading (S_4); (*I*) paired inspiratory–dynamic-expiratory CT shows normal cartilaginous wall configuration; (*J*) during expiration, the excessive collapse of the posterior membrane is noted (*large arrow*), consistent with EDAC. The findings extended to mainstem bronchi, resulting in extent grading of E4. (*K*) After stent insertion, there was maintained airway patency with no AC (S_1). (*L*) Follow-up bronchoscopy shows AC distal to the left and right bronchial arms of the Y silicone stent, consistent with migration of choke points.

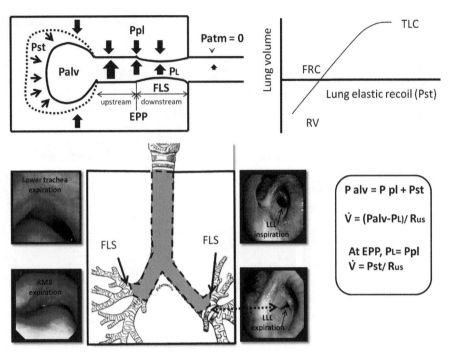

Fig. 4. Expiratory flow limitation theory and affect bronchoscopic EDAC. (*Upper panel, left*) The alveolar pressure (Palv) causes air to flow during expiration and is approximately equal to the recoil pressure of the lungs (Pst) plus the pleural pressure (Ppl): Palv = Ppl + Pst. During forced expiration, the intraluminal pressure (P_L) eventually becomes equal to pleural pressure (Ppl) at a point called the EPP. In the upstream segment (alveolarward from the EPP), the transmural pressure (Ptm = P_L–Ppl) is positive, but in the downstream segment (mouthward from the EPP), it is negative within the intrathoracic airways. At a given lung volume, driving pressure upstream from the EPP would be equal to lung elastic recoil (Pst), whereas downstream from the EPP, airways would be compressed during expiration. This region of compression of intraluminal caliber is referred to as a flow-limiting segment (FLS) or choke point In emphysema, for instance, the reduced elastic recoil and increased resistance of the upstream segment result in decreased transluminal pressure and consequent increased AC; in morbid obesity, the reduced elastic recoil from restriction and increased pleural pressures also results in EDAC. (*Upper panel, right*) As lung volume decreases from total lung capacity (TLC) toward residual volume (RV), the elastic recoil (Pst) decreases as well, and pleural pressure (Ppl) increases during forced expiration. (*Lower panel, left*) Thus, the EPP migrate upstream, resulting in a lengthening of the increasingly narrow downstream segment (note compressed trachea and right mainstem bronchus [RMB]). This situation increases airway resistance and prevents further increases in expiratory airflow, causing the EPP to become fixed when airflow becomes constant. FLS move peripherally during exhalation to the lobar/segmental and at most subsegmental bronchi (note left lower lobe bronchus open during inspiration but nearly completely closed during exhalation in a patient flow limited at rest).

which is the slope of the curve describing *A* as a function of transmural pressure (Ptm = P_L–Ppl), and the density (ρ) of the gas, according to Equation 2.[36] A functional definition for choke points is as follows: the most downstream (mouthward) points where the airway pressure does not change with driving pressure. Intraluminal airway catheters can be used to localize choke points by measuring airway pressure during induced flow limitation by decreasing the downstream pressure. This concept has led to the development of intraoperative location of the choke point techniques that might predict response to stent insertion.[37]

From Equation 2, it can be seen that $\dot{V}$ ws decreases when *A* becomes smaller, and Caw and ρ become larger, as would be the case for a hypercompliant intrathoracic airway during expiration as seen in TBM. Increasing central airway compliance increases airway resistance and decreases maximum expiratory flow, which contributes to the airflow limitation in TBM, characterized by hypercompliant airways. Results from studies of airflow limitation in theoretic, experimental models and clinical studies show that when the collapsing trachea is supported by a rigid tube, airflow improves and the choke point could migrate from the central airway toward the periphery.[38–40] In addition, $\dot{V}$ ws indirectly depends on the lung elastic recoil pressure (Pst) and the pressure loss (Pfr) upstream from the choke point, because a decreased pressure head (defined as Pst–Pfr) makes the distending transmural pressure (Ptm) smaller and, accordingly, makes A smaller (see **Fig. 4**). This theory is in accordance with the EPP theory. The choke point is the equivalent of the juncture of upstream and FLS according to EPP theory. Wave speed theory supplements EPP theory by addressing pressure-area relationships at the choke point and predicting values of maximal flow.

The EPP and wave speed theories and experiments support the concept that upstream and downstream segments are connected by a discrete airway segment, the choke point, which dissipates all increases in driving pressure and limits flow. Clinical application of these concepts improves our understanding of the impact of structural wall changes on flow dynamics in disease processes. For example, chronic inflammation and remodeling in asthma affect mechanical properties of the airway wall.[41] Using esophageal balloons to measure pleural pressure and airway pressure probes, airway compliance can be determined at multiple anatomic points. Long-lasting asthma was found to cause less compliant central airways, suggesting that chronic inflammation and remodeling of the airway wall may result in stiffer dynamic elastic properties of the asthmatic airway.

Applied Physiology

EPP theory and wave speed theory explain EDAC during forced expiration in healthy individuals

The flow-limitation theories show that increasing pleural pressures during forced expiration result in greater dynamic airway compression downstream from the EPP and adjacent choke points. Clinical studies show sex and age differences in the degree of dynamic collapse.[24] Dynamic CT investigations showed that regardless of age, men tend to have greater inspiratory and expiratory force-generating capacity. Maximum expiratory pressure is 30% to 50% greater among men compared with women throughout adulthood.[42] If the effort is maintained throughout expiration, greater compression of the downstream airway segment might be expected in men than in women. Although the mean % collapse is similar for men (55% ± 23%) and women (52% ± 17%), only men (older men had both greater CSA at TLC and smaller CSA during dynamic exhalation than younger men) showed a significant positive correlation between % collapse and age.

However, both sexes showed % collapse of more than 50% in healthy individuals.[24] These results suggest that sex and age differences should be considered when assessing patients for suspected pathologic collapse and support the fact that the 50% cutoff for defining abnormality results in false-positive findings without consequence on flow.[12,17,24]

EPP theory and wave speed theory explain EDAC in COPD

Two abnormalities in COPD contribute to early AC during expiration: decreased elastic recoil at all lung volumes (emphysema) and inflammatory narrowing of the airways (bronchitis). These processes determine the major site of increased resistance to be in the small airways (ie, airways of <2 mm diameter).[43] In the presence of small airway obstruction, EPP and the choke points were shown to be further upstream (toward the alveoli) than in normal individuals.[44] The destruction of lung tissue decreases the number and elasticity of the radial attachments from the parenchyma to the airway, and thus decreases airway stability. Experimental studies applying wave speed theory in canine models of emphysema show that the main reduction in maximum flow is explained by the decrease in elastic recoil; the other contributing factors are increases in frictional resistance from alveoli to sublobar bronchi and changes in airway compliance.[45] A decrease in airway stability in emphysema decreases the maximum flow by decreasing CSA for a given transmural airway pressure, and by relatively increasing airway compliance. Alternatively, altered bronchial pressure-area behavior could result from a relative increase in peribronchial interstitial pressure. Thus, for a given intraluminal pressure P_L, airway CSA in emphysema would be smaller than in healthy lungs, because the transmural pressure (P_L–peribronchial pressure) would be less (see **Fig. 4**). This reduction in CSA in COPD has not been proved to be caused by cartilage abnormalities and thus cannot be considered true malacia. Physiologic and morphologic studies of determinants of maximal expiratory flow in COPD show that airway collapsibility did not correlate with the amount of airway cartilage, inflammation, or airway wall thickness.[46] Decreased cartilage volume in COPD has been described by several investigators[47–49] but was not found by others.[50] Because the mechanical properties of airway cartilage have not been investigated, it cannot be excluded that these properties would relate in airway collapsibility. Some investigators[51] reported that the proteolytic enzyme, papain, could weaken airway cartilage but not destroy it, because its histologic appearance remained unchanged.

A clinical study[52] addressed the question whether expiratory flow limitation is caused primarily by narrowing of the central airways or by the more peripheral airways in patients who have COPD and concurrent abnormal degrees of central AC. The investigators analyzed the degree of central airway collapsibility by using a semiquantitative analysis of bronchoscopic images and related it to expiratory flow limitation in patients with what the investigators named TBM. However, all patients had invagination of the posterior membranous portion, which caused tracheal narrowing; the tracheal collapse was not caused by softening of the cartilaginous rings, thus making the entity studied consistent with a diagnosis of EDAC. Simultaneous pressure measurements in the trachea and esophagus were performed to identify expiratory flow limitation during quiet breathing and to determine the critical transmural pressure required for maximum expiratory flow. The investigators found that 15% of patients with EDAC were not flow limited during quiet breathing, 53% were flow limited throughout exhalation, and 30% were flow limited only during the latter part of the exhalation. Patients with flow limitation at rest had more tracheal narrowing (EDAC) than those without, but the severity of expiratory flow limitation was not closely related to tracheal collapsibility. AC during quiet breathing was unrelated to FEV_1 (forced expiratory volume in first second of expiration). Twenty-three patients (28%) were flow limited during quiet exhalation at transmural pressures that did not cause central AC. In these patients, the tracheal collapse was less than 50% during quiet exhalation and increased to more than 50% only during forced exhalation, when the pleural pressures increased, suggesting that tracheal collapse to more than 50% narrowing during forced exhalation is not responsible for limiting maximum expiratory flow. The important finding of this study was that EDAC was mostly seen in patients with tidal expiratory flow limitation. These data are relevant when considering interventions addressing EDAC, especially if symptomatic central airway narrowing exists without significant documented airflow obstruction. It could be argued that even in patients with EDAC during tidal exhalation, given the expiratory flow limitation at rest, EDAC represents the airway downstream (mouthward) from the choke points and is not responsible for pressure decrease and flow limitation. The way to show whether EDAC is flow limiting is to measure the degree of pressure decrease along the collapsing segment.[37]

However, the success of stent insertion or tracheoplasty is assessed not just by improvement in airflow but also by relief of symptoms such as cough and dyspnea and reduced frequency of infection. This finding is especially relevant for those patients with central AC in which collapse of the posterior membrane is noted and there is concurrent collapse of the cartilaginous wall, namely those patients with crescent-type malacia or a combination of malacia and EDAC. For this purpose, the use of intraluminal airway pressure catheter measurements distal and proximal to the narrowed airway during tidal breathing allows intraoperative estimation of the physiologic benefits of a particular interventional procedure.[37]

The evidence that the degree of central AC in COPD is independent of disease severity and does not correlate significantly with physiologic parameters is reproducible.[6,11] Dynamic CT studies suggest that the incidental identification of excessive expiratory tracheal collapse (measured at 1 cm above the aortic arch [midtrachea] and 1 cm above the carina [lower trachea]) in COPD is not clinically significant. One study evaluated 100 adults meeting GOLD (Global Initiative for Chronic Obstructive Lung Disease) criteria for COPD who underwent PFT, 6-minute walk test (6MWT), Saint George's Respiratory Questionnaire (SGRQ), and spirometry gated low-dose CT at TLC and during dynamic exhalation with spirometric monitoring (CT was performed during a forced expiratory maneuver: participants took a deep breath and then blew out hard and fast [similar to a forced vital capacity [FVC] maneuver in the PFT laboratory]). The mean FEV_1 was 64% predicted, and percentage expiratory collapse was 59% ± 19% for tracheal measurement and 61 ± 18% for lower tracheal measurements. Twenty percent of the study participants met study criteria for excessive expiratory collapse, which was defined as a reduction of more than 80% in the tracheal lumen during forced expiration. Consistent with the bronchoscopic study described earlier,[52] there was no significant correlation between percentage expiratory tracheal collapse and pulmonary function measures, total SGRQ score, or 6MWT distance. The SGRQ symptom subscale was only weakly correlated with percentage collapse of the midtrachea (R = 0.215, $P = .03$).[6]

Bronchoscopic and dynamic CT studies highlight the fact that clinically significant EDAC that interferes with flow or symptoms should not be defined by forced expiratory maneuvers. The lack of association between the severity of tracheal collapse and GOLD stage of COPD was also described by other investigators, who studied 71 patients with COPD,[11] but these latter investigators reported a higher prevalence of excessive expiratory tracheal collapse (53%), likely because they used a lower threshold for diagnosis (>50%). Thus, the incidental detection of excessive expiratory tracheal collapse in a population with COPD of different degrees of airflow obstruction may not be clinically relevant, especially in the absence of other comorbidities. The resistance of the upstream segment based on EPP theory affects flow and determines the location of the choke points and the downstream compressed airway segment. From a clinical standpoint, severity of bronchial wall thickness, responsible for increased Resistance of the upstream segment (Rus), was significantly higher in patients with EDAC and correlated with the degree of maximal AC.[11] Based on the mechanisms of flow limitation outlined earlier, central AC is a consequence of:

1. Increased pleural pressures, as seen during forceful expiratory maneuver or cough
2. Hypercompliant central airway during expiration, with relatively low pleural pressures, as seen with weakened or destroyed cartilage (TBM) or decreased drive pressure in the setting of peripheral airway obstruction (EDAC in COPD)
3. Increased resistance in the segment upstream from the choke point, as seen in chronic bronchitis, asthma, and bronchiectasis, which leads to EDAC
4. Decreased elastic recoil and early formation of choke points at high lung volumes during exhalation responsible for EDAC in emphysema

Such central AC could occur in patients with or without COPD, may not be flow limiting, and possibly not associated with impaired functional status. From a flow dynamic perspective, detection of expiratory tracheal or mainstem bronchial collapse at the level of the posterior membrane should trigger a search for causes of airflow obstruction within the lung (COPD, bronchiolitis, asthma), not the central airways.[35]

EPP theory and wave speed theory explain EDAC in obesity

Obesity can cause low lung volumes and restrictive ventilatory impairment. Individuals with a body mass index (BMI, calculated as weight in kilograms divided by the square of height in meters) greater than 40 kg/m² have reduced TLC, functional residual capacity (FRC), and vital capacity. In otherwise healthy obese individuals with BMI greater than 40 kg/m², expiratory flow limitation is common in the supine position.[27]

Pleural pressure in obese individuals at relaxation volume is greater than normal, often becoming positive. This finding was shown in obese supine and paralyzed individuals undergoing general anesthesia[28] and also in conscious obese individuals.[29] Based on the EPP theory, the increased pleural pressure throughout the chest in these individuals explains the EDAC that is often encountered during bronchoscopy or dynamic CT, because transmural pressure (P_L–Ppl) is decreased, and during exhalation the airway collapses at the posterior membrane portion, causing EDAC (see **Fig. 4**).

Pathophysiology: key points

1. Healthy volunteers performing forced expiratory maneuvers and patients with morbid obesity, COPD, and other obstructive ventilatory disorders have EDAC as a result of interactions between pleural pressures, elastic recoil, airway compliance, and peripheral airway resistance.
2. EDAC documented on bronchoscopy or dynamic CT may not interfere with flow, regardless of the degree of AC.
3. EDAC may not correlate with severity of ventilatory impairment or QOL measures.

FUNCTIONAL EVALUATION
Pulmonary Function Testing

Spirometry in patients with central AC may reveal obstructive ventilatory impairment but does not correlate with severity of the airway narrowing.[52] Spirometry measurements are not necessarily representative of the degree of symptomatic improvement after interventions such as stent insertion or tracheoplasty,[53,54] suggesting that interventions either improve other factors (cough, secretion management) or do improve pulmonary mechanics but not airflow as measured by FEV_1% predicted. However, the flow-volume curve contour in COPD correlates with pulmonary mechanics,[55] and 2 different types of flow-volume loops are identified: AC and scooped-out patterns (**Fig. 5**). AC pattern is characterized by a decrease in flow rate from the peak flow to an inflection point less than 50% of peak flow rate. The inflection point occurs within the first 25% of expired vital capacity. The inspiratory limb of the curve showing no evidence of obstruction can be seen in almost 40% of patients with COPD,[25] and it correlates with the bronchoscopic finding of EDAC.[26] The groups of patients with the 2 distinct flow-volume

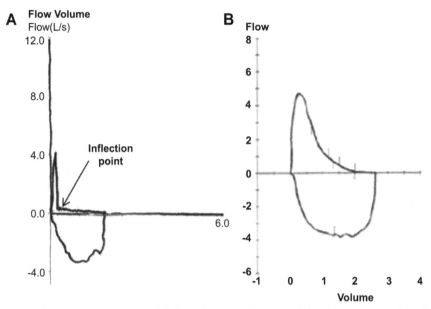

Fig. 5. Flow-volume loop patterns in COPD. (*A*) The AC pattern shows a sudden decrease in peak expiratory flow, defined as a 50% decrease within 25% of FVC. (*B*) The scooped-out pattern is without an initial spike and is characterized by a more curvilinear reduction in flow rate over the vital capacity.

loops patterns cannot be distinguished from clinical symptoms.[55] Results of studies show higher resistance to flow in AC group at high and mid lung volumes but comparable resistance to flow at lower lung volumes in both groups. The RV and FRC were higher in the AC group, indicating a more severe hyperinflation, despite comparable loss of elastic recoil, consistent with functional closure of small airways caused by intrinsic airway abnormality. The degree of hyperinflation was found to have no correlation with the peak flow or the flow rate at the inflection point in the AC group. At the peak flow, the mean pleural pressure was similar in the 2 groups; below peak, the AC group had considerably higher maximal pressure compared with the non-AC group, and this was sustained through 75% of expired vital capacity. These data suggest that AC pattern seems to be determined by a combination of loss of elastic recoil and peripheral AC, findings supporting the EPP theory. Flow oscillations on the flow-volume loop have also been described in patients with ECAC. These oscillations take on a saw-tooth appearance, defined as a reproducible sequence of alternating decelerations and accelerations of flow.[56]

Impulse oscillometry (IOS) is an effort-independent test during which brief pressure pulses generated by a loudspeaker mounted in series with a pneumotachygraph are applied during tidal respiration, and recordings are used to provide an estimate of total respiratory system impedance. Measurements of resistance (R) and reactance (X) at different frequencies might differentiate between central and peripheral components of airway obstruction. Increased R at a low oscillation frequency (5 Hz) reflects an increase in total respiratory resistance suggestive of airway obstruction such as that found in patients with COPD, whereas an increase at a higher frequency (20 Hz) reflects more specifically increased central airway resistance such as that found in patients with central airway obstruction.[57] The IOS maneuver does not cause respiratory fatigue and may be better tolerated by patients with irritable, inflamed airways such as those with ECAC. However, preliminary reports suggest that IOS data from ECAC are similar to those from patients with COPD, resulting in increased resistance at 5 Hz, marked frequency dependence in resistance, more negative reactance at 5 Hz, and increased resonant frequency.[58] Normalization or improvement of IOS data after treatment of ECAC confirms that the IOS pattern is caused by the central AC and not peripheral obstruction.[58] Furthermore, because in EDAC the predominant site of flow limitation is in the periphery, higher R5 and R5 to R20 values are expected than with TBM, for which the main site for flow limitation is the central airways, and thus higher R20 is expected. These findings need to be confirmed in future studies.

Functional Bronchoscopy

Functional bronchoscopy consists of physiologic measurements during bronchoscopy and performance of dynamic bronchoscopy. This latter technique refers to bronchoscopy performed during various respiratory maneuvers with the patient having received at most only anxiolytics. The patient can thus follow commands and cooperate during the procedure with respiratory maneuvers and changes in body position. For instance, a patient with malacia and orthopnea may not have the bronchoscopic findings of malacia unless the bronchoscopy is performed in a supine position. Similarly, a patient with a history of tracheostomy and dyspnea when bending over or during neck flexion may have posttracheostomy stomal stricture, with malacia revealed only when the lesion becomes intrathoracic and increased pleural pressures during exhalation result in further narrowing of the airway lumen and cause flow limitation, inability to raise secretions, or trigger coughing spasms. Conversely, if the lesion is at the thoracic inlet, symptoms may occur only during inspiration if the lesion becomes extrathoracic, such as when the patient performs neck extension.

Intraluminal pressure, changes in pressure over the length of a stenosis, and airflows can be superimposed over the bronchoscopic image in real time using a technique of endospirometry.[59] Dynamic changes can be studied during quiet breathing, forced breathing maneuvers, coughing, and neck flexion/extension, and the impact on pressure change responsible for symptoms can be determined. Results from studies show that intraluminal pressure monitoring allows the detection of the FLS responsible for flow limitation. With the use of airway catheters in dogs[60] and in humans,[34,36] the FLS could be located by measuring airway pressure (P_L) during induced flow limitation generated by either an increase in pleural pressure or a decrease in downstream pressure.

Because assessment of the FLS requires forced expiratory vital capacity maneuvers, detecting flow limitation by measuring P_L cannot be performed during bronchoscopy if patients cannot follow instructions, such as those patients undergoing general anesthesia. However, a simple and well-tolerated bronchoscopic technique has been proposed and studied in this setting, using P_L measurements: a double-lumen airway catheter capable of simultaneously measuring P_L at 2 sites in the trachea can be used to assess tracheal obstruction.[37] When the catheter is positioned with the 2 holes located on each side of a stenosis, the 2 pressures plotted against each other show a line with a slope less than 45° caused by resistance difference between the 2 points. If the 2 holes are simultaneously located proximal from or distal to the narrowing, pressures between these sites are in phase, and if plotted against each other, show a straight line with a slope of 45°. By measuring airway pressure proximal and distal to the narrow airway segment and plotting the 2 pressures against each other during quiet tidal breathing, the site of maximum obstruction and the degree of narrowing can be physiologically assessed, allowing intraoperative prediction of the procedural outcomes.

Bronchoscopy allows direct visualization of the airway mucosa, can be performed in critically ill patients at the bedside, is not associated with ionizing radiation, and allows assessment of response to noninvasive positive pressure ventilation (NIPPV) when this is considered a treatment alternative.[61] For this purpose, a full face mask can be used and secured to the patient's face with elastic straps.[62] A dual-axis swivel adapter (T-adapter) is also attached to the mask and connected to the ventilator. NIPPV is applied in incremental pressures until the AC is palliated or until the patient becomes uncomfortable (patients have occasionally reported chest tightness, dyspnea, and uncomfortable pressure sensation over the face and choking during bronchoscopic continuous positive airway pressure [CPAP] titration for ECAC), whichever comes first. A CPAP pressure of 0 cm H_2O is usually initiated and titrated upwards. If necessary, as in the evaluation of central AC, procedures are performed in the upright and supine positions as well as on and off CPAP to evaluate the degree of airway narrowing and response to CPAP (**Fig. 6**). In EDAC/TBM, CPAP pressures of 7 to 10 cm H_2O usually assure airway patency but pressures can be increased by 3 cm H_2O incrementally until airway caliber during tidal exhalation is considered satisfactory (eg, at least 50% of that noted during inspiration). Intraluminal pressure monitoring during CPAP is possible (Lutz Freitag, MD, Germany, personal communication, 2012) but has not yet been systematically studied.

Dynamic CT

Low-dose dynamic CT reveals TBM and EDAC when performed according to a central airway protocol, which includes end-inspiratory and dynamic-expiratory imaging.[63] Scout images are captured to determine the area of coverage (trachea, mainstem bronchi, and bronchus intermedius). Scanning is performed in a craniocaudal

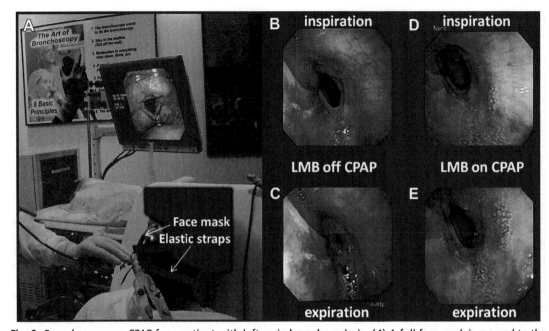

Fig. 6. Bronchoscopy on CPAP for a patient with left main bronchomalacia. (*A*) A full face mask is secured to the patient's face with elastic straps and a dual-axis swivel adapter is attached to the mask and connected to the ventilator. (*B*) Left main bronchial lumen during inspiration at CPAP 0 cm H_2O. (*C*) During tidal expiration, on CPAP 0 cm H_2O, there is near-complete closure of the airway. (*D*) On CPAP of 10 cm H_2O, the inspiratory airway lumen CSA is improved. (*E*) During tidal expiration, on CPAP of 10 cm H_2O, the airway lumen patency is maintained.

direction during both end-expiratory and dynamic-expiratory phases, and the percentage of AC is calculated by subtracting the dynamic-expiratory CSA from the end-inspiratory CSA, divided by the end-inspiratory CSA. Some protocols capture images at 3 different time points during the respiratory cycle: at the end of inspiration, at the end of expiration, and during dynamic exhalation.[63–65] The use of end-inspiratory CT images alone is not useful for detecting TBM or EDAC, because after closing the vocal cords for a breath-hold, the intraluminal airway pressure can become positive, the transmural pressure increased and the airways can be distended. End-expiratory CT images at suspended exhalation may also be misleading for similar reasons; the intraluminal pressure may be higher than during dynamic expiration, and because the expiratory effort has ceased, the pleural pressure is not maximal and the degree of collapse may be diminished. The maximal collapse may not be detected by paired end-inspiratory–end-expiratory CT scans. Therefore, dynamic (cine) CT is used in the assessment of TBM and EDAC as an alternative or complementary test to dynamic bronchoscopy (see **Fig. 3**). Dynamic CT reveals the greatest degree of collapse and is now routinely used in radiology.[6,12,63–65] Image acquisition performed

during dynamic exhalation accentuates AC because images are captured during forced expiratory maneuver, not tidal expiration. The abnormal collapse detected does not reflect the patient's airway dynamics during tidal respiration. In addition to showing potentially a nonpathologic process and causing false-positive diagnosis, dynamic CT also requires additional technologist training. Supervision and coaching of patients is necessary, not always feasible in very dyspneic, uncooperative, or critically ill patients. If patients start coughing, the degree of AC is accentuated even further.[66] Three-dimensional reconstruction images are useful for obtaining a perspective on the extent and degree of collapse, but the axial images are used for accurate measurements of CSA. In general, 3 anatomic levels for each respiratory cycle time point are examined (the aortic arch, main carina, and intermediate bronchus), but there is inconsistency among studies in regards to the number and location of anatomic sites chosen for airway lumen measurements.[6,7,11,12,63–67]

Dynamic CT was shown to reveal similar degree of AC to bronchoscopy.[63,68] Given its noninvasiveness, dynamic CT can be used as the initial test when TBM or EDAC is suspected. However, most investigators use dynamic CT as an adjunct not an alternative to bronchoscopy in preoperative planning[69] or posttherapy monitoring. CT measurements of forced expiratory tracheal collapse are highly reproducible over time and thus can be used for monitoring after intervention and progression of disease.[70] Dynamic CT has been used for general preoperative imaging to assess the degree of narrowing and craniocaudal extent of AC, to define intrinsic (eg, cartilage thickening in relapsing polychondritis) or extrinsic (eg, compression by mediastinal masses or vascular structures) abnormalities and to plan stent insertion by allowing measurement of the airway caliber.[71] CT has been used to follow up patients after stent placement to assess stent patency, detect complications such as migration, formation of granulation tissue, mucus obstruction, or choke point migration. CT was also used in the preoperative evaluations of patients being considered for tracheoplasty to confirm extent, severity, and airway shape because patients with crescent-type TBM are most likely to benefit from reinforcement of the posterior membrane.[72,73] CT allows exclusion of other diseases requiring different interventions, such as a paratracheal mass or relapsing polychondritis. Postoperative evaluation after tracheoplasty can be performed using CT, which reveals changes in the degree of expiratory collapse and potentially detects the rare but severe complications of this procedure, such as airway dehiscence, mediastinal hematoma, or abscess.[74] In addition to noninvasiveness, the main advantage over bronchoscopy is the ability to evaluate the structures around the airways potentially responsible for malacia (ie, goiter, aortic aneurysm, double aortic arch) and assess the changes of lung parenchyma that may cause or be associated with central AC (ie, emphysema, bronchiolitis, air trapping). The disadvantages include the lack of details about the mucosa, the necessary patient cooperation with respiratory maneuvers, and exposure to ionizing radiation. Lower-dose techniques allow a 23% radiation dose reduction compared with the standard technique. These techniques can be used for central airway imaging because of the inherent contrast between central airways and adjacent soft tissue without compromising diagnostic information.[68,75] Advances in CT technology allow now faster image acquisition. The 320-detector row scanner covers 16 cm craniocaudal volume per rotation and allows real-time dynamic imaging of trachea. This technique has already been used for diagnosis of EDAC and assessment of response to CPAP.[20]

However, from a physiologic standpoint, dynamic CT findings of excessive AC during forced exhalation have been considered of uncertain physiologic significance.[6,12,17,24] Recent dynamic CT studies are in agreement with the physiologic understanding of EDAC based on the flow-limitation theories. Although the previous definition of abnormal collapse greater than 50% cross-sectional luminal collapse is still used by investigators,[11] symptomatic collapse, which may require interventions, is usually 95% to 100%.[53,54] Advances in imaging resulted in changing of our understanding of the pathologic central AC. Initial radiographic definition of cross-sectional diameter reduction of 50% or greater during coughing on bronchography dating from more than 45 years ago[13] is now known to be inadequate because 80% of normal healthy individuals meet this criterion during forced exhalation.[12] The different degrees of AC noted on imaging studies led to radiologic subtyping of the 50% or greater criterion according to severity.[2,14] Results of studies show that the % expiratory decrease in CSA should not be the only criterion, because there is overlap in degree of expiratory collapse among healthy volunteers and patients with central airway disease[12,16]; furthermore, the degree of collapse greater than 50% is not uncommon in COPD and may not be responsible for flow limitation.[6]

Results of studies show the presence of the highly collapsed central airways in COPD using dynamic-expiratory or end-expiratory CT scans[11,76–78] and the lack of significant physiologic impairment resulting from EDAC. For instance, one study aimed to reveal the correlations between tracheal volumetric measures, including collapsibility, and lung volume measures on inspiratory and end-expiratory CT scans and to evaluate the relationship between tracheal collapsibility and lung function. The study included 85 smokers (normal lung function [n = 14]; GOLD stage 1 [n = 14]; stage 2 [n = 38]; stage 3 [n = 11]; stage 4 [n = 8]) who underwent PFTs and chest CT at full inspiration and end-expiration. Tracheal volume and collapsibility, expressed as expiratory/inspiratory (E/I) ratios of these volumes, were found to be related to lung volume and collapsibility. The highly collapsed trachea on end-expiratory CT did not indicate more severe airflow limitation or air trapping in smokers because only weak correlation was found with FEV_1/FVC or RV/TLC ratios, respectively.[67] The tracheal collapsibility negatively correlated with FEV_1/FVC and FEV_1% predicted, suggesting that the highly collapsed trachea on end-expiratory scans indicated less severe airflow limitation in the individuals analyzed in this study. These findings add to the body of evidence that the collapsed trachea on end-expiratory scans in the form of EDAC is not a morbid finding and should be distinguished from the abnormally collapsed trachea in TBM.

These observations are relevant for future radiologic and physiologic studies of tracheal collapse in COPD or TBM.[67] In addition to COPD, using dynamic CT, EDAC was also shown in 69% adult patients with cystic fibrosis.[79] Based on data from dynamic CT studies, radiology literature suggests the need for more rigorous criteria for diagnosing clinically relevant EDAC, with potentially separate diagnostic threshold levels for the trachea and right and left bronchi.[12,17] Correlation of forced expiratory CT findings of EDAC with symptoms and pulmonary function testing is necessary in the decision-making process before considering EDAC a cause of a patient's symptoms and subsequently proceed with interventions.

The increasing use of dynamic CT for TBM and EDAC led to recognition of several morphologic types of central AC. Similar to bronchoscopic classifications, numerous descriptive terms have been proposed, but no 1 system has been universally adopted. CT classification is based on morphology on inspiratory and expiratory images. For instance, on inspiratory images, the normal trachea is generally oval or round. In patients with the most common type of TBM (the crescent type), even during inspiration, the anterior wall of the cartilage is flattened and the shape of the trachea has been described on CT scans as lunate, in which the coronal/sagittal diameter ratio is greater than 1.[80–82] A second type is the saber-sheath morphology, usually associated with COPD.[83] Some patients with this type of tracheal configuration have malacia as well,[84] but this can occur in the presence of normal inspiratory tracheal morphology. A biconvex, fish-mouth pattern has also been described.[72] Based on expiratory images, the terms used in the radiology literature include crescent, characterized by marked anterior bowing of posterior wall, or the so-called frown sign[82] and circumferential, characterized by isotropic reduction in airway cross section.

Dynamic Magnetic Resonance Imaging

The use of magnetic resonance imaging (MRI) has been rarely reported in adults with TBM and EDAC,[85,86] but it is used to diagnose and monitor response to stabilization techniques for pediatric TBM.[87–89] MRI studies reveal similar results with those from dynamic CT analyses of central AC. For instance, in 1 study, a significantly higher collapse was found in patients with COPD compared with volunteers, with 70% of patients with COPD showing a collapse of more than 50%.[85] Contrary to CT scanning, MRI has the advantage of avoiding radiation and offering superior contrast resolution and more definitively

characterizes soft tissue masses. MRI can delineate tracheal and main bronchial patency and their close anatomic relationship with the adjacent vascular structures. Modern MRI allows central airway imaging with adequate resolution.[85,90] As with CT, contrast agents are still used, but in the case of MRI, intravenous gadolinium contrast-based agents are generally recommended unless contraindications exist. Images can be affected by respiratory and cardiac motion artifact, which makes interpretation of intrathoracic MRI images more difficult. Mainstem bronchi trajectories are oblique and bias the accuracy of CSA measurement. Increased acquisition times often require the patient to stay still for at least several minutes at a time, which may not be possible in dyspneic, uncooperative, or critically ill patients.[91] The MRI examination takes about 15 minutes. Three dynamic measurements can be performed in the coronal, oblique, and transverse orientation, respectively. Minimal and maximal cross-sectional luminal diameters and tracheal lumen area can be calculated. In 1 study, the median degree of tracheal collapse was found to be 43% in volunteers and 64% in smokers. The maximal CSA of the upper tracheal lumen as well as the expiratory collapse was larger in patients with COPD than in normal individuals.[85] Similar to data from CT studies, a significant proportion of patients with COPD (70%) and 30% of volunteers showed a collapse of more than 50%. Overall, however, the high spatial (submillimeter) and temporal resolution (10 frames/s) of dynamic CT cannot yet be obtained by MRI techniques.[92]

MRI has been used to assess focal malacia associated with laryngotracheal stenosis[93,94] or diffuse malacia from relapsing polychondritis.[95] The dynamic (cine) MRI has been particularly useful to define pediatric TBM.[96] MRI is established as the standard modality for imaging the pediatric mediastinal airway.[96] Ventilation and perfusion mapping and quantification are also possible and may have a role in the future MR imaging of patients with TBM and EDAC.

High-Frequency Endobronchial Ultrasonography

High-frequency endobronchial ultrasonography (EBUS) using a 20-MHz radial scanning probe was shown to identify the hypoechoic and hyperechoic layers that correlate with the laminar histologic structures of the central airways.[97] Cartilage abnormalities (weakness, fracture, edema) was described in patients with malacia caused by tuberculosis, relapsing polychondritis, lung cancer, and compression by vascular rings.[97–99]

EBUS could potentially distinguish between TBM and EDAC because in the latter it seems that the cartilage is intact, and the posterior membrane is thinner than normal, likely because of atrophy of elastic fibers.[99] The instability of the posterior tracheal wall is in agreement with the known loss of elastic fibers, which enables inflation and collapse during respiration. Cartilage abnormalities in the central airways of patients with COPD and ECAC have not been systematically studied with EBUS. This finding is relevant because based on wave speed theory and EPP theory, the CSA at the choke point is determined by the pleural pressures, resistance of the upstream airways and compliance of the airway. It is relevant for treatment to know if the airway compliance is increased because of the reduced stiffness from weakened cartilage. However, the pathologic hallmarks of COPD are destruction of the lung parenchyma, which characterizes emphysema; inflammation of the peripheral airways, which characterizes bronchiolitis, and inflammation of the central airways, which characterizes chronic bronchitis. In patients with chronic bronchitis, inflammation was found to be present in the airway wall and in the mucous glands, particularly in cartilaginous bronchi larger than 2 mm in diameter. However, there is no mention of cartilaginous destruction in biopsy studies of patients with COPD.[100] More studies are needed, but there is potential for high-frequency EBUS to be used as a surrogate of histology in patients with ECAC.

Vibration Resonance Imaging

Vibration response imaging (VRI) is a noninvasive imaging tool using piezoacoustic sensors to transform analog signals from the chest into dynamic grayscale images similar to the process involved in ultrasound imaging. VRI has been reported in the evaluation of patients with asthma, COPD, aspiration of foreign objects, and central airway obstruction undergoing bronchoscopic interventions.[101] The experience in patients with ECAC is limited,[58] but the disappearance of floating and fluttering dynamic imaging pattern after stent insertion is consistent with previous studies showing improvement in patients with other forms of central airway obstruction after bronchoscopic interventions.[101] Because sounds at frequencies of 100 to 250 Hz are mainly generated in the central airways and frequencies of 500 to 650 Hz in the terminal bronchioles, the differential analysis of VRI might allow localization of pathologic processes in different compartments of the lung.[101] TBM and EDAC may provide

different dynamic grayscale images, because in TBM, the FLS are predominantly central, whereas they are peripheral in EDAC, although these hypotheses remain to be studied. Given its noninvasiveness, this modality could potentially be used for telemedicine monitoring of symptomatic patients.

Evaluation: key points

1. Spirometry values do not correlate with the degree of AC.

2. Expiratory flow-volume curve may show a sudden decrease in peak flow very early during a forced expiratory maneuver (also known as AC pattern) or flow oscillation (also known as saw-tooth pattern).

3. Dynamic and functional bronchoscopy are performed to distinguish and classify TBM and EDAC, to determine choke point location, and subsequently to decide on the need for and type of treatment.

4. Low-dose paired inspiratory–dynamic-expiratory CT is complementary to bronchoscopy by providing information about the adjacent vasculature, mediastinal masses, or parenchymal changes that may explain the cause of ECAC.

5. Low-dose paired inspiratory–dynamic-expiratory CT results in false-positive findings of EDAC if the 50% cutoff is used to define abnormal collapse.

6. Dynamic MRI can be used to detect ECAC and has lower resolution than CT scanning but is preferred in the pediatric population because of lack of ionizing radiation.

7. High-frequency EBUS may be used as a surrogate of histology to identify structural airway wall changes in ECAC.

TREATMENT

Functional impairment attributable to ECAC warrants evaluation for treatment. Patients with incidental abnormal AC on bronchoscopy or CT scanning performed for other reasons should not undergo interventions.[3,102] Functional impairment in ECAC may result from at least 3 causes: dyspnea, cough, mucus retention.[9,14,53] EDAC is also associated with higher morbidity and poorer survival in elderly patients who have undergone bronchial and bronchovascular sleeve resections for lung cancer.[21] Therefore, as for other pulmonary disorders, QOL and functional impairment scales may be appropriate to measure the impact of respiratory symptoms on overall health, daily life, and perceived well-being in patients suffering from ECAC. This evaluation typically involves PFTs, 6MWT, and determination of Karnofsky performance status, American Thoracic Society Dyspnea Score, and respiratory-affected QOL based on the SGRQ.

Significant impairment of the patient's functional status and QOL is necessary before considering potential intervention. However, there are no controlled studies to support 1 therapy versus another. Research is limited by ethical issues. For instance, a randomized trial of tracheobronchoplasty versus sham surgery is obviously not feasible, but it is possible to design a randomized study of rigid bronchoscopy and rigid bronchoscopy plus Y-stent placement for diffuse and severe EDAC. The disease process, before invasive interventions, has to be clearly defined and quantified in terms of morphology of ECAC, extent, severity of narrowing, and impact on functional class and QOL scores (**Fig. 7**).

Cause-Based Treatment Strategies

Treatment of the primary cause of AC may or may not improve the degree of airway narrowing or symptoms. The invasive nature of alternative strategies (stents, tracheoplasty) justifies an initial attempt at medical treatment of the cause of EDAC/TBM. For instance, reversibility of EDAC can occur after properly treating chronic bronchitis with bronchodilators, steroids, and antibiotics. In 1 study,[55] the AC pattern on the flow-volume loop characterizing EDAC showed complete reversibility in a few (3/20) patients after 3 weeks. From a physiologic standpoint, based on EPP theory, this finding is relevant because the AC pattern can normalize after treating bronchitis (Rus component) without a concomitant normalization of elastic recoil. On the other hand, bronchodilators may increase airway wall compliance, suggesting that increased compressibility of the large airways causes the EPP to become fixed at a point nearer the thoracic outlet. The increased length of the upstream segment (Rus) and decreased CSA at the EPP would thus offset the advantage gained by increased caliber of upstream airways with respect to maximal expiratory flow rates.[103] This finding may explain why some patients with EDAC caused by COPD do not improve after bronchodilators. Some patients may have worsened maximum expiratory flow rates.[104,105]

Treatment of emphysema itself could lead to improvement in EDAC, further supporting the argument that EDAC is not a primary tracheobronchial disorder. Improvement in expiratory flows after lung volume reduction surgery is largely caused by increases in recoil pressure (Pst). Placement of the endobronchial valves results in less hyperinflation (improved Pst), and bronchoscopic follow-up may show improved EDAC (Hugo Oliveira, MD, Brazil, personal communication, 2008), but this hypothesis needs to be tested in emphysema treatment trials. For patients with a known cause of cartilage inflammation such as relapsing polychondritis, treatment with immunosuppressive therapy is offered first unless the airway is critically narrowed and the patient in extremis (see **Fig. 7**). However, results of studies and clinical experience suggest that once malacia has developed, antiinflammatory agents may not restore cartilage integrity.[106] For patients with disease refractory to medical treatment, strategies aimed at restoring airway patency are offered based on the degree of airway narrowing, craniocaudal extent, and, most importantly, impact on symptoms, predicted response, and expected complications (see **Fig. 7**).

NIPPV

Application of positive airway pressure serves as a pneumatic stent,[107] because the intraluminal pressure is increased, thus improving the airway stiffness and expiratory flow based on wave speed theory (Equation 2). Alternatively, flow may be improved simply because lung volumes are higher during positive pressure ventilation. The higher elastic recoil, based on the EPP theory, improves the maximum expiratory flow (Equation 1). Data from pediatric TBM confirm this concept. CPAP significantly increased maximal expiratory flow at FRC in healthy infants and infants with tracheomalacia.[108] This increase in flow at FRC was secondary to the increase in lung volume with CPAP, because maximal expiratory flows measured at the different levels of CPAP were not different when compared at the same lung volumes. The optimal level of CPAP in infants with severe tracheomalacia may be related to increasing the lung volume to a level at which the infant is not flow limited during tidal breathing, without also significantly increasing the work of breathing through a decrease in pulmonary compliance at increased lung volumes.

From a clinical standpoint, regardless of its mechanism of action, CPAP was shown to improve dyspnea, cough, and secretion management in selected patients with TBM. The amount of pressure necessary to maintain airway patency can be determined by performing bronchoscopy assisted by NIPPV.[61] Adjunctive NIPPV decreases pulmonary resistance and can be used to improve spirometry values, sputum production, atelectasis, and exercise tolerance, but its long-term efficiency has not been clearly shown.[23,109,110] NIPPV has been used in adults with TBM from relapsing polychondritis and tracheomalacia from long-standing compression by a large goiter or thyroid cancer, wherein the cartilaginous rings of the trachea are considerably weakened or destroyed, leading to softening and floppiness of the trachea. NIPPV was also effective and safe in the management of stridor and airway compromise after early extubation of patients with postthyroidectomy tracheomalacia.[111] In 1 study, 6 patients developed stridor and airway compromise, which resolved immediately with the initiation of NIPPV without further respiratory support being required and without complications.[111]

Application of noninvasive positive expiratory pressure (PEP) may improve expiratory flow and cough efficiency in patients with ECAC. This finding was shown in a study of 40 children with TBM.[112] Patients and 21 age-matched controls performed spirometry followed by cough spirometry with PEP of 0, 5, 10, 15, and 20 cm H_2O using an adjustable PEP valve. Cough expiratory flow between 75% and 25% of vital capacity (CEF25-75) for each curve was calculated to represent the effectiveness of cough at midlung volume. In the TBM group, CEF25-75 increased by a mean of 18.8%, 1.7%, and 0.5% at PEP of 5, 10, and 15 cm H_2O, respectively, but decreased by 2.4% at PEP of 20 cm H_2O. In the control group, the CEF25-75 decreased at all levels of PEP, with worse flow at higher PEP levels.[112] This study[112] suggests that the use of adjustable PEP valve increases flow during cough spirometry and may provide a useful adjunct to chest physiotherapy. It also shows the importance of scientifically choosing PEP levels, because higher levels (ie, 20 cm H_2O) may worsen expiratory flow.

Bronchoscopic Interventions

Some patients with EDAC improve QOL after insertion of a central airway stabilization by stent. However, this situation is not explained by improvement in airflow as measured by FEV_1.[53] One explanation for improved symptoms is that central airway stability makes the flow less turbulent, similar to heliox, which was shown to improve exercise capacity in patients with moderate to severe COPD.[113] In the short-term (10–14 days), airway stabilization using silicone stents in patients with various forms of ECAC was shown to improve respiratory symptoms, QOL, and functional status.[53,114] In 1 large study, 45 of 58 patients (77%) reported symptomatic improvement; QOL scores improved in 19 of 27 patients (70%); dyspnea scores improved in 22 of 24 patients (91%); and functional status scores improved in 18 of 26 patients (70%).[53] Stents may also improve outcomes for patients with Mounier-Kuhn syndrome[115] and have been used in patients with malacia from relapsing polychondritis, with variable results.[39,116,117] Of 8 patients with bronchoscopically detected TBM in a study of patients with relapsing polychondritis, only 3 were treated (2 by stent insertion and 1 by tracheostomy and removal of previously placed stents).[118] Metal stents have been used in the past with variable success in patients with TBM. Advantages include placement by flexible bronchoscopy, dynamic expansion, and maintenance of airway mucociliary function with uncovered stents. However, in some studies, metal stents had to be removed because of stent mechanical failure or because of stent-related complications. Stent fracture and fatal hemorrhage from perforation have been reported; in the United States, metal stents are no longer recommended for use in benign central airway disease if other alternatives are available.[119,120]

To potentially detect stent-related adverse effects or migrated choke points requiring further interventions, follow-up bronchoscopy or dynamic CT has been used in clinical studies.[121] Stent-related adverse events are common and usually occur within the first few weeks after stent insertion (median time 4 weeks).[53,114] These results seem to justify follow-up imaging 4 to 6 weeks after stent insertion (see **Fig. 7**). Sometimes, follow-up detects distally migrated choke points after stent insertion.[39,40] Placing a stent at the site of maximal collapse during exhalation might result in migration of the choke point toward the periphery of the lung[122] and has been addressed in patients with central airway obstruction caused by lung cancer and also in patients with malacia from relapsing polychondritis. Additional stents may be required if patients are still symptomatic and the choke points are still in the central airways. In 1 series, bilevel positive airway pressure was used after stent insertion for patients whose choke points had migrated to the small bronchi, as documented on CT.[39] Rather than inserting more foreign material into an already inflamed airway, it may be more reasonable to use adjuvant NIPPV. If stent insertion does not improve symptoms and there is no migration of the choke points, then stent removal is advisable to avoid complications. Stent migration, obstruction by mucus and granulation tissue, infection, fracture, and airway perforation are well described in the literature.[3] The distinction between stent-related adverse events and symptoms related to TBM may be difficult to assess based on clinical grounds, so any new onset or worsening of symptoms should prompt bronchoscopy or CT scanning (see **Fig. 7**).

Yttrium aluminum perovskite (YAP) laser treatment has been anecdotally reported to improve lung function and symptoms in EDAC caused by Mounier-Kuhn syndrome; laser was applied with the intention of stiffening the posterior membrane by devascularization and subsequent

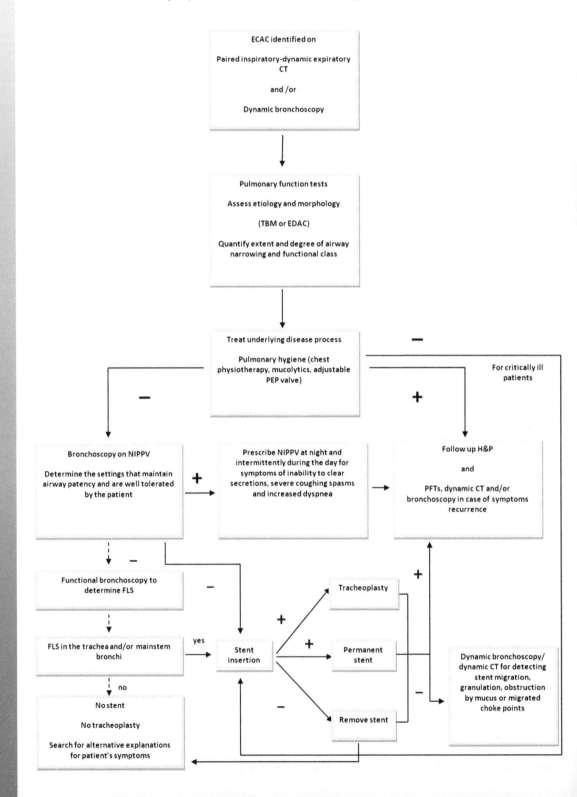

retraction of tissues.[123] Its wavelength is double that of the yttrium aluminum garnet laser, allowing for tissue devascularization and coagulation at low power (15–20 W) in a discontinuous mode.[124] The depth of penetration using YAP laser is estimated at 3 mm and may reach the submucosal tissues, triggering a fibrotic process[125] that may stiffen the posterior membrane. Concerns remain about posterior membrane perforation and relapse of disease with the need for repeated interventions.

Surgical Interventions

Cervical tracheoplasty, resection/reconstruction, or tracheostomies are usually performed for extrathoracic tracheal malacia. Tracheal resection has been proposed for focal tracheomalacia, with good outcome and low mortality in experienced centers.[126] However, this procedure was performed for posttracheostomy-related malacia and not for extensive disease. Open surgical interventions for intrathoracic disease include airway splinting and tracheostomy. Splinting (tracheoplasty) has been used to consolidate and reshape the airway wall, whereas tracheostomy is performed to maintain a stable airway and potentially bypass the malacic segment. Tracheostomy provides invasive ventilatory support if necessary, but it can be complicated by secondary tracheomalacia and stenosis and should not be considered a first-line treatment in elective cases. Before proposing membranous tracheoplasty, a stent trial has been used to identify those patients who are likely to benefit from surgery in the long-term. When performed on this protocol, membranous tracheoplasty seemed to provide a favorable outcome in uncontrolled studies.

This procedure reinforces the membranous portion of the trachea in severe diffuse ECAC.[54,127] The thoracic airways are splinted from the thoracic inlet to the distal left mainstem bronchus and distal bronchus intermedius. The outcomes of membranous tracheoplasty are promising, but complications are not insignificant; for instance, 1 study evaluated 66 patients with severe diffuse crescent-type TBM and EDAC (disease affecting trachea and bilateral mainstem bronchi).[128] However, the 2 entities were grouped together under TBM and results were not reported separately. Thirty-seven patients had complete sets of preoperative and postoperative measurements of FEV_1, and no significant difference was shown before and after the procedure. Twenty-two of 37 patients had improved FEV_1, with a mean increase of 234 mL, whereas 15 of 37 patients showed no improvement or frank worsening of their postoperative FEV_1, with a mean decrease of 235 mL, and 1 patient also had the same FEV_1 values preoperatively and postoperatively. This study confirms earlier physiologic findings that stabilization of the collapsing tracheal and bronchial airway may not improve airflow but may result in improvements in short-term (3-month) QOL measurements. The median length of stay in the hospital after this surgical intervention was

Fig. 7. Management algorithm for diffuse ECAC. Once identified on dynamic CT or dynamic bronchoscopy, PFTs are performed (if not performed previously) to assess if there is any associated impact on maximum expiratory flow or dynamic hyperinflation. A clear categorization as TBM or EDAC is performed and cause is searched for. The extent, degree of narrowing, and impact on functional status and QOL are then evaluated to determine if treatment is warranted. The cause of the process (when known) should be medically treated first, if possible. In addition to disease-specific treatment, chest physiotherapy, mucolytics, adjustable positive expiratory pressure valves can be used to improve secretion management. If the underlying cause is treated and the patient improves, a follow-up strategy with clinical examination, PFTs, and CT/bronchoscopy is warranted in case of symptom recurrence. If this fails and the patient is critically ill (unable to be weaned from invasive or noninvasive ventilatory support), the airway has to be stabilized and stent insertion is performed. If the patient is not critically ill, then NIPPV-assisted bronchoscopy is performed to determine if positive pressure application maintains airway patency. If the airway patency is maintained during NIPPV application, then those particular settings can be prescribed for nighttime NIPPV and intermittent use during the day as triggered by symptoms. If the patient does not respond to NIPPV, 1 strategy involves a so-called stent trial. If there is improvement (objectively documented), tracheoplasty is offered to operable patients; if patients are not surgical candidates, a permanent stent insertion is an alternative understanding if there is a high risk for stent-related adverse effects. Alternatively, functional bronchoscopy can be performed to localize the FLS amenable to stabilization techniques (stent insertion or tracheoplasty). If the FLS are in the trachea or mainstem bronchi, then a stent trial is performed (an algorithm to proceed directly with tracheoplasty has not yet been studied). If the FLS are not in the central airways, then stent insertion or tracheoplasty should not be offered, because they are unlikely to improve flow and alternative explanations for patient's symptoms should be investigated. After stent insertion or tracheoplasty, a follow-up bronchoscopy or dynamic CT should be performed within 4 to 6 weeks to assess airway patency and potential adverse events. H&P, history and physical examination; +, improvement and –, lack of improvement after a specific intervention; dashed line, an alternative strategy, depending on availability/expertise with technique.

8 days (range, 4–92 days), of which 3 days (range, 0–91 days) were in the intensive care unit. Two patients (3.2%) died postoperatively and overall complications were seen in 38% of patients and included a new respiratory infection, pulmonary embolism, and atrial fibrillation. Six patients (10%) required reintubation and 9 (14%) received a postoperative tracheotomy, including 4 tracheotomies intraoperatively immediately after the tracheobronchoplasty in anticipation of the need for frequent therapeutic aspiration bronchoscopy and tracheal suctioning, which was needed in 47 of 66 patients. A less invasive approach used video-assisted thoracoscopic surgical tracheobronchoplasty combined with airway stent placement for the treatment of 2 cases of TBM.[129] The anecdotal evidence and concurrent use of stents raise questions about the long-term benefits of the combined modality.

Treatment strategies: key points

1. Asymptomatic ECAC, regardless of the degree of AC, should not be treated.

2. Treatment of the underlying cause must be attempted before considering more invasive interventions.

3. NIPPV-assisted bronchoscopy allows titration of applied pressures that maintain airway patency during expiration.

4. Intraluminal airway pressures measurements localize the choke points and may predict response to interventions.

5. Focal disease can be treated by resection or reconstruction or bypassed with an indwelling tracheostomy tube.

6. Significantly impaired patients with severe and diffuse EDAC or crescent TBM may benefit from membranous tracheoplasty.

7. Inoperable patients with refractory symptoms may benefit from silicone stent insertion.

8. Most patients with ECAC and indwelling airway stents require frequent bronchoscopic interventions to manage stent-related mucus obstruction, migration, and granulation tissue.

SUMMARY

TBM is characterized as weakened or destroyed cartilage in the central airways, resulting in expiratory flow limitation. EDAC is characterized by excessive bulging of the posterior membrane inside the central airway lumen. ECAC is a syndrome that includes both TBM and EDAC. Depending on the degree of AC, anatomic site, and respiratory maneuver used for defining it, EDAC is seen in normal individuals, those with morbid obesity, and those with a variety of obstructive ventilatory disorders. A careful physiologic assessment of the impact of ECAC on airflow and functional status is warranted before treatment. Identification of the flow-limiting airway segments can be obtained by performing functional bronchoscopy before invasive interventions. Even when the central AC is identified as responsible for symptoms, we suggest a conservative approach with medical treatment and NIPPV before committing patients to potentially harmful effects resulting from airway stents or open surgical procedures.

REFERENCES

1. World Health Organization. The WHO family of international classifications. Available at: http://www.who.int/classifications/en/. Accessed May 22, 2006.

2. Murgu SD, Colt HG. Description of a multidimensional classification system for patients with expiratory central airway collapse. Respirology 2007;12:543–50.

3. Murgu SD, Colt HG. Tracheobronchomalacia and excessive dynamic airway collapse. Respirology 2006;11:388–406.

4. Park JG, Edell ES. Dynamic airway collapse. Different from tracheomalacia. Rev Port Pneumol 2005;11:600–2.

5. Kalra A, Abouzgheib W, Gajera M, et al. Excessive dynamic airway collapse for the internist: new nomenclature or different entity? Postgrad Med J 2011;87:482–6.

6. Boiselle PM, Michaud G, Roberts DH, et al. Dynamic expiratory tracheal collapse in COPD: correlation with clinical and physiological parameters. Chest 2012;142(6):1539–44.

7. Aquino SL, Shepard JA, Ginns LC, et al. Acquired tracheomalacia: detection by expiratory CT scan. J Comput Assist Tomogr 2001;25:394–9.

8. Stern EJ, Graham CM, Webb WR, et al. Normal trachea during forced expiration: dynamic CT measurements. Radiology 1993;187:27–31.

9. Nuutinen J. Acquired tracheobronchomalacia. A clinical study with bronchological correlations. Ann Clin Res 1977;9:350–5.

10. Masaoka A, Yamakawa Y, Niwa H, et al. Pediatric and adult tracheobronchomalacia. Eur J Cardiothorac Surg 1996;10:87–92.

11. Sverzellati N, Rastelli A, Chetta A, et al. Airway malacia in chronic obstructive pulmonary

disease: prevalence, morphology and relationship with emphysema, bronchiectasis and bronchial wall thickening. Eur Radiol 2009;19:1669–78.

12. Boiselle PM, O'Donnell CR, Bankier AA, et al. Tracheal collapsibility in healthy volunteers during forced expiration: assessment with multidetector CT. Radiology 2009;252:255–62.

13. Rayl JE. Tracheobronchial collapse during cough. Radiology 1965;85:87–92.

14. Johnson TH, Mikita JJ, Wilson RJ, et al. Acquired tracheomalacia. Radiology 1973;109:576–80.

15. Feist JH, Johnson TH, Wilson RJ. Acquired tracheomalacia: etiology and differential diagnosis. Chest 1975;68:340–5.

16. Thiriet M, Maarek JM, Chartrand DA, et al. Transverse images of the human thoracic trachea during forced expiration. J Appl Physiol 1989;67:1032–40.

17. Litmanovich D, O'Donnell CR, Bankier AA, et al. Bronchial collapsibility at forced expiration in healthy volunteers: assessment with multidetector CT. Radiology 2010;257:560–7.

18. Brouns M, Jayaraju ST, Lacor C, et al. Tracheal stenosis: a flow dynamics study. J Appl Physiol 2007; 102:1178–84.

19. Jokinen K, Palva T, Sutinen S, et al. Acquired tracheobronchomalacia. Ann Clin Res 1977;9:52–7.

20. Joosten S, MacDonald M, Lau KK, et al. Excessive dynamic airway collapse co-morbid with COPD diagnosed using 320-slice dynamic CT scanning technology. Thorax 2012;67:95–6.

21. Bölükbas S, Bergmann T, Fisseler-Eckhoff A, et al. Short- and long-term outcome of sleeve resections in the elderly. Eur J Cardiothorac Surg 2010;37:30–5.

22. Represas Represas C, Fernández-Villar A, García-Tejedor JL, et al. Excessive dynamic airway collapse: a new disease. Rev Clin Esp 2010;210: 53–5.

23. Tamura Y, Sakatani K, Yamakoshi N, et al. A case of severe COPD associated with tracheo-bronchial stenosis, treated with non-invasive positive pressure ventilation. Nihon Kokyuki Gakkai Zasshi 2008;46:915–20.

24. O'Donnell CR, Litmanovich D, Loring SH, et al. Age and gender dependence of forced expiratory central airway collapse in healthy volunteers. Chest 2012;142(1):168–74.

25. Healy F, Wilson AF, Fairshter RD. Physiologic correlates of airway collapse in chronic airflow obstruction. Chest 1984;85:476–81.

26. Campbell AH, Faulks LW. Expiratory air-flow pattern in tracheobronchial collapse. Am Rev Respir Dis 1965;92:781–91.

27. Baydur A, Wilkinson L, Mehdian R, et al. Extrathoracic expiratory flow limitation in obesity and obstructive and restrictive disorders: effects of increasing negative expiratory pressure. Chest 2004;125:98–105.

28. Behazin N, Jones SB, Cohen RI, et al. Respiratory restriction and elevated pleural and esophageal pressures in morbid obesity. J Appl Physiol 2010; 108:212–8.

29. Steier J, Jolley CJ, Seymour J, et al. Obese patients develop an intrinsic positive end expiratory pressure (PEEP) when supine. Am J Respir Crit Care Med 2008;177:A275.

30. Mead J, Turner JM, Macklem PT, et al. Significance of the relationship between lung recoil and maximum expiratory flow. J Appl Physiol 1967;22:95–108.

31. Dawson SV, Elliott EA. Wave-speed limitation on expiratory flow–a unifying concept. J Appl Physiol 1977;43:498–515.

32. Macklem PT, Fraser RG, Brown WG. The detection of the flow-limiting bronchi in bronchitis and emphysema by airway pressure measurements. Med Thorac 1965;22:220–30.

33. Macklem PT, Wilson NJ. Measurement of intrabronchial pressure in man. J Appl Physiol 1965; 20:653–63.

34. Smaldone GC, Smith PL. Location of flow-limiting segments via airway catheters near residual volume in humans. J Appl Physiol 1985;59:502–8.

35. Baram D, Smaldone G. Tracheal collapse versus tracheobronchomalacia: normal function versus disease. Am J Respir Crit Care Med 2006;174: 724 [author reply: 724–5].

36. Pedersen OF, Brackel HJ, Bogaard JM, et al. Wave-speed-determined flow limitation at peak flow in normal and asthmatic subjects. J Appl Physiol 1997;83:1721–32.

37. Nishine H, Hiramoto T, Kida H, et al. Assessing the site of maximal obstruction in the trachea using lateral pressure measurement during bronchoscopy. Am J Respir Crit Care Med 2012;185: 24–33.

38. Pedersen OF, Ingram RH Jr. Configuration of maximum expiratory flow volume curve: model experiments with physiological implications. J Appl Physiol 1985;58:1305–13.

39. Miyazawa T, Nishine H, Handa H, et al. Migration of the choke point in relapsing polychondritis after stenting. Chest 2009;136:81S.

40. Miyazawa T, Miyazu Y, Iwamoto Y, et al. Stenting at the flow-limiting segment in tracheobronchial stenosis due to lung cancer. Am J Respir Crit Care Med 2004;169:1096–102.

41. Brackel HJ, Pedersen OF, Mulder PG, et al. Central airways behave more stiffly during forced expiration in patients with asthma. Am J Respir Crit Care Med 2000;162(3 Pt 1):896–904.

42. Enright PL, Kronmal RA, Manolio TA, et al. Respiratory muscle strength in the elderly. Correlates and reference values. Cardiovascular Health Study Research Group. Am J Respir Crit Care Med 1994;149(2 Pt 1):430–8.

43. Hogg JC, Macklem PT, Thurlbeck WM. Site and nature of airway obstruction in chronic obstructive lung disease. N Engl J Med 1968;278:1355–60.

44. Despas PJ, Leroux M, Macklem PT. Site of airway obstruction in asthma as determined by measuring maximal expiratory flow breathing air and a helium-oxygen mixture. J Clin Invest 1972;51:3235–43.

45. Mink SN. Expiratory flow limitation and the response to breathing a helium-oxygen gas mixture in a canine model of pulmonary emphysema. J Clin Invest 1984;73:1321–34.

46. Tiddens HA, Bogaard JM, de Jongste JC, et al. Physiological and morphological determinants of maximal expiratory flow in chronic obstructive lung disease. Eur Respir J 1996;9:1785–94.

47. Tandon MK, Campbell AH. Bronchial cartilage in chronic bronchitis. Thorax 1969;24:607–12.

48. Nagai A, West WW, Paul JL, et al. The National Institutes of Health Intermittent Positive-Pressure Breathing trial: pathology studies. I. Interrelationship between morphologic lesions. Am Rev Respir Dis 1985;132:937–45.

49. Nagai A, Thurlbeck WM, Konno K. Responsiveness and variability of airflow obstruction in chronic obstructive pulmonary disease. Clinicopathologic correlative studies. Am J Respir Crit Care Med 1995;151(3 Pt 1):635–9.

50. Dunnill MS, Massarella GR, Anderson JA. A comparison of the quantitative anatomy of the bronchi in normal subjects, in status asthmaticus, in chronic bronchitis, and in emphysema. Thorax 1969;24:176–9.

51. Moreno RH, McCormack GS, Brendan J, et al. Effect of intravenous papain on tracheal pressure-volume curves in rabbits. J Appl Physiol 1986;60:247–52.

52. Loring SH, O'Donnell CR, Feller-Kopman DJ, et al. Central airway mechanics and flow limitation in acquired tracheobronchomalacia. Chest 2007;131:1118–24.

53. Ernst A, Majid A, Feller-Kopman D, et al. Airway stabilization with silicone stents for treating adult tracheobronchomalacia: a prospective observational study. Chest 2007;132:609–16.

54. Majid A, Guerrero J, Gangadharan S, et al. Tracheobronchoplasty for severe tracheobronchomalacia: a prospective outcome analysis. Chest 2008;134:801–7.

55. Jayamanne DS, Epstein H, Goldring RM. Flow-volume curve contour in COPD: correlation with pulmonary mechanics. Chest 1980;77:749–57.

56. Vincken WG, Cosio MG. Flow oscillations on the flow-volume loop: clinical and physiological implications. Eur Respir J 1989;2:543–9.

57. Pornsuriyasak P, Ploysongsang Y. Impulse oscillometry system in diagnosis of central airway obstruction in adults: comparison with spirometry and body plethysmography. Chest 2009;136:123S.

58. Handa H, Miyazawa T, Murgu SD, et al. Novel multimodality imaging and physiologic assessments clarify choke-point physiology and airway wall structure in expiratory central airway collapse. Respir Care 2012;57:634–41.

59. Murgu SD, Colt HG. Bronchoscopic treatment of post tracheostomy tracheal stenosis with chondritis. Expert commentary by Lutz Freitag. In: Colt HG, Murgu SD, editors. Bronchoscopy and central airway disorders. Philadelphia: Elsevier; 2012. p. 105–18.

60. Pedersen OF, Thiessen B, Lyager S. Airway compliance and flow limitation during forced expiration in dogs. J Appl Physiol 1982;52:357–69.

61. Murgu SD, Pecson J, Colt HG. Bronchoscopy on non invasive positive pressure ventilation: indications and technique. Respir Care 2010;55:595–600.

62. BronchAtlas bronchoscopy on CPAP for OSA.wmv. Available at: http://www.youtube.com/watch?v=-MP-WdVcCxY. Accessed July 19, 2012.

63. Lee KS, Sun MR, Ernst A, et al. Comparison of dynamic expiratory CT with bronchoscopy for diagnosing airway malacia: a pilot evaluation. Chest 2007;131:758–64.

64. Baroni RH, Feller-Kopman D, Nishino M, et al. Tracheobronchomalacia: comparison between end-expiratory and dynamic expiratory CT for evaluation of central airway collapse. Radiology 2005;235:635–41.

65. Ferretti GR, Jankowski A, Perrin MA, et al. Multidetector CT evaluation in patients suspected of tracheobronchomalacia: comparison of end-expiratory with dynamic expiratory volumetric acquisitions. Eur J Radiol 2008;68:340–6.

66. Hein E, Rogalla P, Hentschel C, et al. Dynamic and quantitative assessment of tracheomalacia by electron beam tomography: correlation with clinical symptoms and bronchoscopy. J Comput Assist Tomogr 2000;24:247–52.

67. Yamashiro T, San José Estépar R, Matsuoka S, et al. Intrathoracic tracheal volume and collapsibility on inspiratory and end-expiratory CT scans correlations with lung volume and pulmonary function in 85 smokers. Acad Radiol 2011;18:299–305.

68. Lee EY, Strauss KJ, Tracy DA, et al. Comparison of standard-dose and reduced-dose expiratory MDCT techniques for assessment of tracheomalacia in children. Acad Radiol 2010;17:504–10.

69. De Wever W, Vandecaveye V, Lanciotti S, et al. Multidetector CT-generated virtual bronchoscopy: an illustrated review of the potential clinical indications. Eur Respir J 2004;23:776–82.

70. Boiselle PM, O'Donnell CR, Loring SH, et al. Reproducibility of forced expiratory tracheal collapse:

assessment with MDCT in healthy volunteers. Acad Radiol 2010;17:1186–9.

71. Lee KS, Lunn W, Feller-Kopman D, et al. Multislice CT evaluation of airway stents. J Thorac Imaging 2005;20:81–8.

72. Baroni RH, Ashiku S, Boiselle PM. Dynamic CT evaluation of the central airways in patients undergoing tracheoplasty for tracheobronchomalacia. AJR Am J Roentgenol 2005;184:1444–9.

73. Wright CD. Tracheomalacia. Chest Surg Clin N Am 2003;13:349–57.

74. Lee KS, Ashiku SK, Ernst A, et al. Comparison of expiratory CT airway abnormalities before and after tracheoplasty surgery for tracheobronchomalacia. J Thorac Imaging 2008;23:121–6.

75. Zhang J, Hasegawa I, Feller-Kopman D, et al. 2003 AUR Memorial Award. Dynamic expiratory volumetric CT imaging of the central airways: comparison of standard-dose and low-dose techniques. Acad Radiol 2003;10:719–24.

76. Ederle JR, Heussel CP, Hast J, et al. Evaluation of changes in central airway dimensions, lung area and mean lung density at paired inspiratory/expiratory high-resolution computed tomography. Eur Radiol 2003;13:2454–61.

77. Ochs RA, Petkovska I, Kim HJ, et al. Prevalence of tracheal collapse in an emphysema cohort as measured with end-expiration CT. Acad Radiol 2009;16:46–53.

78. Lee CJ, Lee JH, Song JW, et al. Correlation of tracheal cross-sectional area with parameters of pulmonary function test in COPD. Tuberc Respir Dis (Seoul) 1999;46:628–35.

79. McDermott S, Barry SC, Judge EE, et al. Tracheomalacia in adults with cystic fibrosis: determination of prevalence and severity with dynamic cine CT. Radiology 2009;252:577–86.

80. Lomasney L, Bergin CJ, Lomasney J, et al. CT appearance of lunate trachea. J Comput Assist Tomogr 1989;13:520–2.

81. Boiselle PM, Feller-Kopman D, Ashiku S, et al. Tracheobronchomalacia: evolving role of dynamic multislice helical CT. Radiol Clin North Am 2003; 41:627–36.

82. Boiselle PM, Ernst A. Tracheal morphology in patients with tracheomalacia: prevalence of inspiratory lunate and expiratory "frown" shapes. J Thorac Imaging 2006;21:190–6.

83. Gupta PP, Yadav R, Verma M, et al. High-resolution computed tomography features in patients with chronic obstructive pulmonary disease. Singapore Med J 2009;50:193–200.

84. Fukai I, Yamakawa Y, Kiriyama M, et al. Saber-sheath malacic trachea remodeled and fixed into a normal shape by long-term placement and then removal of gianturco wire stent. Ann Thorac Surg 2003;76:597–8.

85. Heussel CP, Ley S, Biedermann A, et al. Respiratory lumenal change of the pharynx and trachea in normal subjects and COPD patients: assessment by cine-MRI. Eur Radiol 2004;14:2188–97.

86. Suto Y, Tanabe Y. Evaluation of tracheal collapsibility in patients with tracheomalacia using dynamic MR imaging during coughing. AJR Am J Roentgenol 1998;171:393–4.

87. Ley S, Loukanov T, Ley-Zaporozhan J, et al. Long-term outcome after external tracheal stabilization due to congenital tracheal instability. Ann Thorac Surg 2010;89:918–25.

88. Weber TR, Keller MS, Fiore A. Aortic suspension (aortopexy) for severe tracheomalacia in infants and children. Am J Surg 2002;184:573–7 [discussion: 577].

89. Simoneaux SF, Bank ER, Webber JB, et al. MR imaging of the pediatric airway. Radiographics 1995; 15:287–98 [discussion: 298–9].

90. Ley-Zaporozhan J, Ley S, Kauczor HU. Morphological and functional imaging in COPD with CT and MRI: present and future. Eur Radiol 2008;18:510–21.

91. Kuo GP, Torok CM, Aygun N, et al. Diagnostic imaging of the upper airway. Proc Am Thorac Soc 2011;8:40–5.

92. Heussel CP, Hafner B, Lill J, et al. Paired inspiratory/expiratory spiral-CT and continuous respiration cine-CT in the diagnosis of tracheal instability. Eur Radiol 2001;11:982–9.

93. Cansiz H, Yener M, Tahamiler R, et al. Preoperative detection and management of tracheomalacia in advanced laryngotracheal stenosis. B-ENT 2008; 4:163–7.

94. Türkmen A, Altan A, Turgut N, et al. Comparison of percutaneous dilatational tracheostomy with surgical tracheostomy. Middle East J Anesthesiol 2008; 19:1055–67.

95. Murgu SD, Colt HG. Stent insertion for diffuse circumferential tracheobronchomalacia caused by relapsing polychondritis. In: Colt HG, Murgu SD, editors. Bronchoscopy and central airway disorders; A patient-centered approach. Expert commentary by Teruomi Miyazawa and Noriaki Kurimoto. Philadeplhia: Elsevier; 2012. p. 139–52.

96. Faust RA, Rimell FL, Remley KB. Cine magnetic resonance imaging for evaluation of focal tracheomalacia: innominate artery compression syndrome. Int J Pediatr Otorhinolaryngol 2002;65:27–33.

97. Kurimoto N, Murayama M, Yoshioka S, et al. Assessment of usefulness of endobronchial ultrasonography in determination of depth of tracheobronchial tumor invasion. Chest 1999; 115:1500–6.

98. Miyazu Y, Miyazawa T, Kurimoto N, et al. Endobronchial ultrasonography in the diagnosis and treatment of relapsing polychondritis with tracheobronchial malacia. Chest 2003;124:2393–5.

99. Murgu S, Kurimoto N, Colt H. Endobronchial ultrasound morphology of expiratory central airway collapse. Respirology 2008;13:315–9.

100. Turato G, Zuin R, Saetta M. Pathogenesis and pathology of COPD. Respiration 2001;68: 117–28.

101. Becker HD, Slawik M, Miyazawa T, et al. Vibration response imaging as a new tool for interventional-bronchoscopy outcome assessment: a prospective pilot study. Respiration 2009;77:179–94.

102. Carden KA, Boiselle PM, Waltz DA, et al. Tracheomalacia and tracheobronchomalacia in children and adults: an in-depth review. Chest 2005;127: 984–1005.

103. Bouhuys A, van de Woestijne KP. Mechanical consequences of airway smooth muscle relaxation. J Appl Physiol 1971;30:670–6.

104. Prendiville A, Green S, Silverman M. Paradoxical response to nebulized salbutamol in wheezy infants, assessed by partial expiratory flow-volume curves. Thorax 1987;42:86–91.

105. Panitch HB, Keklikian EN, Motley RA, et al. Effect of altering smooth muscle tone on maximal expiratory flows in patients with tracheomalacia. Pediatr Pulmonol 1990;9:170–6.

106. McAdam LP, O'Hanlan MA, Bluestone R, et al. Relapsing polychondritis: prospective study of 23 patients and a review of the literature. Medicine 1976; 55:193–215.

107. Wiseman NE, Duncan PG, Cameron CB. Management of tracheobronchomalacia with continuous positive airway pressure. J Pediatr Surg 1985;20: 489–93.

108. Davis S, Jones M, Kisling J, et al. Effect of continuous positive airway pressure on forced expiratory flows in infants with tracheomalacia. Am J Respir Crit Care Med 1998;158:148–52.

109. Ferguson GT, Benoist J. Nasal continuous positive airway pressure in the treatment of tracheobronchomalacia. Am Rev Respir Dis 1993;147: 457–61.

110. Adliff M, Ngato D, Keshavjee S, et al. Treatment of diffuse tracheomalacia secondary to relapsing polychondritis with continuous positive airway pressure. Chest 1997;112:1701–4.

111. Chi SY, Wu SC, Hsieh KC, et al. Noninvasive positive pressure ventilation in the management of post-thyroidectomy tracheomalacia. World J Surg 2011;35:1977–83.

112. Sirithangkul S, Ranganathan S, Robinson PJ, et al. Positive expiratory pressure to enhance cough effectiveness in tracheomalacia. J Med Assoc Thai 2010;93(Suppl 6):S112–8.

113. Palange P, Valli G, Onorati P, et al. Effect of heliox on lung dynamic hyperinflation, dyspnea, and exercise endurance capacity in COPD patients. J Appl Physiol 2004;97:1637–42.

114. Murgu SD, Colt HG. Complications of silicone stent insertion in patients with expiratory central airway collapse. Ann Thorac Surg 2007;84: 1870–7.

115. Odell DD, Shah A, Gangadharan SP, et al. Airway stenting and tracheobronchoplasty improve respiratory symptoms in Mounier-Kuhn syndrome. Chest 2011;140:867–73.

116. Sarodia BD, Dasgupta A, Mehta AC. Management of airway manifestations of relapsing polychondritis: case reports and review of literature. Chest 1999;116:1669–75.

117. Dunne JA, Sabanathan S. Use of metallic stents in relapsing polychondritis. Chest 1994;105: 864–7.

118. Ernst A, Rafeq S, Boiselle P, et al. Relapsing polychondritis and airway involvement. Chest 2009; 135:1024–30.

119. Bolot G, Poupart M, Pignat JC, et al. Self-expanding metal stents for the management of bronchial stenosis and bronchomalacia after lung transplantation. Laryngoscope 1998;108: 1230–3.

120. US Food and Drug Administration. FDA Public Health notification: complications from metallic tracheal stents in patients with benign airway disorders. Available at: http://www.fda.gov/Medical Devices/Safety/AlertsandNotices/PublicHealth Notifications/ucm062115.htm. Accessed July 20, 2012.

121. Murgu SD, Colt HG. Treatment of adult tracheobronchomalacia and excessive dynamic airway collapse: an update. Treat Respir Med 2006;5: 103–15.

122. Lehman JD, Gordon RL, Kerlan RK Jr, et al. Expandable metallic stents in benign tracheobronchial obstruction. J Thorac Imaging 1998;13: 105–15.

123. Dutau H, Maldonado F, Breen DP, et al. Endoscopic successful management of tracheobronchomalacia with laser: apropos of a Mounier-Kuhn syndrome. Eur J Cardiothorac Surg 2011;39:e186–8.

124. Dumon MC, Cavaliere S, Vergnon JM. Bronchial laser: techniques, indications, and results. Rev Mal Respir 1999;16:601–8.

125. Ellis PD. Laser palatoplasty for snoring due to palatal flutter: a further report. Clin Otolaryngol Allied Sci 1994;19:350–1.

126. Grillo HC. Surgical treatment of postintubation tracheal injuries. J Thorac Cardiovasc Surg 1979; 78:860–75.

127. Wright CD, Grillo HC, Hammoud ZT, et al. Tracheoplasty for expiratory collapse of central airways. Ann Thorac Surg 2005;80:259–67.

128. Gangadharan SP, Bakhos CT, Majid A, et al. Technical aspects and outcomes of

tracheobronchoplasty for severe tracheobroncho-malacia. Ann Thorac Surg 2011;91:1574–80 [discussion: 1580–1].

129. Tse DG, Han SM, Charuworn B, et al. Video-assisted thoracoscopic surgical tracheobronchoplasty for tracheobronchomalacia. J Thorac Cardiovasc Surg 2011;142:714–6.

130. Gilkeson RC, Ciancibello LM, Hejal RB, et al. Tracheobronchomalacia: dynamic airway evaluation with multidetector CT. Am J Roentgenol 2001;176:205–10.

131. Mair EA, Parsons DS. Pediatric tracheobronchomalacia and major airway collapse. Ann Otol Rhinol Laryngol 1992;101:300–9.

Tracheobronchial Stenosis
Causes and Advances in Management

Jonathan Puchalski, MD, MEd[a],*, Ali I. Musani, MD[b]

KEYWORDS

- Tracheobronchial stenosis • Systemic therapy • Bronchoscopy • Bioabsorbable stenting

KEY POINTS

- Tracheobronchial stenosis results from malignant and benign causes.
- Treatment includes systemic therapy in addition to endoscopic or surgical approaches.
- Balloons, heat therapy, and stenting are useful for stenosis involving the proximal airways. These therapies may provide immediate improvement in dyspnea.
- Surgical resection of limited benign and malignant stenosis has a high success rate and may provide long-lasting results.
- New surgical therapies, as well as developments in bioabsorbable stenting, hold promise for the future treatment of tracheobronchial symptomatic stenosis.

INTRODUCTION

Airway stenosis may involve the glottis, subglottis (below the vocal cords but above the inferior cricoid), or tracheobronchial tree. It may be congenital or acquired, caused by benign or malignant diseases, focal or diffuse, and present with various symptoms. Patients with significant stenosis may present with dyspnea, wheezing, or stridor. Stridor occurs when the airway diameter in an adult diminishes to approximately 6 mm. Given that congenital and pediatric stenosis may often have different causes and require different treatments, this article focuses primarily on adult stenosis of the tracheobronchial tree.

EVALUATION

Beyond the physical examination, evaluation often includes a combination of physiologic, radiographic, and endoscopic assessments. Pulmonary function tests may show a delay in reaching peak expiratory flow, a truncation of peak expiratory and peak inspiratory flow, and/or an abrupt decrease in expiratory flow at the end of expiration. There may be flattening of the inspiratory and expiratory phases in the presence of fixed upper airway obstruction. A chest radiograph may detect tracheal disease although multiplanar computed tomography (CT) is useful for characterization of disease extent, exact configuration, and for planning treatment. This airway CT is different from neck or chest CT scans with thinner cuts that allow for three-dimensional reconstruction. Often called virtual bronchoscopy, the three-dimensional external and internal airway images have a high sensitivity and specificity compared with rigid bronchoscopy.[1] For dynamic collapse, such as in tracheobronchomalacia, inspiratory and expiratory CT imaging may demonstrate the characteristic crescent changes seen with collapse of the posterior membrane.

Subsequent evaluation is typically done via endoscopy. Defining the injury and assessing the

Disclaimer and Financial Disclosures: None.
[a] Thoracic Interventional Program, Division of Pulmonary, Critical Care and Sleep Medicine, Yale University School of Medicine, 15 York Street, Room 100, Laboratory of Clinical Investigation (LCI), New Haven, CT 06510, USA; [b] Interventional Pulmonology, Division of Pulmonary, Critical Care and Sleep Medicine, National Jewish Health, University of Colorado, Denver, 1400 Jackson Street, Denver, CO 80206, USA
* Corresponding author.
E-mail address: jonathan.puchalski@yale.edu

Clin Chest Med 34 (2013) 557–567
http://dx.doi.org/10.1016/j.ccm.2013.05.002

presence of active inflammation and edema are essential. Bronchoscopic biopsies may secure the pathologic diagnosis. Recent studies demonstrate that measuring lateral airway wall pressure on each side of the stenosis and plotting pressure-pressure curves can quantitatively assess the site of maximal obstruction and degree of stenosis. The investigators suggest these measurements estimate the need for additional procedures more than bronchoscopy alone and demonstrated that the cross-sectional area, dyspnea scale, pulmonary function tests, pressure difference, and angle of the pressure-pressure curve improved after interventional procedures.[2] An understanding of potential causes is also required to guide therapy.

CAUSES AND PATHOGENESIS

Although dynamic obstruction, such as occurs with vocal cord dysfunction or tracheobronchomalacia, causes similar symptoms, this article focuses on stenosis that is fixed. Tracheobronchial stenosis may be predominantly intraluminal, such as postintubation tracheal stenosis, or from extrinsic compression, caused by a tumor. Glottic, subglottic, and high tracheal stenosis may require significantly different stabilization and treatment than carinal or bronchial stenosis. Furthermore, therapeutic approaches may be different depending on whether the disease is benign or malignant, and the extent of disease. The more common conditions causing tracheobronchial stenosis are listed in **Box 1** and shown in **Figs. 1** and **2**.

FOCAL BRONCHIAL DISEASES

Both malignant and benign diseases may cause focal narrowing of the tracheobronchial tree. Within the trachea, malignancy predominates. Primary tracheal malignancies include squamous cell carcinoma and adenoid cystic carcinoma, among others. Non–small cell lung cancer and small cell lung cancer are obvious causes of obstruction due either to extrinsic airway compression, intrinsic airway tumor, or a combination of both. When confined to the trachea or mainstem bronchi, surgical resection may be curative. Metastatic disease from a variety of conditions may cause obstruction from endobronchial deposits or massive adenopathy. Breast, colorectal, renal cell, and melanoma are the most common extrathoracic malignancies to metastasize to the lungs. When the disease is advanced, various endoscopic modalities may complement chemotherapy or radiation therapy. Typically, bronchoscopic management includes a combination of opening the airway (balloons), debulking the tumor (heat or cold therapy), and

---

Box 1
Common causes of tracheobronchial stenosis

Cause of Tracheal or Bronchial Stenosis

Focal inflammation
  Tracheostomy
  Intubation
  Trauma
  Burns
  After transplant

Systemic inflammation
  Wegener granulomatosis
  Relapsing polychondritis
  Sarcoidosis
  Amyloidosis
  Inflammatory bowel disease
  Others

Infectious
  Tuberculosis
  Aspergillus
  Others

Dynamic collapse
  Focal malacia
  Diffuse tracheobronchomalacia

Miscellaneous
  Saber sheath trachea
  Tracheobronchopathia osteochondroplastica
  Broncholithiasis
  Idiopathic

Malignancy
  Adenoid cystic carcinoma
  Squamous cell carcinoma
  Lung cancer: non–small and small cell
  Metastatic disease

---

stabilizing the airway for the longer term (stenting). These treatment modalities are described later.

The most common causes of benign iatrogenic stenosis include intubation, tracheostomy, and lung transplant. Mucosal ischemia followed by granulation tissue and fibrosis often creates 1.5 to 2.5 cm of stenosis after intubation or tracheostomy with cuffed tubes.[3] With low-pressure cuffs and maintaining a pressure less than 30 mm Hg, the incidence after intubation has decreased to 1%, whereas after tracheostomy, stenosis

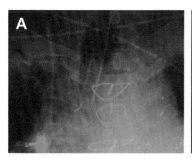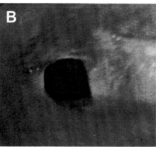

Fig. 1. Iatrogenic causes of benign tracheal stenosis. (A) Overinflation of the endotracheal tube may lead to mucosal ischemia and subsequent stenosis. Cuffed tracheostomy tubes pose a similar risk. Tracheal stenosis from these focal insults may look like that shown in (B).

approaches 10% to 15% and bronchial anastomotic stenosis after transplant occurs in up to 15%.[3]

A variable degree of stenosis has been reported in up to 90% of patients with tuberculosis.[3] Airway involvement from tuberculosis likely evolves in stages, from submucosal tubercules to ulceration and necrosis. Subsequent healing can lead to fibrosis, often with long segments of circumferential stenosis. Stenosis of the airways can also occur from adjacent lymphadenopathy. Prebronchoscopic sputum results are often negative despite active disease, and CT findings may be nonspecific.[4]

Aside from tuberculosis, other infectious organisms can cause tracheobronchial stenosis. *Klebsiella rhinoscleromatis* is an encapsulated gram-negative bacterium endemic in tropical and subtropical areas; it causes rhinoscleroma, a slowly progressive granulomatous disease. Nodules or

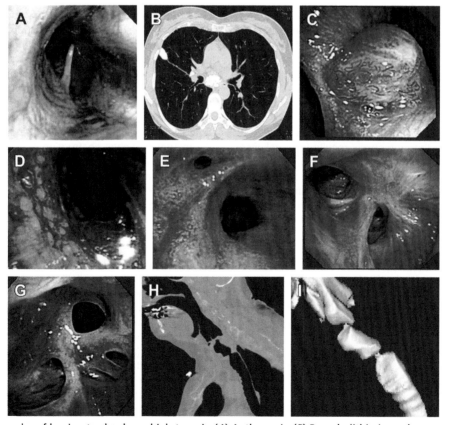

Fig. 2. Examples of benign tracheobronchial stenosis. (A) Anthracosis. (B) Broncholithiasis, as shown on CT scanning. (C) Endoscopic image of the adjacent mucosal reaction. (D) Tuberculosis with submucosal granulomas. (E) Bronchial stenosis caused by Wegener granulomatosis. (F) Posttransplant bronchial stenosis. (G) Complex webbed stenosis of unknown cause. (H) Sagittal and (I) three-dimensional reconstruction of focal benign tracheal stenosis.

masses that form in the granulomatous phase may cause partial obstruction (pseudoepitheliomatous hyperplasia) and the final sclerotic phase may result in fibrosis. Biopsy or cultures assist in establishing the diagnosis.[4] Fungi, particularly *Aspergillus*, may cause tracheobronchitis in immunocompromised hosts, such as those with AIDS, underlying malignancy, or after transplant. Epithelial ulceration and submucosal inflammation occurs and may lead to strictures, whereas deeper bronchial wall necrosis may lead to bronchial or bronchovascular rupture and death.[3]

Bronchial anthracofibrosis demonstrates characteristic bronchoscopic findings in the absence of known pneumoconiosis or smoking.[3] It is hypothesized that the black pigments are derived from anthracotic material in the adjacent lymph nodes, with possible perforation of the nodes or penetration of carbon particles into the mucosa. Healing with a fibrotic response may lead to bronchial narrowing or obstruction. A CT scan may demonstrate mediastinal and hilar lymphadenopathy and endoscopy may reveal smooth bronchial narrowing. Atelectasis may accompany these findings. Biopsy should be performed to exclude malignancy.[4]

Tracheobronchopathia osteochondroplastica spares the posterior membrane and typically appears as submucosal nodules extending into the tracheobronchial lumen. Histologically, these are submucosal osteocartilaginous growths that leave the mucosal surface intact.[5] Treatment options for severe airway compromise include surgical or laser resection, radiation, or stent placement.

Broncholithiasis typically results from calcification of a lymph node caused by previous infection with organisms such as *Tuberculosis* or *Histoplasmosis*. The lymph node may erode into the airway in which case the patient may cough up calcified material. Alternatively, the lymph node may cause compression of the airways. Interventional or surgical approaches may be necessary depending on the compromise of the airways.

Idiopathic tracheal stenosis occurs almost exclusively in middle-aged women. A weblike or complex stenosis develops mostly in the area of the cricoid. Although endoscopic therapy is efficacious, late recurrences are frequent and the disease requires ongoing follow-up.[4]

SYSTEMIC DISEASES

Relapsing polychondritis is associated with recurrent inflammation of cartilaginous structures of the nose, external ear, peripheral joints, and airways. Up to 50% of patients may develop airway involvement, often starting at the larynx or subglottic space and progressing to involve more of the tracheobronchial tree. An inflammatory infiltrate develops in the cartilage and perichondrial tissue. The ensuing airway inflammation may lead to airway strictures, whereas collapse of the cartilaginous support may also lead to tracheobronchomalacia. The diagnosis may be made by meeting specific clinical criteria, whereas a chest CT may demonstrate attenuation of the airway walls (classic smooth thickening of anterior and lateral walls with characteristic sparing of the posterior membrane). Cartilaginous destruction may lead to the need for tracheobronchial stenting.[4]

Wegener granulomatosis is characterized by necrotizing granulomatous vasculitis, which may lead to subglottic, tracheal, or bronchial stenosis. It has been reported that 10% to 20% of patients with Wegener granulomatosis develop laryngotracheostenosis.[6] Granulomatous inflammation and vasculitis are seen in the mucosa and submucosa early in the disease, whereas fibrosis ensues later. Bronchoscopy may demonstrate ulcerative tracheobronchitis, inflammatory stenosis, or noninflammatory stenosis.[5] Steroids and immunosuppressant therapy are the mainstay but bronchoscopic intervention may be required. Surgery may also be required, including laryngotracheal reconstruction, albeit with increased risk of postprocedural repeated dilation.[6]

Bronchial involvement is more common than tracheal involvement in sarcoidosis. Bronchial wall thickening caused by granulomas and peribronchial interstitial fibrous tissue may result in smooth or irregular luminal narrowing. Lobar or segmental bronchial obstruction may occur from airway wall fibrosis, granulomatous inflammation, or lymph node compression. As with the inflammatory diseases described earlier, when systemic therapy fails to control disease, bronchoscopic interventions may be required.

Tracheobronchial amyloidosis may be present as an isolated manifestation with tracheal deposition of amyloid, or in conjunction with systemic amyloidosis. Pathologically, the amyloid is deposited in proximity to the tracheal gland acini and the blood vessel walls. The glands eventually atrophy and the amyloid produces irregular plaques and nodules in the mucosa. On occasion, masses may appear (amyloidomas) that may be radiographically difficult to distinguish from neoplasms. Biopsies are diagnostic, and Congo Red staining may highlight the amyloid. Radiation therapy may sometimes be required in addition to the interventional techniques described later.[3,5]

Rare causes of airway stenosis include inflammatory bowel disease; either ulcerative colitis or Crohn disease may produce airway inflammation.

Airway disease may present as ulcerative tracheitis and tracheobronchitis, bronchiectasis, and small airway disease such as obliterative bronchiolitis.[4] As with the aforementioned conditions, airway interventions may be required if systemic therapy is insufficient.

VENTILATORY STRATEGIES BEFORE INTERVENTIONS FOR AIRWAY STENOSIS

Flexible and rigid bronchoscopy are performed to evaluate and treat airway stenosis. Whereas the flexible scope can be inserted in an unventilated patient, via a laryngeal mask airway or through the endotracheal tube, it contributes to obstruction because of its size. The rigid bronchoscope requires general anesthesia but allows ventilation through its side port. Intravenous short-acting agents such as remifentanil and propofol may be combined with narcotics, neuromuscular blockers, or inhaled agents during induction and throughout the procedure while maintaining strict airway control. With mid tracheal lesions, a decrease in respiratory rate or exhalational times may be necessary to minimize inspiratory pressures.

Many anesthesiologists use jet ventilation at low (20 breaths/min) or high (150 breaths/min) frequency. This may be performed with a catheter through the rigid bronchoscope, a laryngoscope, and a small (eg, 5.0 mm) endotracheal tube, or even via a transcricothyroid membrane catheter.[7] A series of 44 patients with severe upper airway obstruction demonstrated successful ventilation after transtracheal catheters placed under local anesthesia via the cricothyroid membrane or below the first or second trachea rings. Although minor complications occurred infrequently, they did not experience the major pressure-related problems reported elsewhere (pneumothorax, massive surgical emphysema, pneumomediastinum, and cardiovascular instability). The anesthesiologists adjusted the driving pressure or frequency when higher pressures were observed.[8] Other techniques include high-frequency positive pressure ventilation, high-frequency oscillatory ventilation, or cardiopulmonary bypass if adequate oxygenation cannot be maintained.

BRONCHOSCOPIC INTERVENTIONS FOR AIRWAY STENOSIS

As mentioned earlier, the therapeutic options for airway stenosis depend on the cause of the obstruction. Patients with systemic diseases and clinically significant airway stenosis, benign yet inoperable disease, or advanced malignancy may require bronchoscopic interventions. Various bronchoscopic techniques are possible to relieve the obstruction. Although these procedures are expected to have an immediate impact when the appropriate patient is selected, long-term follow-up is essential to monitor the response to treatment and determine whether repeat procedures are necessary. This section focuses on airway balloons, heat modalities, and bronchial stenting to provide immediate relief for significant stenosis.

Airway dilation may be accomplished through rigid and flexible bronchoscopy. The rigid bronchoscope may core through areas of stenosis with the shear mechanics of the rigid scope providing dilation. A metal bougie dilator provides a similar effect. When this is not possible, balloon expansion may be useful. The benefits of balloons include the avoidance of surgery and other sophisticated techniques or equipment. Compliant balloons, such as the angioplasty balloon catheter (Fogarty), may be best for a fleshy or necrotic intraluminal tumor that easily compresses. More rigid balloons, such as the controlled radial expansion (CRE) balloon (Boston Scientific) may be used to dilate tight areas of stenosis. These balloons expand from 6 mm to 20 mm (using different balloon catheters) while being manually inflated. Care must be taken to avoid tearing the airways or rupturing them by using too large a balloon or careless dilation. In a recent study, patients demonstrated a subjective improvement in symptoms as well as 1-month sustained improvement in pulmonary function tests. However, for those who required more than 1 procedure, most required stenting. Combining their results with a literature review encompassing 340 patients and 554 balloon dilation procedures, the processes most amenable to balloon dilation were those with fixed stenosis; those with active inflammation, calcification, carcinoma, or in whom the surrounding cartilage was destroyed (malacia) were less responsive.[9]

Ablative techniques are frequently used to reestablish airway patency. These include heat and cold therapies. Circumferential weblike stenosis may benefit from incisions with an electrocautery knife (**Fig. 3**). Imagining the face of a clock, 3 small incisions (at 9 o'clock, 12 o'clock, and 3 o'clock) can be made with the knife and subsequent balloon dilation performed. The knife creates 1- to 2-mm incisions generating weak points such that the balloon will dilate the airway with targeted rather than sporadic and uncontrolled mucosal tearing. Recent analysis of the reusable electrode knife in the cut mode demonstrated improved symptoms, improved pulmonary function tests, and less fibrin production than laser therapy in a similar group of patients. Less than half of the

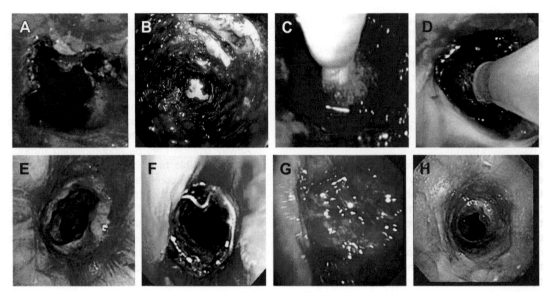

Fig. 3. Treatment options for tracheal stenosis. (*A*) Electrosurgical knife applied at the 3 o'clock position. (*B*) Results of cautery to reopen suprastomal stenosis. (*C*) Angioplasty balloon dilation. (*D*) The more rigid CRE balloon dilation. (*E*) Inflammatory tracheal stenosis. (*F*) This unique stenosis was treated with a hybrid stent before surgical resection. (*G*) Complete stenosis of the subglottic space. (*H*) Silicone stent after reestablishing patency.

patients in this small analysis required repeat intervention for weblike stenosis.[10]

Additional heat modalities used for treatment of tracheobronchial stenosis include electrocautery, argon plasma coagulation (APC) and laser therapy. These techniques are discussed elsewhere in this issue on interventional pulmonology and thus discussion here is kept brief. With cautery, an electric current is used to generate heat. Several devices may be used to apply this current, including the knife, a probe, and snare/cutting loop. Unlike the knife described earlier, the probe is blunt. The user sets the wattage (eg, 20–40 W) and depth of penetration; these combined with the time of topical impact determine the depth of mucosal destruction. In contrast, APC uses an argon gas charged with an electric current to achieve thermal tissue destruction. The argon gas flows flexibly around angles such that APC is suitable for bronchial segments that take off at acute angles to major airways. APC is a noncontact mode of thermal coagulation and as such, helps clear blood and mucus while performing superficial coagulation. Cerebral gas embolism has been reported as a unique complication of this procedure. Both electrocautery and APC offer advantages of ease and lower cost compared with laser therapy.[11]

The most common type of lasers used in the airways are the neodymium–yttrium-aluminum-garnet (Nd-YAG) and carbon dioxide (CO_2) lasers. The Nd-YAG provides tissue vaporization and coagulation. It has deeper thermal energy than the CO_2 laser and may penetrate up to 10 mm.[12] The CO_2 laser has more precise cutting abilities. The development of the flexible fiber CO_2 delivery system allows for the flexible bronchoscope to be used to ablate and cut with this laser. This contrasts with the typical microscope-mounted CO_2 laser, which requires general anesthesia. The laser is typically in pulse mode at 5 to 10 W delivered to 2 to 3 wedges separated by tissue to avoid circumferential mucosal denuding. Postoperative dexamethasone may be given to minimize upper airway edema when this ablation is performed high in the airway.[13] All heat therapies require that a patient receive less than 40% inspired oxygen to avoid airway fires during the procedure.

Mitomycin C may be an adjunct to radial incisions made with laser or cautery. Pledgets of cotton soaked in mitomycin C are topically applied to the areas of stenosis. This is believed to impede the inflammatory response.[14,15] A prospective, randomized, double-blind placebo-controlled trial of 26 patients with laryngotracheal stenosis of various causes suggested that 2 applications 3 to 4 weeks apart delayed but did not prevent the recurrence of stenosis in benign disease.[15] A retrospective analysis of 67 procedures in 36 patients also demonstrated a longer symptom-free interval than when endoscopy was used without mitomycin C.[16] To our knowledge, there is no Cochrane review or meta-analysis of the effects of mitomycin C and thus its use requires further investigation before claiming efficacy.

In contrast to heat and medical therapies, contact and spray cryotherapy have been described. Contact cryotherapy uses a probe whereby extreme cold is alternated with internal body temperature to create a freeze-thaw cycle. Its efficacy is debatable as results have been variable. Spray cryotherapy uses a 7-French catheter and nitrogen as a base cryogen. Approximately 25 W (J/s) of energy is transferred, similar to laser therapy, but there is no risk of airway fire with the latter. Early results with spray cryotherapy are encouraging but further studies are needed to document its efficacy and safety.[17]

Airway stenting is an important strategy for managing various types of tracheobronchial obstruction. Stents are also discussed in other articles in this issue. Airway stenting may be used either temporarily or chronically. Several different types of stents exist (see **Fig. 3**), although metal stents have a US Food and Drug Administration black box warning for benign disease in part because of their predisposition to form granulation tissue. For benign conditions, silicone stents are preferred. These stents may be tubular, a Y-configuration that covers portions of the trachea and mainstem bronchi, an hourglass configuration with wider ends and a narrower center, or may be customized. On the other hand, metal stents are tubular. The advantage of metal stents is that, unlike silicone stents, they can be placed with the flexible bronchoscope. The metal stents may be completely covered, partially covered, or uncovered. Metal stents are more expensive than silicone stents. Both are susceptible to migration, granulation tissue formation, mucus plugging, and other complications.

Practice management varies, but any patient who has a stent placed requires appropriate follow-up. The duration a stent should remain in place is not known and likely depends on the clinical scenario. Patients with malignant stenosis often die with the stent in place; benign stenosis may require long-term placement. Factors predicting the ability to remove stents in tuberculosis included the lack of complete lobar atelectasis and performing stent placement within 1 month of the development of any atelectasis. Stents were left in place for 12.5 months in those patients whose stenosis was successfully treated by the temporary silicone stent.[18] A patient with relapsing polychondritis and a silicone stent for 16 years has been described recently.[19] Thus, the exact duration of stent placement varies according to each patient.

RESULTS OF AIRWAY INTERVENTIONS

For idiopathic tracheal stenosis, initial success is high, but recurrence is typical. In a retrospective study of 23 patients with idiopathic stenosis treated at 9 institutions, the stenosis recurred in 30% of patients at 6 months, 59% at 2 years, and 87% at 5 years. A combination of therapies was frequently used.[20] Improvements that result from airway interventions in malignant disease likely deserve distinction from interventions for benign disease because of the systemic effects of cancer. A few studies have investigated quality of life and dyspnea after airway interventions for cancer. Amjadi and colleagues[21] used the validated European Organization for Research and Treatment of Cancer Quality of Life Questionnaire (EORTC QLQ-C30) and included 20 patients over 6 months. Using a combination of the therapies described earlier, more than 80% of airway caliber was restored in 80% of patients and 85% of patients demonstrated an improvement of dyspnea scores at 24 hours that extended to 30 days. Quality-of-life response was variable, likely because of the impact of symptoms such as pain from metastases and other factors that are not influenced by airway therapy. A separate retrospective cohort study of 37 patients with high-grade symptomatic central airway obstruction evaluated exercise capacity, lung function, and quality of life. More than 90% of patients had restoration of airway patency (>50% of airway restored). Statistically significant improvements in the 6-minute walk test were noted up to 180 days. Dyspnea scores, resting Borg, forced expiratory volume in 1 second, and forced vital capacity were improved at day 30. An improvement in quality of life was seen in 43% of patients. The median survival was 166 days and the 6-month survival rate was 46%.[22]

FUTURE ENDOBRONCHIAL THERAPY

Biodegradable airway stents are under investigation and have been placed in humans. Polydioxanone is a semicrystalline biodegradable polymer that has some shape memory and degrades over time by random hydrolysis. The degradation time has not been exactly defined. Four children received 11 polydioxanone tracheal stents and 3 of the 4 are alive and in good clinical condition 12 months after the first stents were placed. It was difficult to predict the amount of radial force needed to maintain an airway without causing granulation tissue or creating risks for erosion, and to predict the rate of degradation.[23] Twenty biodegradable stents have been placed in 6 patients after lung transplant who developed bronchial stenosis at the anastomosis. These stents were also made of polydioxanone; 5 of the 6 patients were alive and intervention free up to 44 months after the first stent was placed.[24] Various ongoing studies in animal models of this and other materials (polycaprolactone[25]) may lead to clinically applicable biodegradable airway stents in the future.

SURGICAL MANAGEMENT

Surgery is possible for localized malignancy as well as benign stenosis that affects less than half of the trachea. The aforementioned interventional procedures may play an important preoperative role to establish airway patency and enhance safety and ease of perioperative ventilation. Other preoperative interventions include aggressive treatment of gastroesophageal reflux, evaluating for the presence of aspiration, and preoperative treatment of patients colonized with methicillin-resistant Staphylococcus aureus.

The location of stenosis may dictate the type of surgical procedure performed. The main types of therapeutic procedures for subglottic stenosis include laryngotracheal resection and anastomosis, laryngoplasty without segmental resection and with or without bone or cartilage grafting, or endoscopic procedures. The Cotton-Meyer grading scale describes the degree of stenosis and resection is accomplished using a single-stage laryngotracheal reconstruction (LTR) or double-stage LTR procedure. Cricotracheal resection may be performed when the larynx is spared.[26] Pearson described the technique of anterolateral cricoid cartilage resection and primary thyrotracheal anastomosis with preservation of the recurrent laryngeal nerve in 1975. Grillow subsequently described the use of a flap of posterior membranous trachea in cases of circumferential subglottic stenosis.[27] A recent meta-analysis demonstrated that laryngotracheal resection was more effective than the other 2 techniques, especially in the absence of glottic involvement. The random-effect pooled success rate of LTR was greater than 95%, that of laryngoplasty was 76%, and that of endoscopy highly variable (40%–82%). The investigators concluded that laryngoplasty is suitable for resection of long segments or subglottic stenosis with glottis involvement. Patients with less than 1 cm of stenosis and without framework destruction may be reasonable candidates for endoscopic management as a first modality, with surgery reserved for failure.[28]

Significant advances in tracheal surgery occurred in the 1950s and refinements in the techniques led to resection of longer segments. The main principles of resection include meticulous dissection to preserve the blood supply of the trachea and recurrent laryngeal nerves, as well as avoidance of excessive anastomotic tension. As with laryngotracheal involvement, the types of tracheal surgery depend on the location of the stenosis. Cotton and Fearon introduced the costal cartilage augmentation procedure in 1976 that has become known as LTR and other open techniques have been adopted, including the anterior cricoid split, tracheal resection with end-to-end reanastomosis, and slide tracheoplasty.[1]

In slide tracheoplasty, a long stenotic segment is divided transversely at its midpoint and the upper and lower stenotic segments divided longitudinally, anteriorly, and posteriorly. The splayed upper and lower segments are then slid together to produce a trachea with quadrupled cross-sectional area.[29]

Tracheal resection with reanastamosis is seen as a procedure of choice given its high success rate (71%–95%) and minimal morbidity.[30] It can be accomplished using a neck collar incision for high stenosis or median sternotomy for mid to lower tracheal stenosis. After dissection from the surrounding tissue, reanastomosis may be end-to-end tracheal, cricotracheal, or thyrotracheal, depending on the location of the stenosis. Securing sutures between the skin of the chin and anterior chest may maintain neck flexion to avoid excess tension at the anastomosis during the early preoperative period.[31] Early extubation, avoidance of systemic corticosteroids, and use of absorbable submucosal sutures may limit complications.[30] Pericardial patches, rib grafting, and other techniques have also been described to facilitate resection. Over 40 years and 503 patients with postintubation stenosis, results were good in 87.5% of patients. All benign and 70% of malignant tumors were resectable. Recent perioperative mortality was 3% and anastomotic complications occurred in 15%. Multivariate analysis demonstrated that length of resection, diabetes, redo resections, laryngeal involvement, pediatric age, and presence of tracheostomy were important prognostic factors for complications.[32]

Further distally into the airways, carinal resections are feasible although complicated. Typically, either a median sternotomy or right thoracotomy is performed and the neocarina is fashioned from the 2 divided main bronchi. The longer bronchus is usually anastomosed end to end with the trachea and the shorter bronchus attached to the sidewall of the longer bronchus with end-to-end anastomosis. Bronchial resections for malignant or benign stenosis are also performed. A bronchial sleeve resection begins with bronchotomy of the proximal airway followed by anastomosis with the lower airways. The diseased segment is removed, tension-free anastomosis is attempted, and occasional pedicled pleura or pericardium can be used between the bronchial anastomosis and vasculature.[33]

FUTURISTIC SURGICAL APPROACHES

Autografts, allografts, bioengineered tracheal platforms, and tracheal transplants may become more prominent in the future. The innate complexity and compromising blood supply of the trachea make a single tissue graft of the trachea rarely sufficient to achieve adequate function. Autografts include a patient's own tissue to reconstruct the airways; for example, resection of bronchi and replacement in the trachea, or muscle flaps to bridge defects resulting from tracheobronchial reconstruction. The grafts must have rigidity, epithelium, and adequate vascular supply.

Seguin and colleagues[34] demonstrated that functional tissue could be regenerated in sheep after replacement of the trachea with a cryopreserved aortic allograft. The use of cryopreserved specimens would offer advantages for use in tissue banks, for permanent storage, and by limiting the need for immunosuppression. It has been shown that respiratory epithelial cells and cartilage can regenerate in animal models of aortic allografts and that the allograft progressively transforms into a structure resembling tracheal tissue. Airway stenting was mandatory in pigs to prevent collapse of the initially compliant graft, and the investigators concluded that long-term stenting was necessary to provide stability as the neotrachea formed.[35] Tracheal replacement using bioabsorbable scaffolds[36] have been described. These studies are still mostly limited to animals.

Composite tissue grafts may include costal cartilage for support, mucosal grafts (buccal, palate) for epithelium, and pedicled flaps or free tissue transfer flaps for blood supply. Prosthetic scaffolds, such as a mesh, have been combined with free tissue flaps in advanced efforts to reconstruct the airway. An overview of unique surgical approaches to tracheal reconstruction is recommended.[37] A tissue-engineered tracheal allograft has been described, using a cadaveric trachea decellularized and with human leukocyte antigens removed, and with autologous bronchial epithelial cells harvested, cultured, and implanted on the internal surface of the trachea. Bone marrow–derived mesenchymal stem cells were harvested and differentiated toward chondrogenesis and implanted on the external surface of the tracheal graft. Although it revascularized well, there are concerns about the dependability of neovascularization of free grafts.[37]

Tracheal transplant is a challenge because of the vascular supply of the trachea, constant movement of the trachea, and constant exposure to bacteria. Only a few reports of tracheal transplant exist. The current concepts of tracheal transplantation include vascularization, growth of epithelium, and use of a chimeric product that includes donor tissue (cartilage, respiratory mucosa) and recipient tissue (membranous trachea, forearm fascia, forearm skin, and buccal mucosa). In this approach, the donor trachea is implanted in the forearm and allowed to vascularize, then epithelialized with recipient mucosal graft, and ultimately transposed into the trachea. Immunosuppressants are gradually withdrawn to allow anastomotic repopulation of recipient blood vessels and respiratory epithelium, and the recipient buccal mucosa and recipient forearm blood vessels preserve the airway lumen in the mid portion. This fascinating work is well worth reading.[38]

SUMMARY

Tracheobronchial stenosis results from malignant and benign causes. Treatment includes systemic therapy in addition to endoscopic or surgical approaches. Balloons, heat therapy, and stenting are useful for stenosis involving the proximal airways. These therapies may provide immediate improvement in dyspnea. Surgical resection of limited benign and malignant stenosis has a high success rate and may provide long-lasting results. New surgical therapies, as well as developments in bioabsorbable stenting, hold promise for the future treatment of tracheobronchial symptomatic stenosis.

REFERENCES

1. Brigger MT, Boseley ME. Management of tracheal stenosis. Curr Opin Otolaryngol Head Neck Surg 2012;20(6):491–6.
2. Nishine H, Hiramoto T, Matsuoka S, et al. Assessing the site of maximal obstruction in the trachea using lateral pressure measurement during bronchoscopy. Am J Respir Crit Care Med 2012;185(1):24–33.
3. Grenier PA, Beigelman-Aubry C, Brillet PY. Nonneoplastic tracheal and bronchial stenoses. Radiol Clin North Am 2009;47(2):243–60.

4. Grenier PA, Beigelman-Aubry C, Brillet PY. Nonneoplastic tracheal and bronchial stenoses. Thorac Surg Clin 2010;20(1):47–64.

5. Prince JS, Duhamel DR, Levin DL, et al. Nonneoplastic lesions of the tracheobronchial wall: radiologic findings with bronchoscopic correlation. Radiographics 2002;22(Spec No):S215–30.

6. Wester JL, Clayburgh DR, Stott WJ, et al. Airway reconstruction in Wegener's granulomatosis-associated laryngotracheal stenosis. Laryngoscope 2011;121(12):2566–71.

7. Morrison MP, Meiler S, Postma GN. Ventilatory techniques for central airway obstruction. Laryngoscope 2011;121(10):2162–4.

8. Ross-Anderson DJ, Ferguson C, Patel A. Transtracheal jet ventilation in 50 patients with severe airway compromise and stridor. Br J Anaesth 2011;106(1):140–4.

9. Shitrit D, Kuchuk M, Zismanov V, et al. Bronchoscopic balloon dilatation of tracheobronchial stenosis: long-term follow-up. Eur J Cardiothorac Surg 2010;38(2):198–202.

10. Amat B, Esselmann A, Reichle G, et al. The electrosurgical knife in an optimized intermittent cutting mode for the endoscopic treatment of benign web-like tracheobronchial stenosis. Arch Bronconeumol 2012;48(1):14–21.

11. Bolliger CT, Sutedja TG, Strausz J, et al. Therapeutic bronchoscopy with immediate effect: laser, electrocautery, argon plasma coagulation and stents. Eur Respir J 2006;27(6):1258–71.

12. Puchalski J, Feller-Kopman D. The pulmonologist's diagnostic and therapeutic interventions in lung cancer. Clin Chest Med 2011;32(4):763–71.

13. Zozzaro M, Harirchian S, Cohen EG. Flexible fiber CO_2 laser ablation of subglottic and tracheal stenosis. Laryngoscope 2012;122(1):128–30.

14. Cortes de Miguel S, Cabeza Barrera J, Gallardo Medina M, et al. Topical endotracheal mitomycin C as a complementary treatment for endoscopic treatment of recurrent laryngotracheal stenosis. Farm Hosp 2011;35(1):32–5.

15. Smith ME, Elstad M. Mitomycin C and the endoscopic treatment of laryngotracheal stenosis: are two applications better than one? Laryngoscope 2009;119(2):272–83.

16. Simpson CB, James JC. The efficacy of mitomycin-C in the treatment of laryngotracheal stenosis. Laryngoscope 2006;116(10):1923–5.

17. Fernando HC, Sherwood JT, Krimsky W. Endoscopic therapies and stents for benign airway disorders: where are we, and where are we heading? Ann Thorac Surg 2010;89(6):S2183–7.

18. Lim SY, Park HK, Jeon K, et al. Factors predicting outcome following airway stenting for post-tuberculosis tracheobronchial stenosis. Respirology 2011;16(6):959–64.

19. Nakayama T, Horinouchi H, Asakura K, et al. Tracheal stenosis due to relapsing polychondritis managed for 16 years with a silicon T-tube covering the entire trachea. Ann Thorac Surg 2011;92(3):1126–8.

20. Perotin JM, Jeanfaivre T, Thibout Y, et al. Endoscopic management of idiopathic tracheal stenosis. Ann Thorac Surg 2011;92(1):297–301.

21. Amjadi K, Voduc N, Cruysberghs Y, et al. Impact of interventional bronchoscopy on quality of life in malignant airway obstruction. Respiration 2008;76(4):421–8.

22. Oviatt PL, Stather DR, Michaud G, et al. Exercise capacity, lung function, and quality of life after interventional bronchoscopy. J Thorac Oncol 2011;6(1):38–42.

23. Vondrys D, Elliott MJ, McLaren CA, et al. First experience with biodegradable airway stents in children. Ann Thorac Surg 2011;92(5):1870–4.

24. Lischke R, Poxniak J, Vondrys D, et al. Novel biodegradable stents in the treatment of bronchial stenosis after lung transplantation. Eur J Cardiothorac Surg 2011;40(3):619–24.

25. Liu KS, Liu YH, Peng YJ, et al. Experimental absorbable stent permits airway remodeling. J Thorac Cardiovasc Surg 2011;141(2):463–8.

26. Smith LP, Zur KB, Jacobs IN. Single- vs double-stage laryngotracheal reconstruction. Arch Otolaryngol Head Neck Surg 2010;136(1):60–5.

27. Marulli G, Rizzardi G, Bortolotti L, et al. Single-staged laryngotracheal resection and reconstruction for benign strictures in adults. Interact Cardiovasc Thorac Surg 2008;7(2):227–30 [discussion: 230].

28. Yamamoto K, Kojima F, Tomiyama K, et al. Meta-analysis of therapeutic procedures for acquired subglottic stenosis in adults. Ann Thorac Surg 2011;91(6):1747–53.

29. Grillo HC. The history of tracheal surgery. Chest Surg Clin N Am 2003;13(2):175–89.

30. Marques P, Leal L, Spratley J, et al. Tracheal resection with primary anastomosis: 10 years experience. Am J Otolaryngol 2009;30(6):415–8.

31. Shiraishi T, Yanagisawa J, Higuchi T, et al. Tracheal resection for malignant and benign diseases: surgical results and perioperative considerations. Surg Today 2011;41(4):490–5.

32. Blasberg JD, Wright CD. Surgical considerations in tracheal and carinal resection. Semin Cardiothorac Vasc Anesth 2012;16(4):190–5.

33. Yu JA, Weyant MJ. Techniques of bronchial sleeve resection. Semin Cardiothorac Vasc Anesth 2012;16(4):196–202.

34. Seguin A, Radu D, Holder-Espinasse M, et al. Tracheal replacement with cryopreserved,

decellularized, or glutaraldehyde-treated aortic allografts. Ann Thorac Surg 2009;87(3):861–7.

35. Makris D, Holder-Espinasse M, Wurtz A, et al. Tracheal replacement with cryopreserved allogenic aorta. Chest 2010;137(1):60–7.

36. Tsukada H, Gangadharan S, Garland R, et al. Tracheal replacement with a bioabsorbable scaffold in sheep. Ann Thorac Surg 2010;90(6): 1793–7.

37. Rich JT, Gullane PJ. Current concepts in tracheal reconstruction. Curr Opin Otolaryngol Head Neck Surg 2012;20(4):246–53.

38. Delaere PR. Tracheal transplantation. Curr Opin Pulm Med 2012;18(4):313–20.

Pediatric Interventional Bronchoscopy

Leonardo L. Donato, MD[a],*, Thi Mai Hong Tran, MD[b],
Clement Ammouche, MD[a], Ali I. Musani, MD[c]

KEYWORDS

- Pediatric interventional bronchoscopy • Endoscopy-assisted tracheal intubation
- Bronchial blockers • Tracheoesophageal fistula management • Endoscopic sealing
- Bronchoscopic laser • Airway stents • Balloon catheter dilatation

KEY POINTS

- Pediatric interventional bronchoscopy (IB) procedures are difficult to standardize because of a lack of randomized studies.
- Most of the current literature is in the form of retrospective case series and case reports and large, randomized, blinded studies are desperately needed.
- Despite a lack of robust data, there is a rapidly evolving role for the bronchoscopist in the operating room and in the intensive care units.
- Myriad of minimally invasive diagnostic and therapeutic procedures done under the umbrella of IB preclude undesired surgical procedures.
- IB procedures require intense training and a multidisciplinary approach for patient care. With evolving technology, the role of IB is destined to grow.

THE PLACE FOR INTERVENTIONAL BRONCHOSCOPY IN CHILDREN TODAY

Primarily dominated by foreign-body removal, the profile of pediatric interventional bronchoscopy (IB) has changed over the last decades. Improvements of pediatric intensive care medicine and surgical techniques have widened the range of airway lesions that can be managed through bronchoscopy. Fortunately, the equipment has evolved allowing endoscopic interventions in younger children, including neonates and even fetuses. As a consequence, pediatric IB involves various specialties today: pulmonology, neonatology, intensive care medicine, anesthesiology, otorhinolaryngology, maxillofacial surgery, and cardiothoracic surgery. Decision making depends on a multidisciplinary approach including experienced bronchoscopists, skillful anesthesiologists, and appropriately trained supporting staff.

Pediatric IB has rejuvenated the debate on the use of rigid bronchoscope (RB) versus flexible bronchoscope (FB). Basically, RB is cheaper and longer lasting. Disinfection and storage of RB can be properly achieved in any operating room. Ultrathin FBs are expensive and fragile and require extra equipment and staff for maintenance and disinfection. Thus, the overall cost of FB can be prohibitive in developing countries. On the other hand, a wide proportion of endoscopists who can afford FB have limited experience with RB, which is traditionally reserved for otorhinolaryngologists. Some pulmonologists prefer to start by FB through an endotracheal tube or a laryngeal mask airway. However, the size of ultrathin FB working channels seriously limits the instrumentation; and

Disclosure: The authors declare no conflict of interest with any of the companies cited in this article.
[a] Hôpital Hautepierre, Medico-surgical Pediatric Department, University Hospital Strasbourg, Avenue Molière, 67098 Strasbourg, France; [b] Pulmonary Department, Hanoi National Hospital of Pediatrics, 18/879 La Thành, Đống Đa, Hanoi, Vietnam; [c] Department of Interventional Pulmonology, National Jewish Medical and Research Center, National Jewish Health, Molly Blank J211, 1400 Jackson Street, Denver, CO 80206, USA
* Corresponding author. Pediatrie 2, Hopital Hautepierre, Avenue Moliere, 67098 Strasbourg, France.
E-mail address: leonard.donato@chru-strasbourg.fr

chestmed.theclinics.com

the image quality provided by rod lens telescopes is clearly superior. A wider set of accessories can be passed through rigid tubes, which can also fit several instruments at the same time and allow 2 operators to proceed together (4 hands working). Moreover, the rigid tube can be used as a working instrument by itself (ie, for mass debulking or incarcerated foreign body dislodgement). Finally, endoscopists that have access to both RB and FB will take advantage of choosing the most appropriate technique, according to a particular situation or time course in the same patient.[1,2] FB is an indispensible tool for preinterventional and postinterventional evaluation. Flexible bronchoscopy can be performed under conscious sedation, by the bedside, in a very efficient way. On the other hand, RB requires general anesthesia and offers valuable working comfort for some of the most challenging and complex airway procedures.

various surgical procedures. Ultrathin devices are used as guides for these extremely time-sensitive intubations. The Olympus (Olympus Medical Systems Corp, Tokyo, Japan) BF-N20 ultrathin FB (2.2 mm) can be threaded through a Portex (Smiths Medical International Ltd, Hythe, United Kingdom) 2.5 endotracheal tube (ETT); similarly, the Hopkins (Karl Storz GMBH & Co, Tuttlingen, Germany) 2.8-mm rigid telescope can be threaded through a Portex 3 ETT. These instruments have no suction channel, completely occlude the smallest ETTs, and have to be lubricated before insertion. Thus, their manipulation is challenging particularly in preexisting ventilatory compromise and with anatomic abnormalities.

The procedures described later require a high level of training and skills in pediatric bronchoscopy.

Endoscopy-Assisted Tracheal Intubation

Considering bronchoscopic interventions as therapeutic procedures, the pediatric indications can be summarized as follows:

- Restoration of airway patency in which the endoscopist plays a key role:
  - Foreign-body removal
  - Aspiration of endogenous material
  - Endoscopy-assisted tracheal intubation
  - Stenosis dilation/stenting/laser photoresection/electroresection
  - Endoscopic closure of bronchopleural fistula
- Perioperative bronchoscopy in which the endoscopist assists the anesthesiologist or surgeon:
  - Endoscopy-assisted tracheal intubation
  - Selective intubation for single-lung ventilation
  - Detection/repair of tracheoesophageal fistula (TEF)
  - Airway inspection during thoracic surgery

Conventional intubation by direct laryngoscopy can be cumbersome in situations that preclude the proper exposure of the larynx or when there is a tracheal stricture in the proximal trachea. Examples of such situations include the following:

- Mandibulofacial dysostosis and limited mouth aperture (temporomandibular ankylosis, microstomia, facial trauma)
- Pharyngeal malformations or tumors (macroglossia, lymphangioma, teratoma, sarcoma)
- Abnormalities of larynx (epiglottitis, acquired or congenital subglottic stenosis)
- Cervical spine fractures or luxations

The purpose of this article is not to provide guidelines or rules for various pediatric bronchoscopic procedures but to give an overview of the bronchoscopic interventions that are technically feasible in the small-sized pediatric airways.

THE INTUBATING BRONCHOSCOPE

There is a growing demand on securing difficult airways of neonates and infants in the intensive care unit (ICU) and preoperative scenarios for

To anticipate difficult intubation that implies a strong risk for hypoxia and brain damage, anesthesiologists use various predictors. The current literature describes many options: blind intubation guided by breath sounds, gum-elastic bougie guided intubation, retromolar intubation, 2-persons procedure, laryngeal mask airway, optical and video laryngoscopes, and transillumination devices. Yet fiberoptic intubation is increasingly considered as the gold standard, particularly in the cases whereby limited mouth aperture hinders the former methods to be used and when surgeons require nasotracheal intubation (maxillofacial surgery).[3,4] Nevertheless, these procedures are best performed by highly skilled interventional pulmonologists with a wide range of experience in complex airways.[4] This requirement is a serious limitation of current training programs because they only use mannequins with normal anatomy. A lack of proper training and skills may also lead to the damage of very fragile ultrathin bronchoscopes.

Practically, anesthesia is induced via a face-mask while maintaining spontaneous ventilation. The ETT is placed blindly into the nasopharynx, the FB being subsequently passed through while assistants provide tongue retraction with a large forceps to improve larynx exposure. The FB is advanced through the vocal cords up to the main carina; the ETT is then pushed over the FB in a Seldingerlike technique. The proper placement of the ETT's distal tip is achieved under visual control and the FB is withdrawn (**Fig. 1**).

Intubation with FB may be a failure when huge anatomic abnormalities collapse the pharynx or when laryngeal narrowing poses strong resistance, thus requiring a more rigid device to force the way.[5,6] In RB-guided/telescopic intubation, the larynx is approached using a straight-blade laryngoscope and an ETT-covered rigid telescope is advanced through the vocal cords. The telescope is then withdrawn once the main carina

has been reached, while firmly keeping the tube in place with the left thumb (**Fig. 2**). In the authors' experience, this technique has proven to be life saving in many situations, including epiglottitis, subglottic edema, and iatrogenic subglottic webs (**Fig. 3**). While performing RB/telescopic intubation, it is essential to keep the telescope in the same axis as the airway and to restrain the motion when a brief crack is felt to avoid injury to the main carina or the airway wall. Telescopic intubation carries the drawback of an orotracheal intubation only because the rigid instrument cannot pass through the nose for nasal intubation.

In children, endoscopy-assisted tracheal intubation is probably the most frequent procedure among all of the IB procedures available today.

Selective Intubation

Selective intubation (SI) is a frequent pitfall in intubated babies undergoing mechanical ventilation. Chest auscultation can be misleading in younger children, and chest radiographs for confirming

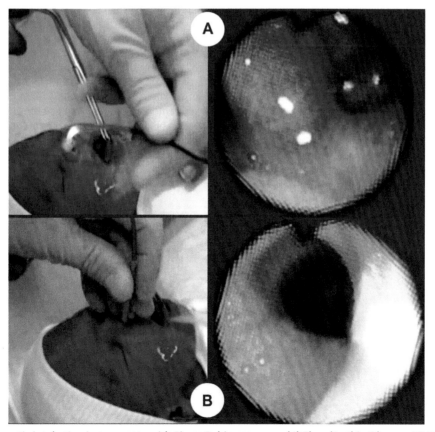

Fig. 1. Fiberoptic intubation in a neonate with Pierre Robin sequence. (*A*) The ultrathin Olympus BF-N20 reaches the larynx through an ETT placed in the pharyngeal position. (*B*) The ETT is advanced over the FB up to the supracarinal position.

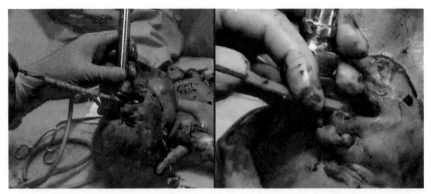

Fig. 2. Telescopic intubation at birth in a boy with cervical teratoma. The ETT is threaded on a 2.8-mm Hopkins rigid telescope and guided through the mouth using a straight-blade laryngoscope. The child was delivered by cesarean section, and the intubation was performed in the operating room within 4 minutes of delivery.

the position of the endotracheal tube are often inaccurate. Proper placement of ETT can be achieved through ultrathin FB examination,[7,8] provided the endoscopist is capable of quickly distinguishing the main carina from a secondary carina.[9] However, SI is useful under some particular circumstances, for instance, in isolating one lung from ventilation in cases of unilateral emphysema or focal hemoptysis.[10] Similarly, a growing indication for SI is video-assisted thoracic surgery (VATS), which requires unilateral ventilation. This technique is particularly useful in children less than 6 to 10 years of age because double-lumen intubation is not feasible for them. Bronchial blockers are also used instead of double-lumen intubations and have proven to be very effective for VATS.[11] The blocker comprises a rounded balloon catheter threaded on a guidewire that makes a loop at its distal tip. Both catheter and FB are

inserted through a multiport adaptor connected to the ETT; airtight valves prevent gas leak. The FB is placed through the wire loop, which guides the catheter into the main stem bronchus on the operative side, and the balloon is inflated under direct vision (**Fig. 4**). Because the procedure carries the risk of tracheal obstruction by balloon retrograde displacement, some investigators recommend to pass the catheter through the lateral hole of the ETT's distal tip and to push the ETT against the main carina to secure the balloon.[12] In the authors' experience, placing the bronchial blocker *after* the child has been positioned laterally, according to the VATS procedure requirements, is usually sufficient, provided large motion of the bronchial axis is avoided. A standard Fogarty (Edwards Lifesciences LLC, Irvine, CA) catheter can also be used instead of the commercial sets that are more expensive.[13]

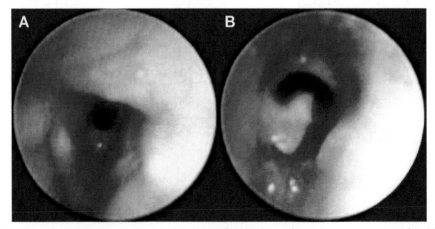

Fig. 3. Subglottic web endoscopic treatment. (*A*) Circumferential membranous scar in a 6-weeks-old girl previously intubated for bronchiolitis. Reintubation attempts under direct laryngoscopy failed. (*B*) Membrane broken by an optical device, with immediate relief of the dyspnea and no more need for intubation.

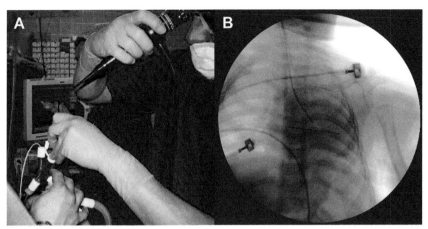

Fig. 4. Bronchial blocker placement in a 9-month-old boy with congenital emphysema undergoing left upper lobectomy by VATS. (*A*) Ultrathin FB and balloon catheter (*yellow*) are inserted through multiport adaptor. (*B*) Selective placement of the balloon (radiolucent) in the left main stem bronchus. The balloon blocks upper and lower lobe ventilation.

THE CHANNELING BRONCHOSCOPE

Two anatomically distinct variants of congenital TEF are described:

- The G-type is long, oblique, and connects the lower esophagus to the pars membranacea of the intrathoracic trachea; it is observed in about 95% of cases and usually associates with esophageal atresia.
- The H-type is short, horizontal, and arises from the cervical trachea, 1 to 2 cm below the vocal cords; it is generally isolated, although associations can be found with the G-type and esophageal atresia.

There is generally no need for perioperative endoscopic evaluation in the G-type because the fistula is detected by dissection during esophageal atresia surgical repair. The H-type TEF is trickier to locate, and the surgeon may need endoscopic assistance to determine the most adequate approach (ie, cervicotomy or thoracotomy).

The TEF postoperative recurrence rate is 5% to 15% in the literature. Although surgical reintervention is usually indicated, various endoscopic sealing methods can be used in selected cases.

Isolated TEF Catheterization

Perioperative bronchoscopy can afford valuable help because esophagograms are often misleading in infants with isolated TEF, particularly in the H-type. A single inspection of the airway may distinguish proximal (cervicotomy) from distal (thoracotomy) fistula. However, sometimes even with bronchoscopic inspection, the findings could be confusing and inconclusive because of borderline forms. In some difficult situations, the orifice is catheterized with a thin radiopaque guidewire. The bronchoscope is withdrawn leaving the catheter in place, and an ETT is subsequently inserted by the catheter side. The diverging point clearly indicates the level of the fistula on the lateral radiograph (**Fig. 5**). Alternatively, a nonendoscopic method has been described as the *bubble test*: an esophageal catheter is placed while patients are ventilated with positive pressure, the external tip of the catheter is plunged into a glass of water, the catheter is then progressively withdrawn, and the level where bubbles are produced is measured.

Endoscopic Closure for Recurrent TEF

The postoperative recurrence of TEF can be difficult to diagnose with contrast-enhanced radiography. The tortuous course of these TEFs usually prevents the catheterization of the channel. TEF recanalization can be demonstrated by endoscopic dye injection and is usually followed by surgical closure in the same anesthetic setting if the leakage is detected (**Fig. 6**).

As an alternative to surgery in patients presenting with complicated recurrent TEF, endoscopic sealing has been proposed by the application of various agents, including collagen glue, fibrin, and cyanoacrylate or sclerosing agents. Relapse is frequent, and multiple procedures are generally needed; thus, the method could be considered as temporary, leaving time for surgical repair to be achieved in better conditions. However, several investigators have published encouraging results

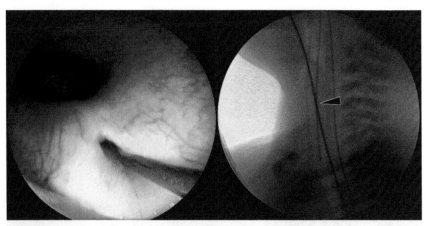

Fig. 5. Perioperative TEF catheterization in a 3-week-old boy with swallowing troubles. A 4F radiopaque catheter threaded into posterior wall defect (cervical fistula). The lateral radiograph shows the level where ETT and catheter separate (*arrowhead*).

when combining mucosal de-epithelialization of the tracheal pouch either by brush abrasion or laser or electrocautery, then subsequent topical application of sealants.[14–17]

THE CALIBRATING BRONCHOSCOPE

Foreign-body removal is another area where IB is considered as the most effective subspecialty with tools and skills set. Martinot and coworkers[1] have proposed an algorithm for choosing RB versus FB for the management of foreign bodies. This topic is not be discussed further in this section.

> IB procedures are usually best suited for segmental stenoses. Choosing the most appropriate method depends on the nature of the lesion.
>
> 1. Mucosal lesions with soft consistency are best treated by laser (eg, weblike lesions, bulky granulomas, mural cysts, and tumors).
>
> 2. Segmental tracheobronchomalacia, extrinsic compression, or postoperative volvulus of the airway may be managed by stenting when surgery or tracheostomy fail to solve the problem.
>
> 3. Fibrocartilaginous rigid stenoses can be dilated by using various procedures (eg, congenital cartilage rings, ischemic stricture, and anastomotic stenosis).
>
> 4. The previously described methods can be combined in case of complex lesions (eg, laser photoresection of mucosal injury and then stenting or stenting of segmental collapse induced by endoscopic dilatation of a fixed stenosis).

Mucosal Lesions of the Lower Airway

Most of these lesions are induced by contact with various foreign materials: ETTs, tracheostomy tubes, stents, stitches, inhaled foreign bodies. Granuloma formation usually resolves by removing the causative agent and giving corticosteroids. If not treated, a cicatricial process occurs with scar membrane formation (web). Granuloma forceps excision can produce heavy bleeding and carries the risk of in-depth mucosal injury with exposure of cartilages, which is a situation that should always be avoided. Tracheobronchial webs can be destroyed either by forcing the way with the

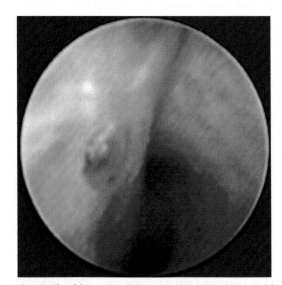

Fig. 6. The blue test. TEF recurrence in a 2-year-old girl operated at birth for type III esophageal atresia. The dye is injected via an esophageal catheter and leaks into the airway through a punctiform defect. Earlier, an esophagogram failed to show the fistula.

bevel of a rigid tube or by pneumatic dilatation[18]; but relapses are frequently observed, and most patients require multiple interventions.

Such recurrences can be prolonged or avoided by using *laser photoresection*. Various laser sources can induce tissue vaporization, coagulation, hemostasis, and necrosis. One of the most popular lasers, YAG, has an in-depth effect that makes it unsuitable for infants and toddlers because of the potential for airway wall perforation and large burns. Inversely, the carbon dioxide (CO_2) laser allows shallow penetration of tissues and precise cutting.[19,20] Despite being the favorite laser type of laryngologists, its use is not very popular among bronchoscopists[15,21] because the CO_2 laser beam is air-transmitted and targeted onto a red light spot, which is easy to aim under laryngeal suspension. But for bronchoscopy purposes, the source has to be connected to a dedicated nonstandard bronchoscopy tube via a set of articulated arms. Protective glasses are required, impairing visibility while lasering. The KTP laser offers an interesting compromise. It is obtained by doubling the frequency of a YAG beam through a crystal of potassium-titanyl-phosphate

(KTP); when set at a low power range (ie, 5 W), the tissue effects are close to the ones of the CO_2 laser. The energy can be modulated to deepen the absorption (eg, carbonization of bulky granuloma or tumor). The KTP beam is transmitted via fiber optics and is compatible with any standard RB or FB equipped with shielded working channels. Coated fibers as thin as 0.6 mm fit the smallest pediatric instruments. It has been suggested that the fiber tip is directed more accurately through FB than by using RB. As a matter of fact, many RB users thread the fiber through the side port of the rigid tube,[15,21,22] which can lead to imprecise targeting. This imprecision is easily solved by taping the fiber onto the outside of the rod lens telescope, so that the bronchoscopist's leading hand can accurately operate the fiber and the telescope at the same time.[23] In young children, interesting results have also been reported with the argon laser.

Weblike diaphragms are treated by radial incisions. In the authors' experience, a single session is usually enough, thus making bronchoscopic laser treatment more effective than pneumatic dilatation (**Fig. 7**). The bronchoscopic laser is

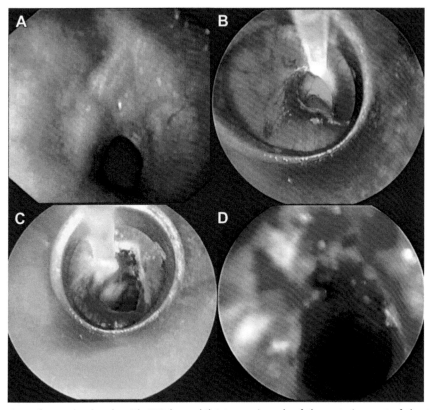

Fig. 7. Resection of a tracheal web with KTP laser. (*A*) Iatrogenic web of the anterior part of the trachea in a 2-year-old girl. (*B*) Laser fiber placed in contact with the membrane. (*C*) Photoresection in progress. (*D*) Web after photoresection.

effective in the removal of large granulomas, ensuring hemostasis, and precise recanalization. Resection of suprastomal granulomas above the tracheostomy site is probably the most frequent indication for the use of laser therapy today, allowing children with tracheostomies to be successfully decannulated.[15,22,24] The laser can also be useful for dislodging incarcerated foreign bodies (**Fig. 8**). Other potential indications include iatrogenic lesions of the central airway,[15,25,26] tracheal cysts and pouches,[21] tracheobronchial angiomas,[27,28] inflammatory pseudotumors and endobronchial tuberculosis,[23,29–31] and various benign and malignant tumors.[31–33] In older children, the use of adult-type lasers, such as YAG, Yttrium Aluminium Perovskite (YAP), and the diode laser, has also been reported. Because equipment is expensive and pediatric indications are not that frequent, the selection of laser type is a matter of availability. Using a KTP, which can be operated either in YAG or KTP mode, is certainly cost-effective. The electrocautery is cheaper but carries the same drawbacks as the YAG laser, namely, large areas of burns.[21,26]

Tracheobronchomalacia and Extrinsic Compression

The conservative approach of wait and watch is justified in most cases with fixed and dynamic airway collapse in children because of a significant growth potential with age.

However, various degrees of intervention are needed in more severe cases, including long-term oxygen therapy; ventilatory support; continuous positive airway pressure tracheostomy; and other surgical procedures, including anterior aortopexy (widely considered as the gold standard for tracheomalacia). Airway stenting is discussed as an alternative when these procedures are not applicable or fail to succeed, in other words, as a rescue indication.

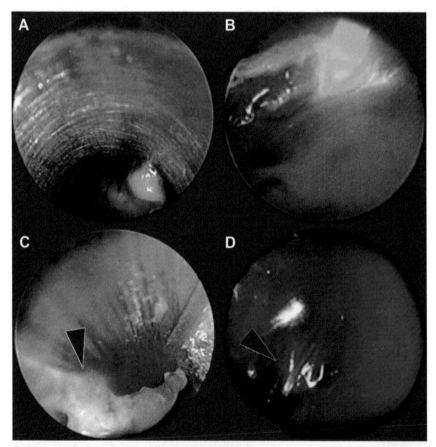

Fig. 8. Resection of airway granuloma with KTP laser. (*A*) Foreign-body induced granulation obstructing intermediate bronchus in an 8-month-old girl. Mechanical debulking was suspended because of bleeding. (*B*) Hemostasis and debulking with laser. (*C*) The granulation tissue adhered to the laser fiber tip (*arrowhead*). (*D*) A small plant spike (*arrowhead*). The foreign body was then successfully removed with a thin forceps under visual control.

Several types of stents can fit the small pediatric airway; these stents are made of metal, silicone, or composite:

- Balloon-expandable metal stents are made of stainless steel tubular meshes. They are threaded onto balloon catheters and are expanded to a desired diameter by inflating the balloon.[34]

- Self-expanding metal stents are made of nitinol, a titanium-based alloy with shape-memory. They are packaged as coils enclosed into a dedicated introducer sheath. These stents are released by pulling-back the external sheath.[35]

- Silicone stents (eg, Dumon stents [Novatech SA, Marseille, France]) are molded, straight tubes with outer studs. Silicone stents can be folded into a dedicated metallic hollow applicator that is placed in the airway via an RB. Once placed through the stenosis, the stent is pushed out with a pusher and pulling the loader tube back.[36]

- Covered metal stents are made of nitinol coils covered with thin polymer sheaths. They are deployed the same way as with uncovered metal stents, either by balloon catheters or by introducer sheaths.[37]

The pediatric literature on airway stents is limited and is mostly in the form of case reports rather than prospective clinical trials. The criteria defined by Sommer and Forte[38] sheds some light on the ideal stent properties; they are compared with the overall results obtained from the few published series in **Table 1**. Uncovered metallic stents are very effective in relieving obstruction of the airways but at the cost of severe complications of granuloma formation, the management of which may require repeated endoscopic interventions.[34,35,39,42] Other complications of these stents include stent fracture and migration to surrounding organs, particularly in the first generation of metal stents. Moreover, mucosal embedding progressively occurs over time, making the removal of these stents hazardous or even impossible.[43] A noteworthy recent publication reports no granulation in 8 infants stented with stainless steel meshes coated with a drug that delays epithelialization.[44] However, the follow-up of patients in this report is short term. All the children are still stented at the end of the study, and possible long-term adverse effects are yet to be seen.

Hence, the US Food and Drugs Administration has issued a black-box warning against the implantation of metal stents in benign conditions.

On the other hand, silicone stents are considered safer for long-term use and are easy to remove, making them a better choice for benign conditions. Nevertheless, silicone stents show frequent migration in pediatric airways.[23,36,42] Covered metal stents have been subsequently developed to combine the properties of uncovered metal stents with those of silicone. The external polyurethane sheath prevents the stent from epithelialization and makes the removal easy. The nitinol expansion force prevents migration in most cases.[37] But because collateral openings may be covered, they cannot be used for right main stem bronchus and carinal reconstruction. A certain degree of granulation, although much less than the uncovered metallic stents, is still observed at the edges of these stents (**Fig. 9**). Long-term follow-up information on residual stenosis is lacking.[45] Encouraging preliminary results have recently been reported with the use of bioresorbable materials,[46] however there is a serious concern about the potential of loosing fragments into the airways.

Rigid Strictures

Postintubation stenosis is frequently observed in premature babies and infants. It is usually found at the level of the cuff or at the distal tip of the ETT. Anastomotic stricture management that occurs following lung transplantation or tracheal surgery has been widely described in adult series. Therapeutic options and results differ from those that are described in subglottic stenosis. Although surgical options exist, conservative measures are usually considered first in these cases because of the underlying conditions (bronchopulmonary dysplasia, poor quality of the ischemic airway wall). Endoluminal pneumatic dilatation can be performed with bronchoscopy or balloons through the stricture. Oval-shaped balloon catheters (angioplasty balloon catheters)[18,47] are clearly more appropriate than round-shaped balloons (Fogarty).[48] An immediate benefit is reported in most patients; but relapse is frequent, and multiple procedures are needed over time. Acquired strictures are complex in nature and can require a combination of methods, including laser photoresection and stent placement.[47] Balloon dilatation is also used in growing children with indwelling uncovered metal airway stents.

Management of congenital tracheal stenosis is quite challenging. These strictures are usually made of full circumference (O-shaped) cartilaginous rings instead of the normal U-shaped rings. According to the number of cartilages involved, these strictures are classified as long-segment stenosis (LSTS), funnel-shaped stenosis that

Table 1
Pediatric airway stents properties

Type of Stent	Insertion	Stability	Compatibility with Collateral Ventilation	Accommodation to Mucociliary Clearance	Biocompatibility	Removal
Uncovered metal stents[34,35,39–41]	Blind,[a] with dedicated introducers	Good	Possible, through the mesh[b]	Satisfactory	Granulation epithelialization[e]	Difficult to impossible
Silicone stents[36]	Blind,[a] with dedicated introducers	Prone to migration	Not possible,[c] lateral orifices covered by the stent	Poor[d] Chest physiotherapy and daily aerosols required	Good[f]	Easy[g]
Covered metal stents[37]	Blind,[a] with dedicated introducers	Good	Not possible,[c] lateral orifices covered by the stent	Poor Chest physiotherapy and daily aerosols required	Satisfactory	Easy[g]

[a] Visual control hindered by introducers when inserted into the bronchoscope; some investigators place metal stents through ETT under fluoroscopic control.
[b] Allows right mainstem bronchus stenting; several stents can be combined.
[c] Use restricted to trachea and left mainstem bronchus; Y-shaped stents not available in the small diameters.
[d] Mucus plugging can occur.
[e] More severe complications have been described, including airway erosions and vascular perforations.
[f] Granulation may develop if the stent is mobile or has been tailored with sharp edges.
[g] Roll-up technique: the proximal edge of the stent is firmly grasped with a forceps, a 360° rotation is applied and the stent is pulled-back.

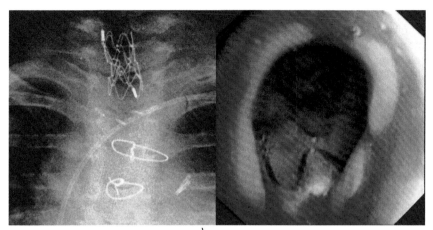

Fig. 9. Covered nitinol stent in a 3-year-old girl with post-tracheostomy stenosis. The radiopaque part of the stent can be seen at the level of third cartilaginous ring. Nonobstructive granuloma formation is visible at the edges of the stent.

usually involves the main carina, and short-segment stenosis (SSTS). Despite the various surgical options available, balloon catheter dilatation is frequently used as an alternative because the cartilaginous rings in these strictures usually have a weak point in the posterior wall.[49] The balloon dilation aims to induce a posterior split in the cartilaginous rings; high pressures are often needed (up to 20–22 atm in some reports), implying the risk for airway wall laceration. The rings are then kept expanded by either an ETT[49–51] or a balloon expandable stent[39,41,44,46] for a certain period of time. Carinal stenosis can be dilated by inflating 2 kissing balloons side by side in both main stem bronchi.[52] Overall, reported results are better in SSTS than in LSTS and in cases whereby stenting is not necessary. In

SSTS, a bronchoscopic laser can be alternatively used to produce a posterior split in the cartilage rings. However, laser can cause damage to the fibromuscular structures at the same time, thus requiring subsequent stent placement.[53,54] The authors have described an alternative method of posterior splitting by direct rigid bronchoscopic bougienage. A serial dilation with increasing diameter of rigid bronchoscopic tubes is performed until a brief crack is felt, indicating cartilage fracture. Because the surrounding fibromuscular structure is compliant, cartilage rings break selectively without injuring the pars membranacea, provided cross-sectional stretching is progressively applied and the tube's forward motion is immediately restrained (**Fig. 10**). In the authors' recent experience of 5 cases of SSTS in neonates and infants,

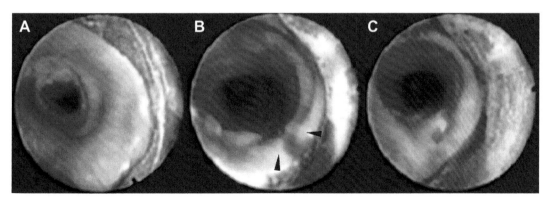

Fig. 10. Rigid bronchoscopic bougienage (dilation) in a 6-week-old girl with SSTS. (*A*) Complete cartilaginous rings of the upper trachea (3 mm inner diameter). (*B*) Serial dilation with increasing diameter of rigid bronchoscopic tubes (diameter gradually increasing from 2.5 mm to 3.5 mm). The arrow points to the fractured cartilage. (*C*) After therapeutic fracture of the cartilaginous rings, the trachea shows normal compliance with minimal bleeding and no damage to the tissue. (*Adapted from* Donato L, Tran TMH, Mihailidou E. Interventional bronchoscopy. In: Priftis KN, Anthracopoulos MB, Eber E, et al, editors. Paediatric bronchoscopy (Progress in Respiratory Research, vol. 38). Basel: Karger; 2010. p. 64–74; with permission of S. Karger AG, Basel.)

4 were successfully treated with rigid broncho-scopic serial dilation without requiring stents. These patients showed normal tracheal growth at a long-term follow-up. In the fifth patient, both rigid tube and balloon dilatation attempts failed to fracture the cartilaginous rings, requiring surgical resection with end-to-end anastomosis. Unfortunately, postoperative anastomotic stricture led to the demise of the patient.[23]

Currently, there is no consensus as to the preferred modality for the management of congenital tracheal stenosis in infants. Most experts consider tracheoplasty as a first option, but in nonsurgical candidates, balloon dilation remains an effective viable option for LSTS.

Funnel-shaped stenosis is usually surgically resected at the same time as the underlying vascular malformation (ring-sling complex), but balloon dilation can be performed if the stricture is isolated.

Patients with SSTS with mild symptoms can be managed conservatively because significant growth is observed in the cross-sectional area over time.[55] Conversely, those who are candidates for early surgery are also at high risk for severe complications. The authors think that selected patients could benefit from therapeutic bronchoscopy before tracheal surgery.

SUMMARY

Pediatric IB procedures are difficult to standardize because of a lack of randomized studies. Most of the current literature is in the form of retrospective case series and case reports. Large, randomized, blinded studies are desperately needed.

Despite a lack of robust data, there is a rapidly evolving role for the bronchoscopist in the operating room and in the ICU. This role is clearly beyond basic diagnostic procedures. As discussed, myriad of minimally invasive diagnostic and therapeutic procedures done under the umbrella of IB preclude undesired surgical procedures. IB procedures require intense training and a multidisciplinary approach for patient care. With evolving technology, the role of IB is destined to grow.

REFERENCES

1. Martinot A, Closset M, Marquette CH, et al. Indications for flexible versus rigid bronchoscopy in children with suspected foreign-body aspiration. Am J Respir Crit Care Med 1997;155:1676–9.
2. Barbato A, Magarotto M, Crivellaro M, et al. Use of the paediatric bronchoscope, flexible and rigid, in 51 European centres. Eur Respir J 1997;10:1761–6.
3. Blanco G, Melman E, Cuairan V, et al. Fiberoptic nasal intubation in children with anticipated and unanticipated difficult intubation. Paediatr Anaesth 2001;11:49–53.
4. Martson PA, Lander TA, Tibesar RJ, et al. Airway management for intubation in newborns with Pierre Robin sequence. Laryngoscope 2012;122:1401–4.
5. Levin R, Kissonn N, Froese N. Fiberoptic and videoscopic indirect intubation techniques for intubation in children. Pediatr Emerg Care 2009;25:479.
6. Michaelson PG, Mair EA. Seldinger-assisted videotelescopic intubation (SAVI): a commonsense approach to the difficult pediatric airway. Otolaryngol Head Neck Surg 2005;132:677–80.
7. Davidson MG, Coutts J, Bell G. Flexible bronchoscopy in pediatric intensive care. Pediatr Pulmonol 2008;43:1188–92.
8. Yoo SY, Kim JH, Han SH, et al. A comparative study of endotracheal tube positioning methods in children: safety from neck movement. Anesth Analg 2007;105:620–5.
9. Bush A. Neonatal bronchoscopy. Eur J Pediatr 1994;153(Suppl 2):S27–9.
10. Holzki J, Kellner M. Life threatening unilateral pulmonary overinflation might be more successfully treated by contralateral selective intubation than by emergency pneumonectomy. Paediatr Anaesth 2003;13:432–7.
11. Hammer GB, Harrison TK, Vricella LA, et al. Single lung ventilation in children using a new pediatric bronchial blocker. Paediatr Anaesth 2002;12:69–72.
12. Ho AM, Karmakar MK, Critchley LA, et al. Placing the tip of the endotracheal tube at the carina and passing the endobronchial blocker through the Murphy eye may reduce the risk of blocker retrograde dislodgement during one-lung anaesthesia in small children. Br J Anaesth 2008;101:690–3.
13. Rehman M, Sherlekar S, Schwartz R, et al. One lung anaesthesia for video assisted thoracoscopic lung biopsy in paediatric patient. Paediatr Anaesth 1999;9:85–7.
14. Richter GT, Rickman F, Brown RL, et al. Endoscopic management of recurrent tracheoesophageal fistula. J Pediatr Surg 2008;43:238–45.
15. Ishman SL, Kerschner JE, Rudolph CD. The KTP laser: an emerging tool in pediatric otolaryngology. Int J Pediatr Otorhinolaryngol 2006;70:677–82.
16. Meier JD, Sulman CG, Almond PS, et al. Endoscopic management of recurrent tracheoesophageal fistula: a review of techniques and results. Int J Pediatr Otorhinolaryngol 2007;71:691–7.
17. Rakoczy G, Brown B, Barman D, et al. KTP laser: an important tool in refractory recurrent tracheoesophageal fistula in children. Int J Pediatr Otorhinolaryngol 2010;74:326–7.

18. Messineo A, Narne S, Mognato G, et al. Endoscopic dilation of acquired tracheobronchial stenosis in infants. Pediatr Pulmonol 1997;23:101–4.

19. Bagwell CE. CO2 laser excision of pediatric airway lesions. J Pediatr Surg 1990;25:1152–6.

20. Monnier P, George M, Monod ML, et al. The role of the CO2 laser in the management of laryngotracheal stenosis: a survey of 100 cases. Eur Arch Otorhinolaryngol 2005;262:602–8.

21. Baring DE, Ansari S, Clement WA, et al. Residual tracheal pouch after repair of tracheaoesophageal fistula: endoscopic KTP laser treatment. J Pediatr Surg 2010;45:1040–3.

22. Sharp HR, Hartley BE. KTP laser treatment of suprastomal obstruction prior to decannulation in paediatric tracheostomy. Int J Pediatr Otorhinolaryngol 2002;66:125–30.

23. Donato L, Tran TM, Mihailidou E. Interventional bronchoscopy. In: Priftis KN, Anthracopoulos MB, Eber E, et al, editors. Paediatric bronchoscopy (Progress in Respiratory Research, vol. 38). Basel (Switzerland): Karger; 2010. p. 64–74 [online videos].

24. Mandell DL, Yellon RF. Endoscopic KTP laser excision of severe tracheostomy-associated suprastomal collapse. Int J Pediatr Otorhinolaryngol 2004; 68:1423–8.

25. Peng YY, Soong WJ, Lee YS, et al. Flexible bronchoscopy as a valuable diagnostic and therapeutic tool in pediatric intensive care patients: a report on 5 years of experience. Pediatr Pulmonol 2011;46: 1031–7.

26. Azizkhan RG, Lacey SR, Wood RE. Acquired symptomatic bronchial stenosis in infants: successful management using an argon laser. J Pediatr Surg 1990;25:19–24.

27. Sierpina DI, Chaudhary HM, Walner DL, et al. An infantile bronchial hemangioma unresponsive to propranolol therapy. Arch Otolaryngol Head Neck Surg 2011;137:517–21.

28. Rameau A, Zur KB. KTP laser ablation of extensive tracheal hemangiomas. Int J Pediatr Otorhinolaryngol 2011;75:1200–3.

29. Breen DP, Dubus JC, Chetaille B, et al. A rare cause of endobronchial tumour in children: the role of interventional bronchoscopy in the diagnosis and treatment of tumours while preserving lung function. Respiration 2008;76:444–8.

30. Eljko B, Martin J, Spomenka M, et al. Inflammatory pseudotumor of the trachea. J Pediatr Surg 2001; 36:631–4.

31. Al-Qathani AR, di Lorenzo M, Yazbeck S. Endobronchial tumors in children: institutional experience and literature review. J Pediatr Surg 2003; 38:733–6.

32. Conforti S, Bonacina E, Ravini M, et al. A case of fibrous histiocytoma of the trachea in an infant treated by endobronchial Nd:YAG laser. Lung Cancer 2007;57:112–4.

33. Li CH, Huang SF, Li HY. Bronchoscopic Nd-YAG laser surgery for tracheobronchial mucoepidermoid carcinoma – a report of two cases. Int J Clin Pract 2004;58:979–82.

34. Filler RM, Forte V, Chait P. Tracheobronchial stenting for the treatment of airway obstruction. J Pediatr Surg 1998;33:304–11.

35. Nicolai T, Huber RM, Reiter K, et al. Metal airway stent implantation in children: follow-up of seven children. Pediatr Pulmonol 2001;31:289–96.

36. Fayon M, Donato L, de Blic J, et al. French experience of silicone tracheobronchial stenting in children. Pediatr Pulmonol 2005;39:21–7.

37. Shin JH, Hong SJ, Park SJ, et al. Placement of covered retrievable expandable metallic stents for pediatric tracheobronchial obstruction. J Vasc Interv Radiol 2006;17:309–17.

38. Sommer D, Forte V. Advances in the management of major airway collapse: the use of airway stents. Otolaryngol Clin North Am 2000;33:163–77.

39. Maeda K, Yasufuku M, Yamamoto T. A new approach to the treatment of congenital tracheal stenosis: balloon tracheoplasty and expandable metallic stenting. J Pediatr Surg 2001;36:1646–9.

40. Furman RH, Backer CL, Dunham ME, et al. The use of balloon-expandable metallic stents in the treatment of pediatric tracheomalacia and bronchomalacia. Arch Otolaryngol Head Neck Surg 1999;125: 203–7.

41. Vinograd I, Keidar S, Weinberg M, et al. Treatment of airway obstruction by metallic stents in infants and children. J Thorac Cardiovasc Surg 2005; 130:146–50.

42. Anton-Pacheco JL, Cabezali D, Tejedor R, et al. The role of airway stenting in pediatric tracheobronchial obstruction. Eur J Cardiothorac Surg 2008;33:1069–75.

43. Lim LH, Cotton RT, Azizkhan RG, et al. Complications of metallic stents in the pediatric airway. Otolaryngol Head Neck Surg 2004;131:355–61.

44. Xu X, Li D, Zhao S, et al. Treatment of congenital tracheal stenosis by balloon-expandable metallic stents in paediatric intensive care unit. Interact Cardiovasc Thorac Surg 2012;14:548–50.

45. Kim JH, Shin JH, Song HY, et al. Benign tracheobronchial strictures: long-term results and factors affecting airway patency after temporary stent placement. AJR Am J Roentgenol 2007;188: 1033–8.

46. Vondrys D, Elliott MJ, McLaren CA, et al. First experience with biodegradable airway stents in children. Ann Thorac Surg 2011;92:1870–4.

47. Hebra A, Powell DD, Smith CD, et al. Balloon tracheoplasty in children: results of a 15-year experience. J Pediatr Surg 1991;26:957–61.

48. Betremieux P, Treguier C, Pladys P, et al. Tracheo-bronchography and balloon dilatation in acquired neonatal tracheal stenosis. Arch Dis Child 1995; 72:F3–7.

49. Messineo A, Forte V, Joseph T, et al. The balloon posterior tracheal split: a technique for managing tracheal stenosis in the premature infant. J Pediatr Surg 1992;27:1142–4.

50. Bagwell CE, Talbert JL, Tepas JJ. Balloon dilatation of long-segment tracheal stenoses. J Pediatr Surg 1991;26:153–9.

51. Tsui KY, Yu HR, Hwang KP, et al. When parents opted not to perform surgery for a long-segment congenital tracheal stenosis child: flexible bronchoscopic balloon tracheoplasty as the primary treatment. Eur J Cardiothorac Surg 2009;36:219–21.

52. McLaren CA, Elliott MJ, Roebuck M. Tracheobronchial intervention in children. Eur J Radiol 2005;53:22–34.

53. Clement WA, Geddes NK, Best C. Endoscopic carbon dioxide laser division of congenital complete tracheal rings: a new operative technique. Ann Thorac Surg 2005;79:687–9.

54. Blackmore K, Kubba H, Clement A. Laser division of congenital complete tracheal rings. Int J Pediatr Otorhinolaryngol 2010;74:1327–30.

55. Cheng W, Manson DE, Forte V, et al. The role of conservative management in congenital tracheal stenosis: an evidence-based long-term follow-up study. J Pediatr Surg 2006;41:1203–7.

The Business of Interventional Pulmonology

Christopher T. Erb, MD, PhD[a], Armin Ernst, MHCM, MD[b,c],
Gaëtane C. Michaud, MS, MD, FRCP(C)[a,*]

KEYWORDS

- Interventional pulmonology • Billing • Coding • Reimbursement • Practice building • Insurance

KEY POINTS

- Future changes are inevitable in funding and reimbursement arrangements.
- Understanding and effectively using the current systems of reimbursement is critical.
- It will be imperative for interventional pulmonology practices to be nimble and adapt to the changing landscape of medical need, legislative mandates, and reimbursement policy.
- Interventional pulmonologists are regularly asked to perform more complicated and advanced procedures, but the reimbursement for time, effort, and skill involved in these procedures has not kept up with reimbursement for other procedural specialties.

INTRODUCTION

Health care finance, in particular, reimbursement for services rendered, is complex and there are multiple means by which physicians are reimbursed for services. To appreciate the potential barriers to procedural reimbursement, it is essential to first understand the means by which care costs are currently being covered and then predict the impact of health care reform on the business of interventional pulmonology (IP).

INSURANCE AND HOW IT IMPACTS REIMBURSEMENT
Private Insurance

Most working Americans obtain health insurance through their employers in the form of an employment benefits package.[1] Employers and employees enjoy a tax advantage as a result of offering and receiving health insurance benefits through the employment relationship. Most employers offer their workers a selection of health insurance plans to choose from; these plans vary in scope of coverage, costs of premiums, and the amount of co-insurance and deductible to be paid by the employee.[2,3] Employers and employees generally share the costs of the insurance. Employer-provided group insurance usually costs less and offers more benefits than individual health insurance plans.

Employer-sponsored health insurance plans are typically either fee-for-service or various types of managed care plans (health maintenance organizations, HMOs, or preferred provider organizations). Fee-for-service insurance is a traditional form of health insurance in which, after providing health care services, the health care provider (or sometimes the patient) sends a bill to the insurance company. A typical fee-for-service plan may pay 80% of a medical bill, leaving 20% to be paid by the individual, known as "co-insurance," or may follow some other kind of prenegotiated payment arrangement. This form of insurance, which was also known as indemnity

[a] Pulmonary, Critical Care and Sleep Medicine, Yale School of Medicine, 20 York Street, New Haven, CT 06510, USA; [b] Pulmonary, Critical Care and Sleep Medicine, Tufts School of Medicine, Boston, MA, USA; [c] Reliant Medical Group, 100 Front Street, 14th Floor, Worcester, MA 01608, USA
* Corresponding author. Pulmonary, Critical Care and Sleep Medicine, Yale School of Medicine, 15 York Street, LCI 100-C, New Haven, CT 06510.
E-mail address: Gaetane.michaud@yale.edu

Clin Chest Med 34 (2013) 583–591
http://dx.doi.org/10.1016/j.ccm.2013.05.005
0272-5231/13/$ – see front matter © 2013 Elsevier Inc. All rights reserved.

insurance, declined sharply in the 1990s as various forms of managed care organizations were introduced into the health insurance marketplace.[4,5]

HMOs are prepaid health insurance plans to which members pay a monthly premium. In exchange, the HMO provides comprehensive coverage, including physician visits, hospital stays, laboratory tests, and therapy. In most HMOs, members are assigned or choose a physician who serves as their primary care physician. The primary care physician monitors the patient's health and provides basic medical care and is also responsible for referring patients to a specialist and other health care professionals as needed. Most HMOs do not require a deductible each year, but they do generally require a small copayment for each medical encounter. Because HMOs receive a fixed fee per member per month, they may focus more on providing preventative health care services, such as immunizations, mammograms, and physicals, and may be more restrictive of more advanced or experimental treatments. They may require "preauthorization" for advanced procedures. Procedures such as electromagnetic navigational bronchoscopy often fall into the category of "experimental" despite the growing evidence to support its use for peripheral nodules and the approval process may be challenging. Preferred provider organizations are a variation on HMOs that are generally less flexible than traditional fee-for-service insurance plans, but more flexible than HMOs in terms of restrictions on where and from whom patients can receive care.[6]

Medicare and Medicaid

Medicare and Medicaid are the 2 most important government-sponsored health insurance programs. Title XVIII of the Social Security Act of 1965 established Medicare. It is a federal health care program that covers most individuals 65 years or older as well as those under age 65 with certain disabilities, and patients of all ages requiring dialysis or renal transplant.

Medicare Part A provides basic coverage for hospital stays, posthospital skilled nursing facility care, home health care, and hospice care and is financed from employee and employer contributions. Medicare Part B is medical insurance, which can be purchased by paying an additional monthly premium. It pays for physician and laboratory costs as well as some outpatient medical services, such as medical equipment and supplies, home health care, and physical therapy. Medicare Part C is an alternative in which individuals with Parts A and B can voluntarily choose to receive all of their health care services from a Medicare-managed care plan provided through private insurance companies.[7,8] Medicare Part D is a voluntary supplemental prescription drug program that requires an additional monthly premium.

For the most part, Medicare makes payments to providers on a fee-for-service basis, but it negotiates deep discounts for many services and procedures compared with most private insurance plans. Some private insurance companies use similar relative value unitlike reimbursement schedules, as discussed in detail later in this article. Newer payment incentives are being proposed that would adjust payments by markers of quality, efficiency, and outcomes.

Medicaid, on the other hand, is a joint federal-state health insurance program for individuals and families with low incomes and limited resources.[9] Although the federal government establishes broad guidelines for the Medicaid program, each state establishes its own eligibility standards, benefit packages, payment rates, and program administration. As a result, there are essentially 56 different Medicaid programs—one for each state, territory, and the District of Columbia. Medicaid programs generally cover physician services, inpatient and outpatient hospital care, nursing facility services, prescription drugs, dental care, physical therapy, rehabilitation services, and hospice care. Medicaid also pays providers primarily on a fee-for-service basis after negotiated discounts. Payment rates vary on a state-by-state basis and may fail to cover the actual cost of an interventional pulmonary procedure.

REIMBURSEMENT FOR PULMONARY PROCEDURES

The most common means of reimbursement in North America is fee-for-service. In essence physicians are paid for each individual service rendered in this model of payment. Alternate means of reimbursement for physicians include relative value units (RVUs), capitation, pay for performance, and salary. In the advent of health care reform and cost containment in the United States and Canada, respectively, alternatives to fee-for-service are being sought and the means by which physicians will be reimbursed for services may be in flux over the next several years. Many provinces of Canada have alternate funding plans, a pay-for-performance-like incentive structure whereby physicians receive a base salary and in addition receive a performance-based incentive. The province negotiates salaries for various physician groups with the health care organization. In the United States, pay for performance, medical home, and accountable care organizations (ACO) are some of the alternatives currently being integrated as part of health care reform.

Pay for Performance

Pay for performance has many faces depending on the type of practice, but essentially it involves incentivizing physicians based on quality and/or efficiency metrics. There is ample evidence to suggest that more advanced training or subspecialization leads to better procedural outcomes, and this form of payment would potentially be favorable to interventional pulmonologists with specialized training who perform a higher volume of certain procedures, such as endobronchial ultrasound for lung cancer staging.[10–12] At present, no metrics or quality benchmarks have been established for interventional pulmonology; however, the AQuIRE initiative by the American College of Chest Physicians was established with this as a primary objective. In a pay-for-performance system, one might anticipate a financial disincentive for performing diagnostic procedures, such as transbronchial needle aspiration (TBNA) with less proficiency than an established minimal diagnostic yield.

Medical Home

With respect to medical home, this strategy takes a more holistic approach whereby the primary care physician plays a central role and manages the entire care team, including any required specialists.[13,14] Under the medical home arrangement, the interventional pulmonologist or thoracic surgeon would be invited to provide an episode of care or procedure for a patient and would be paid from funds controlled by the referring primary care physician. A prespecified sum is paid for the care of the patient and distributed by the medical home as appropriate. Disease-specific medical homes have also been proposed, particularly in the context of a complex chronic disease whereby the central physician would drive the care of the patient. One could imagine a lung cancer medical home with the pulmonologist or medical oncologist becoming a primary care of sorts and managing the disease-specific care of the patient, including testing, counseling, and therapy, provided by the patient's multidisciplinary team. The interventional pulmonologist or thoracic surgeon in this context could be either a team leader or alternatively a member of the multidisciplinary team and be compensated for their portion of the care provided by the service line. The idea of a more comprehensive "medical neighborhood" that would more seamlessly incorporate and integrate subspecialty care into the medical home has also been proposed.[15]

ACO

ACO are a form of managed care designed to promote quality and minimize cost.[16] Although on the surface this may seem similar to a HMO of the 1990s, it is a distinct model. In such a system, a network of physicians or an entire hospital would take responsibility for the care of a group of patients. They would assume both the clinical and the financial burden of their care. Quality metrics would be implemented and the cost of providing the care would be compared with that traditionally paid for by Medicare for the same care. Providers are incentivized if both the quality and the cost reduction targets are met. Incentives are in the form of a predetermined proportion of the cost savings. Models such as these promote cost-effective care and published/unpublished data would suggest that management of pleural disease, mediastinal staging, and lung nodules by intervention pulmonary procedures is cost-effective.[17–21] It is likely on this basis that centers such as Kaiser Permanente have expanded their services to include interventional pulmonary procedures. An ACO model may be advantageous in interventional pulmonology considering the relatively poor fee-for-service procedural reimbursement.

Fee for Service

Most centers in Canada and the United States are fee-for-service. In a fee-for-service model, the interventional pulmonologist, thoracic surgeon, or his/her surrogate negotiates with payers a fee for the procedure or episode of care based on a predetermined fee schedule. The fee schedule assigns an amount according to the current procedural terminology (CPT) code for said procedure. The major concerns with this model are 2-fold: (1) it incentivizes physicians to perform procedures to generate revenue and (2) it may not adequately compensate for physician time or be commensurate with the specialized skill/training necessary to perform the procedure proficiently. In Canada, additional monies may be allocated to physicians based on the time of day the procedure is performed or alternatively the time it takes to perform the procedure. Some interventional pulmonology procedures are subject to a global fee (ie, a single payment for the entire episode of care including the postprocedural management). Thoracoscopy falls into this category. Compensation for the same procedure is highly variable in a fee-for-service model depending on the payer. Self-pay and private insurance tend to reimburse much higher than Medicare or Medicaid for the same service. As stated, reimbursement is subject to discounts negotiated by the care facility and this may be a significant proportion of the billed service.

It is important for interventional pulmonologists to keep in mind the facility fees associated with the procedures as this significantly impacts the true cost of the procedure as well as downstream revenue. Those planning to establish a pulmonary procedure service or interventional pulmonary practice need to consider not simply the initial investment for equipment to perform procedures but also all the many direct and indirect costs. The direct costs of pulmonary procedures would include non-reusable materials, such as forceps, chest tubes, or transbronchial needles, equipment such as bronchoscopes, and labor (ie, the nursing or technical support in the procedure room). Indirect costs on the other hand would take into account the overhead incurred for the bronchoscopy suite and/or operating room. In addition, medicolegal support, maintenance, administration, billings, and collections are all considered indirect costs. The importance of considering all of the costs attributable to a procedure is that these are distributed over the entire patient population served by the interventional pulmonologist and highly influence the potential for downstream revenue generation.[22] There is a minimum number of procedures to be performed by any given institution to break even, and profit will be nonexistent until this threshold is met. Only once this threshold is exceeded does an interventional pulmonary practice become revenue-generating for its sponsoring institution. The breakeven point is individualized but should be considered before establishing a new pleural or bronchoscopy service line.

RVU

The RVU system is a scale used by Medicare and many private insurance companies to determine payments to providers. The scale is adjusted by the amount of physician work, practice expense, and professional liability coverage required to provide a given service.[23] A physician work RVU is assigned based on the amount of time, mental effort, and judgment, as well as technical skill and effort required to perform each service. Despite many advances in technology in interventional pulmonology, many of the assigned RVUs have remained stable. The practice expense component takes into account the nonphysician labor, building space, equipment, and supplies required to run a practice. The practice expense RVU payment value varies by the location where the procedure is being provided: if in a physician office or clinic, more of the infrastructure expense is incurred by the physician practice and the RVU is higher. On the contrary, when performed in a facility such as a hospital-based procedure center, the practice expense RVU is considerably lower because most of the infrastructure expense is embedded in the facility's costs, which in part explains the move in gastroenterology to provide procedural services in outside procedure centers or "surgi-centers."

Each procedure or service is assigned an RVU according to this scale, and payment is commensurate with the RVUs assigned. For example, the standard multiplier in 2013 is $34.023, which is flat from the 2012 value. A geographic practice cost index is applied to each service to account for regional differences in the cost of maintaining a practice and the variation in liability insurance. Physician work and practice expenses account for about 96% of the RVU payment and liability insurance for only 4%. **Table 1** provides a tabular representation of the RVU breakdown for commonly performed IP procedures.

CODING AND BILLING FOR PROCEDURAL SERVICES
CPT Codes

CPT codes are published by the American Medical Association (AMA) and are used to describe procedures and services for purposes of billing public and private health insurance companies.[24] There are 3 categories of CPT codes that are used in

Table 1
Examples of common IP procedures and their assigned RVUs

CPT Code	Procedure	Work RVU	Nonfacility RVU	Facility RVU	Malpractice
31622	Bronch with BAL	2.78	6.48	1.24	0.34
31628	Bronch with TBBx	3.36	6.56	1.40	0.31
31625	Bronch with EBBx	3.80	7.43	1.54	0.30
32555	Thoracentesis w/ U/S	2.27	16.70	0.80	0.23
32557	Chest tube w/ U/S	3.12	24.68	1.07	0.69

Abbreviations: BAL, bronchial alveolar lavage; Bronch, bronchoscopy; EBBx, endobronchial biopsy; TBBx, transbronchial biopsy; U/S, Ultrasound.

distinct ways by insurance companies. Category I codes describe commonly performed services and procedures that are well-established in medical practice in the United States and are Food and Drug Administration (FDA)-approved. Category II codes are used to track performance measures and are added to the main 5-digit category I CPT code but cannot be used alone. Category III codes are assigned to new or emerging technologies and procedures and are considered temporary. They will either lead to a full category I code within 5 years or they will disappear if the procedure does not come into widespread use or achieve FDA approval. Category III codes require documentation of safety and efficacy in the form of trials published in peer-reviewed literature, as well as support from practitioners in the field who are likely to provide the service or perform the procedure in question. Per HIPAA (Health Insurance Portability and Accountability Act) guidelines, insurance companies are not allowed to deny payment of category III codes. A set reimbursement is assigned to each code as well a commensurate RVU. **Table 2** lists commonly used CPT codes and

Table 2
Common CPT codes for pulmonary procedures and their work RVUs

Common CPT Codes for Pulmonary Procedures		
Procedure	CPT Code	Work RVU
Bronchoscopy	31622	2.78
Brushings	31623	2.88
BAL	31624	2.88
EBBx	31625	3.36
TBBx	31628	3.80
ENB	31627	2.00
TBNA	31629	4.09
EBUS	31620	1.42
Tracheal dilatation	31630	3.81
Stent placement	31631	4.36
Removal of FB	31635	3.67
Excision of tumor	31640	4.93
Destruction of tumor	31641	5.02
Therapeutic Aspiration	31645	3.16
Thoracentesis	32555/4 (with/without imaging)	2.27/2.50
Chest tube	32557/6 (with/without imaging)	2.50/3.12
Thoracostomy	32551	3.29
Tunneled pleural catheter	32550	4.17
Pleurodesis/instillation of thrombolytic	32560/32561	1.54/1.39
Pleuroscopy	32601	5.50
Tracheostomy	31600	7.17
Whole-lung lavage	32997	7.31
Pleuroscopy with pleurodesis	32650	10.83
New Codes for Emerging Procedures[25]		
Bronchial valves	31647	4.40
Bronchial thermoplasty	31660	4.25
Supplementary Codes		
Fluoro for Bronch	76496	0.00
Ultrasound guidance	76604	0.55
Moderate sedation	99144-99150	0.00

Abbreviations: BAL, bronchial alveolar lavage; Bronch, bronchoscopy; EBBx, endobronchial biopsy; EBUS, endobronchial ultrasound; ENB, Electronavigational bronchoscopy; FB, foreign body; TBBx, transbronchial biopsy; TBNA, transbronchial needle aspiration.

their accompanying work RVUs for pulmonary procedures. A comprehensive list and explanation of CPT billing codes for all pulmonary and critical care procedures are available from the American College of Chest Physicians.[26]

Modifiers to CPT Codes

A 2-digit modifier code may be added to the stem CPT code to indicate that a procedure was unusual, prolonged, or required some additional service or activity.

The modifier must be supported by documentation in the medical record of the specific circumstances that made the procedure nonstandard. Applying the modifier code will typically lead to higher reimbursement for that particular procedure.

There are 2 types of modifiers: level I, that are 2-digit numerical codes applied to the CPT codes issued by the AMA, and level II, that are alphanumeric codes applied to the Healthcare Common Procedure Coding System (HCPCS) codes issued by CMS.[24] The most common level I modifier codes used by interventional pulmonologists are listed in **Table 3** and include "25" for a "separately identifiable evaluation and management service by the same physician on the same day of the procedure or other service"; this may be applied when the IP physician performs an evaluation and management (E&M) on a patient on the same day that an IP procedure is performed. The modifier is

Table 3
Common CPT code level I modifiers used in interventional pulmonology

Common CPT Code Level I Modifiers Used in Interventional Pulmonology		
Modifier	**Technical Description**	**Common Scenario for Use**
22	Unusual Procedural Service	
25	Significant, separately identifiable evaluation and management service by the same physician on the same day of the procedure or other service	Initial patient evaluation in clinic followed by an interventional procedure on the same day
50	Bilateral procedure	Simultaneous bilateral thoracentesis
51	Multiple procedures	Thoracentesis followed by chest tube
53	Discontinued procedure	Unsuccessful procedure aborted for safety
57	Decision for surgery	Findings during IP procedure lead to plan to refer for surgery
58	Staged or related procedure or service by the same physician during the postoperative period	Conversion from one type of chest tube to another or pleuroscopy followed by chest tube placement
59	Distinct procedural service	Thoracentesis and bronchoscopy on the same day
73	Discontinued outpatient hospital/ ambulatory surgery center procedure before the administration of anesthesia	Patient arrives in ambulatory surgery center procedural center for planned procedure but reveals she has taken aspirin and Plavix that day and procedure is canceled before starting but after setting up
76/77	Repeat procedure by same/another physician	Second attempt at thoracentesis by IP physician after another physician's failed attempt
78	Return to the OR for a related procedure during the postoperative period	Return for adjustment of tracheal stent that has migrated
79	Unrelated procedure or service by the same physician during the postoperative period	Bronchoscopy for staging at one time followed by thoracentesis for relief of effusion at another time
AF	Specialty physician	When IP physician performs a procedure that a physician with less specialized training may also be qualified to perform but data support better outcomes with additional training

added to the E&M code rather than to the procedural code, which is important because the modifier increases the likelihood that both the E&M and the procedure will be reimbursed. The modifier does not guarantee full reimbursement; rather the most reliable strategy is to separate the clinical evaluation from the procedure by 2 business days such that the payer sees these as separate episodes of care. Other useful modifiers in IP practice include "51" for "multiple procedures" if, for example, an initial thoracentesis reveals an empyema and a subsequent chest tube placed the same day; or "57," "decision for surgery," which may be used if an initial thoracentesis reveals a highly loculated effusion and the patient then proceeds to thoracoscopy. The most commonly used level II code used by interventional pulmonologists is likely to be "AF" for specialty physician.

Documentation to Support Procedural Billing

All procedures performed by the interventional pulmonologist must be documented in detail in the medical record, including descriptions of usual circumstances or findings to justify any modifiers that are used.

Payment for image guidance for procedures, such as use of ultrasound for thoracentesis or endobronchial ultrasound for TBNA, requires the IP physician to save the image used to guide the procedure in the medical record. The electronic medical record used by the IP physician should have the capabilities to record, store, and retrieve those images. In addition, when performing procedures with add-on CPT codes, such as TBNA for multiple nodal stations, the aspiration of discreet nodes at multiple levels and the actual nodes sampled must be identified in the procedure report.

Applying for a New CPT Code for a New or Modified Procedure

CPT codes are updated each year by the AMA CPT Editorial Panel, which consists of CPT/HCPAC advisors.[24] New codes are added each year, especially in evolving fields like interventional pulmonology, but it may take several years from the introduction of a new technology in the clinical arena before it is recognized by the AMA CPT Editorial Panel.[27]

Individuals requesting CPT code modifications must submit applications along with supporting materials to the Editorial Panel at least 30 days before the annual meeting to be considered for inclusion in the following year's CPT Code book. Lobbying in the form of direct communication with CPT/HCPAC advisors on behalf of a code change request is not allowed. A detailed description of the application process is available on the AMA's web site.[28]

In order for a new CPT code to be approved, the procedure must meet certain fundamental criteria. It must be approved by the FDA; represent a distinct service that is not already available under a different CPT code or simply be a modification of an existing CPT code; be in widespread use across the United States; and its clinical efficacy must be documented in the peer-reviewed literature. An application to the AMA Editorial Panel for review of a proposed new CPT code must include (1) an executive summary of a literature review including at least 5 references, (2) financial disclosures, (3) review of available data on safety of the proposed procedure, (4) a complete CPT application packet, (5) data on physician work load and practice expenses related to the proposed procedure, (6) prices for supplies and devices, including invoices, and (7) references for those qualified to review the data on behalf of the panel.

SUMMARY

Future changes are inevitable in the funding and reimbursement arrangements discussed in this article. For those interested in establishing, expanding or optimizing their interventional pulmonology practice, understanding and effectively using the current systems of reimbursement are critical. However, it will also be imperative for IP practices to be nimble and adapt to the changing landscape of medical need, legislative mandates, and reimbursement policy. Interventional pulmonologists are regularly asked to perform more complicated and advanced procedures, but the reimbursement for time, effort, and skill involved in these procedures has not kept up with reimbursement for other procedural specialties.[29,30] In fact, in areas such as endobronchial ultrasound, reimbursement has decreased over the past several years.

The Affordable Care Act (ACA), passed in 2010 and currently under review in Congress, promises to introduce new incentives for quality and efficiency by rewarding quality outcomes. Much remains to be seen about how the ACA will affect interventional pulmonology, and many changes can be expected to the law before it is finally implemented.[31] It is expected, for example, that the ACA could benefit "interventionalists" through quality incentives for achieving better outcomes for the procedures they are highly trained to perform, as has been anticipated with the use of intensivist staffing of intensive care units.[32] On the other hand, IP procedures are inherently complex and commonly performed in very sick patients with advanced cancer or end-stage pulmonary disease. One could imagine that the disincentives proposed by the ACA for poor outcomes, complications, and readmissions may discourage interventional pulmonologists from caring for those in greatest need of palliation. On the other hand, it may also result in greater scrutiny and decrease "futile" procedures (ie, those done "just because you can and not because it is the right thing for the patient"). The addition of quality metrics may at some point also bring to light the additional liability of an interventional pulmonary practice, having the potential to in turn impact on professional responsibility premiums, further influencing revenue generation.

As the ACA comes on board in the next several years and introduces new incentives for quality and efficiency, interventional pulmonologists will want to be poised to capitalize on these incentives. Understanding the current landscape of the business of interventional pulmonology is crucial to ensure appropriate preparation and involvement in the direction of the future of the field.

REFERENCES

1. Frostin P. Sources of health insurance and characteristics of the uninsured: analysis of the March 2012 current population survey. EBRI Issue Brief 2012;(376):1–34.
2. Peele P. Employer-sponsored health insurance: are employers good agents for their employees? Milbank Q 2000;78(1):5–21.
3. Gabel J. Job-based health insurance in 2000: premiums rise sharply while coverage grows. Health Aff 2000;19(5):144–51.
4. Gabel J. Withering on the vine: the decline of indemnity health insurance. Health Aff 2000;19(5): 152–7.
5. Iglehart J. The struggle between managed care and fee-for-service practice. N Engl J Med 1994;331(1): 63–7.
6. Weiner JP, de Lissovoy G. Razing a tower of Babel: a taxonomy for managed care and health insurance plans. J Health Polit Policy Law 1993;18(1): 75–103.
7. Baker LC. Association of managed care market share and health expenditures for fee-for-service medicare patients. J Am Med Assoc 1999;281(5): 432–7.
8. Baker LC. The effect of HMOs on fee-for-service health care expenditures: evidence from Medicare. J Health Econ 1997;16:453–81.
9. Rosenbaum S. Medicaid and national health care reform. N Engl J Med 2009;361:2009–12.
10. Silvestri GA, Handy J, Lackland D, et al. Specialists achieve better outcomes than generalists for lung cancer surgery. Chest 1998;114(3):675–80.
11. Yarmus L, Pandian V, Gilbert C, et al. Safety and efficiency of interventional pulmonologists performing percutaneous tracheostomy. Respiration 2012;84:123–7.
12. Mirski MA, Pandian V, Bhatti N, et al. Safety, efficacy, and cost-effectiveness of a multidisciplinary percutaneous tracheostomy program. Crit Care Med 2012;40:1827–34.
13. Rittenhouse DR, Shortell SM. The patient-centered medical home: will it stand the test of health reform? J Am Med Assoc 2009;301(19):2038–40.
14. Rosenthal TC. The medical home: growing evidence to support a new approach to primary care. J Am Board Fam Med 2008;21(5):427–40.
15. Fisher ES. Building a medical neighborhood for the medical home. N Engl J Med 2008;359(12): 1202–5.
16. Ginsburg PB. Spending to save – ACOs and the Medicare shared savings program. N Engl J Med 2011;364:2085–6.
17. Ho C, Clark M, Argaez C. Endobronchial ultrasound for lung cancer diagnosis and staging: a review of the clinical and cost-effectiveness. Ottawa (Canada): Canadian Agency for Drugs and Technologies in Health; 2009.
18. Kunst P, Eberhardt R, Herth F, et al. Combined EBUS real time TBNA and conventional TBNA are the most cost-effective means of lymph node staging. J Bronchol 2008;15:17–20.
19. Harewood GC, Pascual J, Raimondo M, et al. Economic analysis of combined endocscopic and endobronchial ultrasound in the evaluation of patients with suspected non-small cell lunge cancer. Lung Cancer 2010;67:366–71.
20. Steinfort D, Liew D, Conron M, et al. Cost-benefit of minimally invasive staging of non-small cell lung cancer: a decision tree sensitivity analysis. J Thorac Oncol 2010;5(10):1564–70.
21. Medford A, Agrawal S, Free C, et al. A performance and theoretical costs analysis of endobronchial ultrasound-guided transbronchial needle aspiration in a UK tertiary respiratory centre. QJM 2009;102: 859–64.
22. Pastis N, Simkovich S, Silvestri G. Understanding the economic impact of introducing a new procedure: calculating downstream revenue of endobronchial ultrasound with transbronchial needle aspiration as a model. Chest 2012; 141(2):506–12.
23. Dummit LA. The Basics: Relative Value Units (RVUs). Policy Brief. George Washington University: The National Health Policy Forum; 2009.
24. Available at: http://www.cms.gov/Medicare/Coding/MedHCPCSGenInfo/. Accessed July 9, 2013.

25. Alan Plummer L. Coding & billing Quarterly. New York, NY: American Thoracic Society; 2012.

26. ACCP. Coding for chest medicine, 2013. Northbrook, IL: American College of Chest Physicians; 2013.

27. Edell E, Krier-Morrow D. Navigational bronchoscopy: overview of technology and practical considerations – new current procedural terminology codes effective 2010. Chest 2010;137(2):450–4.

28. Applying for CPT Codes. Available at: http://www.ama-assn.org/ama/pub/physician-resources/solutions-managing-your-practice/coding-billing-insurance/cpt.page.Accessed July 9, 2013.

29. Kovitz KL. From the president of the American Association of Bronchology, the future of interventional pulmonology. J Bronchol 2006;13(3):107–8.

30. Manaker S, Ernst A, Marcus L. Affording endobronchial ultrasound. Chest 2008;133(4):842–3.

31. McDonough JE. The road ahead for the Affordable Care Act. N Engl J Med 2012; 367(3):199–201.

32. Logani S, Green A, Gasperino J. Benefits of high-intensity intensive care unit physician staffing under the Affordable Care Act. Crit Care Res Pract 2011; 2011:170814.

Quality-of-life Improvement and Cost-effectiveness of Interventional Pulmonary Procedures

Nicholas J. Pastis, MD[a,b,c,*], Gerard A. Silvestri, MD[a,b,c],
Ray Wesley Shepherd, MD[a,c]

KEYWORDS

- Quality of life • Interventional pulmonology • Cost-effectiveness • Health care resources

KEY POINTS

- For nearly all pulmonary procedures, data exist on quality of life and cost-effectiveness and much of it favors emerging, less invasive technologies.
- Although some studies use rigorous methodology to assess this aspect of care, many do not.
- There are few prospective comparative effectiveness trials that incorporate quality of life and cost data collection at the beginning of the trial for analysis and interpretation at the end.
- Instruments to assess quality of life and cost-effectiveness already exist such that there is no need to reinvent them in the interventional pulmonology space.
- With shrinking health care resources, regulatory agencies and hospitals will demand that new technology not only produce the expected clinical benefit and improve quality of life but that they do so at a reasonable cost compared with existing technologies.

As the breadth of procedural capabilities among interventional pulmonologists (IPs) has expanded, studies have consistently documented the technical success of the procedures. Meanwhile, outcome data on quality of life (QoL) among patients undergoing these procedures has been scant.[1–3] Most studies of interventional pulmonary procedures have reported endoluminal patency, pulmonary function testing, performance scores, or dyspnea scores.[4] These studies have been small and have not been well controlled. Performance status or dyspnea scores reflect patients' perspectives and are probably better surrogate measures, although they are still not validated mechanisms to measure QoL.[5]

Although more than 50 instruments exist for measuring QoL in patients with lung cancer,[5] the European Organization for Research and Treatment of Cancer (EORTC) Quality of Life Questionnaire (QLQ-C30) and its lung cancer–specific supplementary questionnaire (QLC-LC13) are widely used and well documented in studies of

Disclosures: N.J. Pastis has no conflicts of interest to disclose. G.A. Silvestri serves as a consultant to Bronchus Technology, Allegro Diagnostics, and Olympus Corporation. R.W. Shepherd serves as a paid consultation to Boston Scientific.
^a Division of Pulmonary, Critical Care, Allergy, and Sleep Medicine, Medical University of South Carolina, 96 Jonathan Lucas Street, 812 CSB, Charleston, SC 29425, USA; ^b Division of Pulmonary and Critical Care Medicine, Medical University of South Carolina, 96 Jonathan Lucas Street, 812 CSB, Charleston, SC 29425, USA; ^c Division of Pulmonary Disease and Critical Care Medicine, Virginia Commonwealth University Medical Center, Box 980050, Richmond, VA 23298, USA
* Corresponding author. Division of Pulmonary and Critical Care Medicine, Medical University of South Carolina, 96 Jonathan Lucas Street, 812 CSB, Charleston, SC 29425.
E-mail address: pastisn@musc.edu

Clin Chest Med 34 (2013) 593–603
http://dx.doi.org/10.1016/j.ccm.2013.03.005
0272-5231/13/$ – see front matter © 2013 Elsevier Inc. All rights reserved

QoL.[5–10] The questionnaire comprises 5 functional scales (physical, role, emotional, social, and cognitive functioning), 3 symptom scales (fatigue, pain, and nausea/vomiting), a global health status/QoL scale, and multiple single items assessing additional symptoms and perceived financial impact. Such a scale is well suited for interventional pulmonary procedures performed on patients with cancer. However, for patients without malignancy, other QoL scales should be used, for example, the Asthma Quality of Life Questionnaire (AQLQ) to evaluate patients undergoing bronchial thermoplasty.

Cost-effectiveness is a systematic approach to assess the relative value of health care interventions. Constraints on health care spending have led to strong incentives to set priorities among health care expenditures. In general, a clinical intervention can be classified along a spectrum measuring cost and benefit. At one end are interventions that provide benefit at no additional cost, and at the other end are services with a cost but no benefit. In the middle are interventions with potential benefit at some additional cost, and that zone is the focus of cost-effectiveness analysis.[11,12]

To perform a cost-effectiveness analysis, the cost of procedures should be compared with outcomes measured in natural units. However, traditional units such as cost per life saved or life-year gained may not apply to palliative procedures or ones that only improve symptoms in chronic diseases. So it is more appropriate to analyze cost-efficacy for IP procedures in terms of cost per symptom-free day, per day free of emergency room (ER) visit, or per day not requiring expensive intensive care unit (ICU) care.

The subspecialty interventional pulmonology has expanded through endoscopy, guided-bronchoscopy software, and new devices such as bronchial thermoplasty and endobronchial valve therapy. IPs routinely perform invasive pleural procedures and percutaneous tracheostomies safely and effectively.[13] Although the technical success of interventional pulmonary procedures is well documented, this article discusses how these procedures affect QoL and cost-effectiveness.

RELIEF OF CENTRAL AIRWAY OBSTRUCTION

The IP encounters central airway obstruction (CAO) as a result of tumors obstructing the central airways (trachea or main bronchi) or, less commonly, nonmalignant conditions or iatrogenic strictures of the trachea (ie, from prolonged endotracheal tube intubation or tracheostomies). Patients are typically referred because they are inoperable from a cancer standpoint or are unfit for surgery because of extensive medical comorbidities. In the case of lung cancer, CAO is a potentially devastating consequence of up to 30% of patients,[14] and can present with disabling dyspnea, massive hemoptysis, postobstructive pneumonia, or near death from suffocation. Although IP procedures may not alter overall mortality, they can palliate these symptoms to improve QoL.

Rigid bronchoscopy plays a pivotal role in the management of these patients and allows for endobronchial ablation techniques and stent placement. Although flexible bronchoscopy may be used in some cases or may complement rigid bronchoscopy, rigid bronchoscopy is recommended when loss of airway is a concern because it allows for the use of larger instruments, more effective suctioning, and control of the airway for ventilation during the procedure. Because rigid bronchoscopy is combined with ablative techniques and stenting in most cases of CAO, the major studies that relate to QoL typically evaluate rigid bronchoscopy and an ablative technique together. The major benefits of these procedures are relief, prevention, or delay of the following: acute respiratory distress, the need for mechanical ventilation, or death by suffocation. Although patients with benign diseases have a chance for cure, most patients with advanced lung cancer are not candidates for curative resection. In such cases, the goal is to extend and improve QoL by palliating symptoms.

Colt and Harrell[1] evaluated 32 patients admitted to the ICU with acute respiratory failure caused by CAO. There were 19 patients who required emergent endotracheal intubation. The 32 patients underwent rigid bronchoscopy with neodymium-yttrium-aluminum-garnet (Nd:YAG) laser resection and/or silicone stent placement. Partial or total airway patency was achieved in all patients. Although not directly measured, QoL was expected to improve because mechanical ventilation was successfully discontinued in 10 of the 19 patients who were intubated (52.6%), and 20 of 32 patients (62.5%) were transferred to a lower level of care immediately after the intervention.[1]

If health care use can be considered a surrogate for measuring cost-effectiveness, this study showed a favorable impact of rigid bronchoscopy on the following metrics: extubation or decannulation of patients with previously indwelling airways, successful removal of patients from mechanical ventilation, and alteration of the patient's previous level of care (postprocedural transfer to the hospital ward or to the ward of a skilled nursing facility). The daily hospital charge for mechanical ventilation and ICU hospitalization was approximately twice that of a single rigid bronchoscopy procedure with stent placement, and the daily cost of a bed in the ICU was approximately 3.5 times greater than the daily cost of a semiprivate or private room.[1]

Other studies of patients with CAO on mechanical ventilation who underwent rigid bronchoscopies showed favorable results. For example, Stanopoulos and colleagues[15] reported their experience in treating 17 patients on mechanical ventilation for malignant CAO. Patients received mechanical ventilation for 1 to 25 days before intervention. They underwent rigid bronchoscopy with Nd:YAG laser resection, and 9 of the 17 patients were successfully extubated. Median survival was 98 days (range 5–770 days) for successfully extubated patients versus 8.5 days (range 1–15 days) for patients who were unable to be liberated from mechanical ventilation.[15]

In a prospective cohort study by Oviatt and colleagues,[16] exercise capacity, lung function, and QoL were evaluated after interventional bronchoscopy. Patients with high-grade central malignant airway obstruction underwent rigid bronchoscopy with stenting, electrocautery, and/or mechanical resection with the rigid bronchoscope. Unlike other reports suggesting subjective improvements in dyspnea after IP procedures, this study confirmed this improvement by using objective, validated QoL questionnaires.

Thirty-seven patients were assessed with spirometry, 6-minute walk testing (6MWT), and QoL and dyspnea questionnaires (EORTC QLQ-C30 and Lung Cancer Module [LC13]) were performed at baseline and at 30, 90, and 180 days after the procedure. There was an increase in 6MWT by 99.7 m (95% confidence interval [CI] 33.2–166.2 m, $P = .002$), forced expiratory volume in 1 second by 448 mL (95% CI 203–692 mL, $P<.001$), and forced vital capacity by 416 mL (95% CI 130–702 mL, $P = .003$) seen at day 30 compared with baseline. Clinically and statistically significant improvements were noted in composite dyspnea scores at day 30 by both QLQ-C30 (decrease of 39.9, 95% CI 21.4–58.4, $P<.001$) and LC13 (decrease of 28.2, 95% CI 12.9–43.5, $P<.001$) questionnaires. These decreases were on 100-point scales and correlated with "Moderate" to "Very much" in terms of patient-perceived degree of improvement.[16] A change of 5 is considered the minimal clinically important difference.[17]

Amjadi and colleagues prospectively assessed the effect of interventional procedures on the overall QoL of patients with lung cancer with inoperable CAO using the EORTC QLQ-C30. Rigid bronchoscopies were performed and included Nd:YAG laser, cryotherapy, mechanical dilation, and mechanical resection using the tip of the bronchoscope or biopsy forceps, and/or stenting. Among 20 participants analyzed, improvement in airway diameter was achieved in all patients, and more than 80% patency was established in 80% (16/20) of the patients. Dyspnea was assessed by the Borg scale before and 1 day after the procedure. Borg scores improved in 85% of participants ($P = .01$). Thirteen patients achieved an improvement in QoL, although, for the group as a whole, QoL scores remained stable.[18] This study highlights the problem with using dyspnea as a proxy for QoL. Many patients undergoing these procedures for CAO may subsequently deteriorate as a result of nonrespiratory causes such as spread of cancer outside the tracheobronchial tree, loss of appetite, pain, or other comorbidities.

It is important for the interventional pulmonologist to possess a full complement of bronchoscopic approaches to control endobronchial symptoms and improve QoL. Brachytherapy offers several advantages compared with other methods. It can be used to treat endobronchial tumors in areas not accessible to other treatment modalities (ie, upper-lobe bronchi and segmental bronchi). In addition, the biological effect of radiation may allow control of tumor regrowth for a longer period of time than with most other ablative techniques performed via the bronchoscope.[19] In a Cochrane systematic review of all 13 randomized controlled trials on the subject, Cardona and colleagues[20] concluded that x-ray therapy (XRT) was superior to endobronchial brachytherapy (EBBT) for initial palliation of symptoms. However, brachytherapy may be especially useful in patients with endobronchial obstruction who previously received thoracic XRT, in patients who are poor candidates for thoracic XRT because of severe underlying lung disease, or in cases of distal airway obstruction by intraluminal tumor that cannot be easily treated by other ablative procedures or by stenting.

In an analysis by Mallick and colleagues[19] of patients with locally advanced lung cancer who received EBBT, 45 patients completed EORTC QLQ-C30 and LC13 questionnaires. One month following EBBT, there were statistically significant improvements in EORTC QLQ-C30 outcomes relevant to the patient population and the EBBT that was received (physical functioning, role functioning, social functioning, fatigue, and dyspnea) and in LC13 outcomes (dyspnea, cough, and hemoptysis).

With other endobronchial modalities available, brachytherapy may not be the first option to the interventional pulmonologist, but it has a niche and should be considered in special circumstances. It also is a viable option at medical centers without

IPs when the option for the patient to travel is limited.

ENDOBRONCHIAL ULTRASOUND–TRANSBRONCHIAL NEEDLE ASPIRATION

Endobronchial ultrasound (EBUS)–transbronchial needle aspiration (TBNA) has proved to be perhaps the greatest breakthrough for bronchoscopy in the past decade. It can diagnose and stage lung cancer and lymphoma, diagnose sarcoidosis, and evaluate lymph node stations previously inaccessible without mediastinoscopy, which has a small but significant risk of morbidity and mortality.[21–28] In patients undergoing diagnostic and/or staging work-ups, EBUS offers a safer procedure that is minimally invasive and can be performed without general anesthesia or a surgical incision. Serious complications caused by EBUS-TBNA are exceedingly rare, and most studies do not report any.[29]

When used to stage lung cancer, EBUS has been shown to prevent unnecessary thoracotomies. In a multicenter randomized controlled trial, Annema and colleagues[2] evaluated 241 patients with resectable (suspected) non-small cell lung cancer (NSCLC) in whom mediastinal staging was indicated (Assessment of Surgical Staging vs Endoscopic Ultrasound in Lung Cancer: a Randomized Clinical Trial [ASTER trial]). Patients underwent surgical staging or combined endoscopic ultrasound/EBUS with surgical staging only if negative. Thoracotomy was unnecessary in 18% of the mediastinoscopy group versus 7% in the endosonography group.

Using results from the ASTER randomized controlled trial, Sharples and colleagues[30] showed that patients in the endosonography arm had a greater EQ-5D (European Quality of Life-5 Dimensions) utility at the end of staging (0.117; 95% CI 0.042–0.192; $P = .003$). The 6-month cost of the endosonography strategy was £9713 (95% CI £7209 to £13,307) per patient versus £10,459 (£7732 to £13,890) for the surgical arm, mean difference £746 (95% CI -£756 to £2494). The mean difference in quality-adjusted life-year was 0.015 (95% CI -0.023–0.052) in favor of endosonography, and this strategy was more cost-effective than the surgical arm.

In a decision tree sensitivity analysis, Steinfort and colleagues[31] compared the unit cost estimates in Australian dollars (AU$) of EBUS-TBNA with surgical confirmation of negative EBUS results (AU$2961), EBUS-TBNA with no surgical confirmation of negative EBUS results (AU$33,440), conventional TBNA (AU$3754), and mediastinoscopy (AU$8859). EBUS-TBNA (with negative results being surgically confirmed) was the most cost-effective approach compared with other methods for mediastinal staging.

Although conventional TBNA was cheaper to perform than EBUS-TBNA, the lower sensitivity and negative predictive value of conventional TBNA translated into more patients who required confirmatory mediastinoscopies in this study. Although the need for surgical confirmation after negative EBUS-TBNA has been challenged,[29,32–35] the results of this study suggest that it remains cost-effective to confirm negative results, particularly in patients in whom positron emission tomography/computed tomography (CT) suggests lymph node metastasis. However, this issue may vary among institutions and may depend on the mode of noninvasive staging.[36,37]

Other studies have performed cost analysis of the various approaches to mediastinal staging of NSCLC. Despite differing prevalence of lymph node metastasis and differing sensitivity for EBUS-TBNA among the studies, EBUS-TBNA was the most cost-effective approach to mediastinal staging in NSCLC.[38–40]

Despite the cost-effectiveness of EBUS-TBNA, many hospital systems struggle with the decision of whether to initiate an EBUS program because of the capital investment and poor reimbursements. In certain situations, calculating procedural reimbursement alone grossly underestimates the economic impact of EBUS-TBNA. Downstream revenue has been defined by administrators as revenue captured after patients use one hospital service and then use others. Taking potential downstream revenue into account may provide justification for the capital investment. In a report of one medical center's experience, the presence of EBUS-TBNA drew patients to the hospital system from outside the typical referral base, many of whom stayed in the system and led to significant downstream revenue. There may also be intangible benefits such as marketing for the institution and capturing patients into the system who would otherwise have been treated elsewhere.[41]

GUIDED BRONCHOSCOPY

In the National Lung Cancer Screening Trial, lung cancer–specific mortality was reduced through CT screening of at-risk persons.[42] It is predicted that the number of patients diagnosed with pulmonary nodules could increase substantially if lung cancer screening with CT is broadly accepted. Transthoracic needle aspiration (TTNA) has traditionally been the preferred procedure because of a high diagnostic yield (90%). However, the pneumothorax rate is not trivial and has been estimated as high as 25%[43,44] to 43%.[45] More recently, Wiener and colleagues[46] evaluated the population-based risk for complications after TTNA of pulmonary nodules in 15,865 patients. Although hemorrhage was rare, complicating 1% (95% CI, 0.9%–1.2%) of biopsies, the risk of pneumothorax was 15% (95% CI, 14%–16%) and 6.6% (95% CI, 6%–7.2%) of all biopsies resulted in pneumothorax requiring a chest tube.

Guided bronchoscopy includes a variety of techniques (electromagnetic navigation, virtual bronchoscopy, radial EBUS, ultrathin bronchoscope, and guide sheath) and provides an alternative to TTNA for diagnosing pulmonary nodules. In a meta-analysis of 24 guided-bronchoscopy studies (1987 total patients), the pooled diagnostic yield was 70%, and the overall adverse event rate was 1.6% (n = 32) with most being pneumothoraces. Thirty-one patients (1.6%) developed a pneumothorax (range 0%–7.5% across studies), and, of those, 14 (0.7%) required chest tube placement.[47]

Although QoL and cost-effectiveness have not been directly compared between guided bronchoscopy and TTNA, the yield of guided bronchoscopy is reasonable and it can prevent costly and potentially life-threatening pneumothorax, particularly in high-risk patients (ie, those with bullous emphysema or more central nodules). It should at least be considered in such patients as a means to reduce pneumothorax risk and prevent hospitalizations to manage complications. A multicenter, prospective, randomized controlled trial to directly compare guided bronchoscopy with TTNA is needed to help determine the optimal use, cost-effectiveness, and effect on QoL of guided technologies.

BRONCHIAL THERMOPLASTY

Bronchial thermoplasty (BT) is a novel treatment of severe asthma in patients with persistent symptoms despite maximal medical therapy. The procedure involves bronchoscopy in 3 separate sessions to deliver controlled radiofrequency thermal energy to the bronchial walls with the goal of reducing airway smooth muscle mass. Although there are few available data regarding cost-effectiveness specifically, clinical trials to date have shown an improved QoL, reduced symptoms, reduction in the rate of severe exacerbations, fewer emergency department visits, and fewer days lost from school or work.[3,48,49]

Cox and colleagues[48] reported the Asthma Intervention Research (AIR) Trial Study Group data with 112 patients with moderate to severe persistent asthma randomized to BT versus control group. QoL measurements included the AQLQ, Asthma Control Questionnaire (ACQ), symptom scores,

and symptom-free days. At 12 months there were significantly greater improvements in the BT group compared with controls in ACQ (reduction 1.2 ± 1.0 vs 0.5 ± 1.0), AQLQ (1.3 ± 1.0 vs 0.6 ± 1.1), symptom scores (reduction 1.9 ± 2.1 vs 0.7 ± 2.5), and percentage of symptom-free days (40.6% ± 39.7% vs 17.0% ± 37.9%). However, this study lacked a sham arm and was not blinded.

QoL measurements were also among the outcomes reported in the smaller Research in Severe Asthma (RISA) trial of BT in patients with severe symptomatic asthma. Although only 15 patients were treated with BT, the study group showed improved AQLQ and ACQ change from baseline scores versus 17 control patients at 22 weeks and 1-year follow-up. However, there were no significant differences in symptom scores or symptom-free days.[49]

Castro and colleagues[3] published the definitive study on BT by using a randomized, double-blind, sham-controlled design enrolling 288 subjects with severe persistent asthma in the AIR2 study. The primary outcome was the difference in AQLQ scores from baseline to average of 6, 9, and 12 months (integrated AQLQ). The improvement from baseline in the integrated AQLQ score was superior in the BT group compared with sham (BT, 1.35 ± 1.10; sham, 1.16 ± 1.23). Seventy-nine percent of BT and 64% of sham subjects achieved changes in AQLQ of 0.5 or greater. In the posttreatment period (6–52 weeks after BT), the BT group experienced fewer severe exacerbations, emergency department (ED) visits, and days missed from work/school compared with the sham group. Other QoL-related outcomes such as symptom scores, symptom-free days, and ACQ scores did not differ significantly between treatment and control groups.[3] To summarize, the clinical outcomes with BT at 1 year included the following: improved asthma-related QoL; 32% decrease in severe exacerbations; 84% reduction in ER visits for respiratory symptoms; reduction in hospitalization for respiratory symptoms; and fewer days lost from work, school, and other daily activities because of asthma. Improving health-related QoL is an important goal of asthma management,[48,49] and the AQLQ is a validated tool for measuring the impact of asthma and evaluating outcomes of various therapies.[48]

None of the published BT literature has addressed cost-effectiveness specifically. As with other asthma studies, the AIR2 trial found that improved QoL was associated with eliminating costly ED visits.[3,48,49] Patients with severe uncontrolled asthma represent a large percentage of health care use and cost.[48,50] Improved asthma control is not only cost-effective through lowering the economic burden of excessive ED visits and hospitalizations but also through lessening the economic losses to society and the individual caused by lost productivity. Asthma is the fourth leading cause of work absenteeism for adults and results in approximately 15 million missed or less productive workdays per year.[48]

Although it might seem intuitive that reduced ED visits and decreased hospitalizations would improve asthma management cost-effectiveness, this must be balanced with short-term increases in health care use seen in patients having BT who are assessed in appropriate cost analysis–focused studies.

ENDOBRONCHIAL VALVES

The National Emphysema Treatment Trial (NETT) showed improved exercise capacity in patients with severe emphysema undergoing surgical lung volume reduction (LVR) versus medical management in the control group. The major mortality benefit was seen in patients with low baseline exercise capacity and predominantly upper-lobe emphysema.[51] However, the significant morbidity and mortality and prolonged hospital stay with high costs have limited enthusiasm and availability of this surgery over the last decade. This trend has prompted numerous investigations into techniques of bronchoscopic LVR that would potentially be less invasive and show less morbidity and mortality compared with surgical LVR. Studied techniques include blocking devices such as spigots or unidirectional valves, extra-anatomic bypass tracts, sealants, coils, and heated vapor.[52] Although several of these devices and techniques have shown QoL improvements such as improved dyspnea scores or exercise tolerance, few conclusions can be made because none of these techniques at this point have achieved sufficient benefit to obtain approval in the United States for bronchoscopic LVR. There are no clinical trials directly comparing surgical LVR with bronchoscopic techniques regarding cost or other outcomes.

In addition to bronchoscopic LVR, some of these technologies have been applied as experimental treatments for prolonged air leaks in patients having thoracic surgery or other forms of bronchopleural or alveolar-pleural fistula. Varela and colleagues[53] estimated additional hospital costs attributable to prolonged air leak in patients having lobectomy. Prolonged air leak was seen in 23 out of 238 surgical lobectomies, with a mean length of stay of 10 days versus 5 days for those without prolonged air leak. Total additional health care costs attributable to prolonged air leak were estimated to be €39,437.39. The endobronchial valve (Spiration Inc, Redmond, WA) did not meet approval criteria for bronchoscopic LVR but did receive approval by the US Food and Drug Administration as a humanitarian device for prolonged air leaks following lobectomy, segmentectomy, and surgical LVR.[54] A small multicenter series of 7 patients with a median duration of air leak of 4 weeks underwent endobronchial valve placement with a median postprocedure air leak duration of 1 day and hospital discharge in 2 to 3 days in 57% of the patients following the procedure.[55] Although there was no control group, the rapid air leak resolution after a prolonged course suggests an improved length of stay and cost savings. However, additional cost focused studies are necessary to definitively address this issue.

PERCUTANEOUS DILATATIONAL TRACHEOTOMY

Percutaneous dilatational tracheotomy (PDT) has gained favor compared with traditional surgical tracheotomy during the last 15 years and has become the procedure of choice in many institutions. Numerous studies have compared PDT with the surgical technique in terms of complications. Advantages of PDT often cited include less infection and bleeding, smaller incision, faster procedure time, and avoiding transfer of critically ill patients to the operating room. A recent meta-analysis found statistically significant advantages of PDT compared with open surgical techniques for overall complications, procedure length, scarring, and cost.[56]

Although the literature comparing complications of PDT with the surgical technique continues to develop, there has been little examination of PDT as it affects QoL. This omission is understandable because patients having tracheotomy are often critically ill and unable to participate in this type of data collection. Antonelli and colleagues[57] conducted a randomized controlled trial comparing surgical tracheotomy with the Fantoni percutaneous translaryngeal (FTLT) tracheotomy. Although FTLT is an uncommonly performed type of PDT, patients were followed for 1 year and were interviewed using the Short Form 12 Health Survey to rate perceptions of health and QoL. At 1 year, only 27% of the study population was alive and 18 patients having FTLT and 13 patients having surgical tracheotomy were interviewed and examined. There was no statistically significant difference in physical health or emotional health subscores of the Short Form 12 QoL assessment between the 2 groups. Low scores overall were closely related to the tracheostomy still being present. One additional study retrospectively reviewed long-term results after surgical tracheotomy or PDT. This study included a subjective patient standardized questionnaire. Overall patient satisfaction was higher in the PDT group mainly because of superior cosmetic results, with a smaller scar in the PDT group.[58]

Studies of PDT cost-effectiveness have been more common and among some of the first published studies regarding this technique. In 1995, Barba and colleagues[59] compared 21 surgical tracheotomy procedures in the operating room with 27 patients having PDT performed both in the operating room and ICU. Hospital charges were $3400 less for PDT in the ICU compared with surgical tracheotomy in the operating room. In a retrospective review, 65 patients having PDT with the Ciaglia technique (Cook Bloomington, Indiana) without bronchoscopy were compared with surgical controls. Mean patient charges for PDT in the ICU were significantly lower compared with standard surgical tracheotomy in the operating room or PDT performed in the operating room. This finding represented a saving of $1645 for performing PDT or surgical tracheotomy in the ICU.[60]

Financial analysis of PDT has also been performed in specific patient populations. A retrospective review of patients having cardiac surgery examined 59 surgical tracheotomies performed in the operating room and 27 PDT procedures using the Blue Rhino kit (Cook Bloomington, Indiana) performed with bronchoscopy in the ICU. Because the median ICU length of stay was 1 day less for PDT versus surgical tracheotomy in the operating room, the investigators estimated a saving of $84,000 in 1 year based on the volume of PDT at their institution.[61] The shorter ICU length of stay in the PDT group was likely attributable to faster scheduling time outside the operating room.

A meta-analysis of open surgical tracheotomy compared with PDT reviewed 15 published studies for a variety of variables. Four of the studies included cost-effectiveness data with a total of 161 patients in the PDT group and 158 in the open surgical group. The overall pooled result showed a PDT cost advantage of $456.61 compared with the open surgical technique (P<.0001).[62] The overall financial impact of a PDT program at a large university hospital was studied comparing the impact of the formal PDT program compared with the previous PDT practice and with surgical tracheotomy procedures. The analysis did not directly compare the cost of an individual surgical tracheotomy versus PDT and it is possible that the cost-effectiveness of a single PDT in this setting was reduced because of the use of an anesthesiologist at every PDT procedure. However, in analyzing length of stay and estimating back-fill of ICU beds, additional revenue from incremental admissions and surgical procedures could be estimated. The overall net cost-benefit of a designated PDT program to the medical center for 1 year was estimated to be $1,308,949.[62]

Although most cost-effectiveness studies show an advantage of PDT compared with surgical tracheotomy in the operating room, Massick and colleagues[63] compared PDT with bedside surgical tracheotomy and operating room surgical tracheotomy in a randomized prospective trial of 164 patients. Either method of bedside tracheotomy had a significant reduction in cost compared with the operating room procedure. However, open surgical tracheotomy at the bedside was $436 cheaper per procedure than PDT at the bedside. This finding was mostly caused by the additional cost of the bronchoscopy used with PDT. In a more detailed cost analysis, Grover and colleagues[64] also compared PDT in the ICU with surgical tracheotomy in the ICU and surgical tracheotomy in the operating room. Operating room tracheotomy increased cost compared with bedside procedures by $2194 and the open surgical bedside technique resulted in a cost saving of $180 per procedure compared with bedside PDT. This cost saving with the bedside surgical technique was even greater if the additional cost of bronchoscopy associated with PDT was included.

TUNNELED PLEURAL CATHETERS

Tunneled pleural catheters (TPC) are used frequently for recurrent malignant pleural effusions, particularly in patients whose functional status may not be suitable for surgical pleurodesis. There has also recently been increased use in patients with benign pleural disease, although the efficacy and safety in the nonmalignant population are unclear.[65] The primary role of TPCs is to improve dyspnea and possibly lead to pleurodesis and resolution of the effusion in some patients.

Most published TPC studies are case series, one of the largest of which involved 250 TPC procedures in 223 patients. Although there was no control group, symptom control for dyspnea was rated by the patients as complete in 38.8%, partial in 50%, and no improvement in 3.6%. The remainder consisted of failed catheter insertions or lack of follow-up. Thus 96.1% of successfully inserted TPCs resulted in complete or partial symptom control using a strict definition of complete control to avoid bias.[66] In a large systematic review, Van Meter and colleagues[67] reviewed 19 TPC studies with 1370 patients, of whom 1348 had malignant pleural effusions. Although symptom measurements and patient populations were diverse,

95.6% of patients had symptomatic improvement with TPC placement, including patients with trapped lung. One of the studies included used Borg scores and the Guyatt Chronic Respiratory Questionnaire, showing similar symptomatic improvement after treatment with doxycycline pleurodesis via tube thoracostomy compared with TPC placement. There was little reporting among the studies of other specific QoL measurements.

Most recently, the Second Therapeutic Intervention in Malignant Effusion (TIME2) trial compared TPCs with chest tube with talc pleurodesis in 106 patients with malignant pleural effusion included in the primary analysis. There was no significant difference in dyspnea between the two groups in the first 42 days and there was significant improvement in dyspnea in the TPC group at 6 months using a visual analog scale. This study is one of few to also examine specific QoL measurements. There was no significant difference in QoL between the two groups at any time point in follow-up using the EORTC QLQ-30.[68] This study showed that both TPCs and chest tube talc pleurodesis are effective at relieving dyspnea and improving QoL, but TPCs are not superior to talc pleurodesis for these outcomes.

There are limited cost-effectiveness data for TPCs. The ability to perform TPC placement on an outpatient basis suggests that the procedure would be cheaper than inpatient options such as surgical or tube thoracostomy pleurodesis. However, the long-term costs of TPC, including disposable drainage supplies and outpatient follow-up visits, must be considered. Olden and Holloway[69] compared outpatient TPC with talc slurry pleurodesis using a decision analysis cost model showing that talc slurry pleurodesis was slightly less expensive than TPC, but TPC became more cost-effective if life expectancy was less than 6 weeks. Puri and colleagues[70] also used a decision analysis model to compare cost-effectiveness of repeat thoracentesis, TPC, bedside pleurodesis, and thoracoscopic pleurodesis. TPC was the preferred treatment of malignant effusion and limited survival. Bedside pleurodesis was more cost-effective for those with prolonged survival (12 months).

PLEUROSCOPY

Pleuroscopy or medical thoracoscopy is used primarily for parietal pleural biopsy in the setting of unexplained exudative effusions or for chemical pleurodesis of recurrent pleural effusions. Other expanded indications have included treatment of recurrent pneumothorax, sympathectomy, and in the management of parapneumonic effusions.

There has been little formal study of QoL parameters as they relate directly to pleuroscopy, including a lack of randomized trials comparing medical thoracoscopy with surgical thoracoscopy and quality outcomes.

Cost-effectiveness data for medical thoracoscopy are equally limited. Although it seems logical that medical thoracoscopy performed under local or moderate sedation would potentially be more cost-effective than video-assisted thoracoscopic surgery performed under general anesthesia in the operating room, this has not been formally studied. Medical thoracoscopy with aerosolized talc pleurodesis has been compared with chest tube drainage in the setting of primary spontaneous pneumothorax in 108 randomized patients. The cost of hospitalization did not differ between the two groups; however, the total cost favored thoracoscopic pleurodesis because of the greater recurrence rate and need for repeat procedures in the chest tube drainage group over 5 years.[71]

SUMMARY

For nearly all pulmonary procedures, data exist on QoL and cost-effectiveness and much of it favors emerging, less invasive technologies. However, although some studies use rigorous methodology to assess this aspect of care, many do not. Further, there are few prospective comparative effectiveness trials that incorporate QoL and cost data collection at the beginning of the trial for analysis and interpretation at the end. Instruments to assess QoL and cost-effectiveness already exist such that there is no need to reinvent them in the IP space. With shrinking health care resources, regulatory agencies and hospitals will demand that new technology not only produce the expected clinical benefits but that they do so at a reasonable cost compared with existing technologies and improve QoL. These soft end points were historically viewed as an afterthought by clinical investigators. In the future, that will no longer be the case when evaluating new technology in the pulmonary space.

REFERENCES

1. Colt H, Harrell J II. Therapeutic rigid bronchoscopy allows level of care changes in patients with acute respiratory failure from central airways obstruction. Chest 1997;112:202–6.
2. Annema J, van Meerbeeck J, Rintoul R, et al. Mediastinoscopy vs endosonography for mediastinal nodal staging of lung cancer a randomized trial. J Am Med Assoc 2010;304(20):2245–52.
3. Castro M, Rubin A, Laviolette M, et al. Effectiveness and safety of bronchial thermoplasty in the

treatment of severe asthma: a multicenter, randomized, double-blind, sham controlled clinical trial. Am J Respir Crit Care Med 2010;181:116–24.

4. Jantz M, Silvestri G. Effects of interventional procedures on quality of life and pulmonary function. In: Beamis J, Mathur P, Mehta A, editors. Interventional pulmonary medicine. New York: Marcel Dekker; 2004. p. 609–38.

5. Montazeri A, Gillis C, McEwen J. Quality of life in patients with lung cancer: a review of the literature from 1970 to 1995. Chest 1998;113:467–81.

6. Montazeri A, Milroy R, Hole D, et al. Quality of life in lung cancer patients: as an important prognostic factor. Lung Cancer 2001;31:233–40.

7. Montazeri A, Milroy R, Hole D, et al. How quality of life contribute to our understanding of cancer patients' experiences? Qual Life Res 2003;12: 157–66.

8. Gridelli C, Perrone F, Nelli F, et al. Quality of life in lung cancer patients. Ann Oncol 2001;12:S21–5.

9. Aaronson N, Ahmedzai S, Bergman B, et al. The European Organization for Research and Treatment of Cancer QLQ-C30: a quality-of-life instrument for use in international clinical trials in oncology. J Natl Cancer Inst 1993;85:365–76.

10. Bergman B, Aaronson N, Ahmedzai S, et al. The EORTC QLQ-LC13: a modular supplement to the EORTC Core Quality of Life Questionnaire (QLQ-C30) for use in lung cancer clinical trials. EORTC Study Group on Quality of Life. Eur J Cancer 1994;30A:635–42.

11. Weinstein M, Stasson W. Foundations of cost-effectiveness analysis for health and medical practice. N Engl J Med 1977;296:716–21.

12. Finlayson S, Birkmeyer J. Cost-effectiveness analysis in surgery. Surgery 1998;123(2):151–6.

13. Yarmus L, Pandian V, Gilbert C, et al. Safety and efficiency of interventional pulmonologists performing percutaneous tracheostomy. Respiration 2012; 84(2):123–7.

14. Ginsburg RJ, Vokes EE, Ruben A, editors. In: Devita VT, Hellman S, Rosenberg SA, editors. Cancer: principles and practice of oncology. Philadelphia: Lippincott-Raven; 1997. p. 858–911.

15. Stanopoulos I, Beamis J, Martinez F, et al. Laser bronchoscopy in respiratory failure from malignant airway obstruction. Crit Care Med 1993;21:386–91.

16. Oviatt P, Stather D, Michaud G. Exercise capacity, lung function, and quality of life after interventional bronchoscopy. J Thorac Oncol 2011;6(1):38–42.

17. Osoba D, Rodrigues G, Myles J, et al. Interpreting the significance of changes in health-related quality of life scores. J Clin Oncol 1998;16:139–44.

18. Amjadi K, Vodue N, Cruysberghs Y, et al. Impact of interventional bronchoscopy on quality of life in malignant airway obstruction. Respiration 2008;76(4): 421–8.

19. Mallick I, Sharma S, Behera D. Endobronchial brachytherapy for symptom palliation in non-small cell lung cancer–Analysis of symptom response, endoscopic improvement and quality of life. Lung Cancer 2007;55:313–8.

20. Cardona A, Reveiz L, Ospina E, et al. Palliative endobronchial brachytherapy for non-small cell lung cancer. Cochrane Database Syst Rev 2008;(2):CD004284.

21. Garwood S, Judson M, Silvestri G, et al. Endobronchial ultrasound for the diagnosis of sarcoidosis. Chest 2007;132(4):1529–30.

22. Gomez M, Silvestri G. Endobronchial ultrasound for the diagnosis and staging of lung cancer. Proc Am Thorac Soc 2009;15(2):180–6.

23. Vincent B, El-Bayoumi E, Hoffman B, et al. Real-time endobronchial ultrasound-guided transbronchial lymph node aspiration. Ann Thorac Surg 2008;85(1):224–30.

24. Silvestri G. The mounting evidence for endobronchial ultrasound. Chest 2009;136(2):327–8.

25. Herth F, Eberhardt R, Krasnik M, et al. Endobronchial ultrasound-guided transbronchial needle aspiration of lymph nodes in the radiologically and positron emission tomography-normal mediastinum in patients with lung cancer. Chest 2008;133(4):887–91.

26. Herth F, Krasnik M, Vilmann P. EBUS-TBNA for the diagnosis and staging of lung cancer. Endoscopy 2006;38(Suppl 1):S101–5.

27. Herth F, Eberhardt R. Actual role of endobronchial ultrasound (EBUS). Eur Radiol 2007;17(7):1806–12.

28. Herth F, Ernst A, Eberhardt R, et al. Endobronchial ultrasound-guided transbronchial needle aspiration of lymph nodes in the radiologically normal mediastinum. Eur Respir J 2006;28(5):910–4.

29. Varela-Lema L, Fernandez-Villar A, Ruano-Ravina A. Effectiveness and safety of endobronchial ultrasound-transbronchial needle aspiration: a systematic review. Eur Respir J 2009;33:1156–64.

30. Sharples L, Jackson C, Wheaton E, et al. Clinical effectiveness and cost-effectiveness of endobronchial and endoscopic ultrasound relative to surgical staging in potentially resectable lung cancer: results from the ASTER randomised controlled trial. Health Technol Assess 2012;16(18):1–51.

31. Steinfort D, Liew D, Conron M, et al. Cost-benefit of minimally invasive staging of non–small cell lung cancer: a decision tree sensitivity analysis. J Thorac Oncol 2010;5(10):1564–70.

32. Detterbeck F, Jantz M, Wallace M, et al. Invasive mediastinal staging of lung cancer: ACCP evidence-based clinical practice guidelines (2nd edition). Chest 2007;132:202S–20S.

33. Gu P, Zhao Y, Jiang L, et al. Endobronchial ultrasound-guided transbronchial needle aspiration for staging of lung cancer: a systematic review and meta analysis. Eur J Cancer 2009;45:1389–96.

34. Ernst A, Anantham D, Eberhardt R, et al. Diagnosis of mediastinal adenopathy-real-time endobronchial ultrasound guided needle aspiration versus mediastinoscopy. J Thorac Oncol 2008;3:577–82.

35. Krasnik M, Vilmann P, Herth F. EUS-FNA and EBUS-TBNA; the pulmonologist's and surgeon's perspective. Endoscopy 2006;38(Suppl 1):S105–9.

36. Silvestri G, Gould M, Margolis M, et al. Noninvasive staging of non-small cell lung cancer: ACCP evidence-based clinical practice guidelines (2nd edition). Chest 2007;132:178S–201S.

37. Pieterman R, van Putten J, Meuzelaar J, et al. Preoperative staging of non-small-cell lung cancer with positron-emission tomography. N Engl J Med 2000;343:254–61.

38. Medford A, Agrawal S, Free C, et al. A performance and theoretical cost analysis of endobronchial ultrasound-guided transbronchial needle aspiration in a UK tertiary respiratory centre. QJM 2009;102:859–64.

39. Kunst P, Ralph E, Felix HJ. Combined EBUS real time TBNA and conventional TBNA are the most cost-effective means of lymph node staging. J Bronchology Interv Pulmonol 2008;15:17–20.

40. Harewood G, Pascual J, Raimondo M, et al. Economic analysis of combined endoscopic and endobronchial ultrasound in the evaluation of patients with suspected non-small cell lung cancer. Lung Cancer 2010;67:366–71.

41. Pastis N, Simkovich S, Silvestri G. Understanding the economic impact of introducing a new procedure: calculating downstream revenue of endobronchial ultrasound with transbronchial needle aspiration as a model. Chest 2012;141(2):506–12.

42. Aberle D, Adams A, Berg C, et al. Reduced lung-cancer mortality with low-dose computed tomography screening. N Engl J Med 2011;365:395–409.

43. Gould M, Fletcher J, Iannettoni M, et al. Evaluation of patients with pulmonary nodules: when is it lung cancer?: ACCP evidence-based clinical practice guidelines (2nd edition). Chest 2007;132:108S–30S.

44. Rivera M, Mehta A. Initial diagnosis of lung cancer: ACCP evidence-based clinical practice guidelines (2nd edition). Chest 2007;132:131S–48S.

45. Larscheid R, Thorpe P, Scott W. Percutaneous transthoracic needle aspiration biopsy: a comprehensive review of its current role in the diagnosis and treatment of lung tumors. Chest 1998;114:704–9.

46. Wiener R, Schwartz L, Woloshin S, et al. Population-based risk for complications after transthoracic needle lung biopsy of a pulmonary nodule: an analysis of discharge records. Ann Intern Med 2011;155:137–45.

47. Wang J, Nietert P, Silvestri G. Meta-analysis of guided bronchoscopy for the evaluation of the pulmonary nodule. Chest 2011;142(2):385–93.

48. Cox G, Thomson N, Rubin A, et al. Asthma control during the year after bronchial thermoplasty. N Engl J Med 2007;356:1327–37.

49. Pavord I, Cox G, Thomson N, et al. Safety and efficacy of bronchial thermoplasty in symptomatic, severe asthma. Am J Respir Crit Care Med 2007;176:1185–91.

50. Eisner M, Ackerson L, Chi F, et al. Health-related quality of life and future health care utilization for asthma. Ann Allergy Asthma Immunol 2002;89:46–55.

51. Fishman A, Martinez F, Naunheim K, et al. National Emphysema Treatment Trial Research Group: a randomized trial comparing lung-volume-reduction surgery with medical therapy for severe emphysema. N Engl J Med 2003;348:2059–73.

52. Gasparini S, Zuccatosta L, Bonifazi M, et al. Bronchoscopic treatment of emphysema. Respiration 2012;84:250–63.

53. Varela G, Jimenez M, Novoa N, et al. Estimating hospital costs attributable to prolonged air leak in pulmonary lobectomy. Eur J Cardiothorac Surg 2005;27:329–33.

54. Springmeyer S, Bollinger C, Waddell T, et al. Treatment of heterogenous emphysema using the Spiration IBV valves. Thorac Surg Clin 2009;19:247–53.

55. Gillespie C, Sterman D, Cerfolio R, et al. Endobronchial valve treatment for prolonged air leaks of the lung: a case series. Ann Thorac Surg 2011;91:270–3.

56. Higgins K, Punthakee X. Meta-analysis comparison of open versus percutaneous tracheostomy. Laryngoscope 2007;117:447–54.

57. Antonelli M, Michetti V, Di Palma A, et al. Percutaneous translaryngeal versus surgical tracheostomy: a randomized trial with 1-yr double blind follow-up. Crit Care Med 2005;33:1015–20.

58. Hommerich C, Rodel R, Frank L, et al. Long-term results after surgical tracheotomy and percutaneous dilational tracheostomy. A comparative retrospective analysis. Anaesthesist 2002;51(1):23–7.

59. Barba C, Angood P, Kauder D, et al. Bronchoscopic guidance makes percutaneous tracheostomy a safe, cost-effective, and easy to teach procedure. Surgery 1995;118(5):879–83.

60. Cobean R, Beals M, Moss C. Percutaneous dilational tracheostomy: a safe, cost-effective bedside procedure. Arch Surg 1996;131:265–71.

61. Bacchetta M, Girardi L, Southard E, et al. Comparison of open versus bedside percutaneous dilational tracheostomy in the cardiothoracic surgical patient: outcomes and financial analysis. Ann Thorac Surg 2005;79:1879–85.

62. Mirski M, Pandian V, Bhatti N, et al. Safety, efficacy, and cost-effectiveness of a multidisciplinary

percutaneous tracheostomy program. Crit Care Med 2012;40:1827–34.

63. Massick D, Yao S, Powell D, et al. Bedside tracheostomy in the intensive care unit: a prospective randomized trial comparing open surgical tracheostomy with endoscopically guided percutaneous dilatational tracheotomy. Laryngoscope 2001;111: 494–500.

64. Grover A, Robbins J, Bendick P, et al. Open versus percutaneous dilatational tracheostomy: efficacy and cost analysis. Am Surg 2001;67:297–302.

65. Chee A, Tremblay A. The use of tunneled pleural catheters in the treatment of pleural effusions. Curr Opin Pulm Med 2011;17:237–41.

66. Tremblay A, Michaud G. Single-center experience with 250 tunnelled pleural catheter insertions for malignant pleural effusions. Chest 2006;129:362–8.

67. Van Meter M, McKee K, Kohlwes J. Efficacy and safety of tunneled pleural catheters in adults with malignant pleural effusions: a systematic review. J Gen Intern Med 2010;26(1):70–6.

68. Davies H, Mishra E, Kahan B, et al. Effect of an indwelling pleural catheter vs. chest tube and talc pleurodesis for relieving dyspnea in patients with malignant pleural effusion: the TIME2 randomized controlled trial. JAMA 2012;307(22): 2383–9.

69. Olden A, Holloway R. Treatment of malignant pleural effusion: PleurX catheter or talc pleurodesis? A cost-effectiveness analysis. J Palliat Med 2010;13(1):59–65.

70. Puri V, Pyrdeck T, Crabtree T, et al. Treatment of malignant pleural effusion: a cost effectiveness analysis. Ann Thorac Surg 2012;94:374–80.

71. Tschopp J, Boutin C, Astoul P, et al. Talcage by medical thoracoscopy for primary spontaneous pneumothorax is more cost effective than drainage: a randomised study. Eur Respir J 2002;20:1003–9.

Advances and Future Directions in Interventional Pulmonology

Ali I. Musani, MD, FCCP, FACP[a],
Stefano Gasparini, MD, FCCP[b],*

KEYWORDS

- Interventional pulmonology • Bronchoscopy • Endobronchial ultrasound
- Electromagnetic navigation

KEY POINTS

- The term "interventional pulmonology" supersedes the previously used term "thoracic endoscopy," a change that reflects the evolution of a specialty devoted performing highly sophisticated and technologically advanced procedures in the lungs and chest.
- Continuing advances in technology promise to further expand IP's diagnostic and therapeutic frontiers.
- Standardized educational programs to train and test IP physicians will be essential to maintain a high standard of practice in the field.

INTRODUCTION

In the past few decades, new technologies have transformed the way we practice medicine, in general, and minimally invasive medicine and surgery, in particular. Great advances have been made in in the field of interventional pulmonology (IP), especially in the area of bronchoscopy. In fact, we have come so far and have become so dependent on these new modalities that we can't fathom providing patient care without them.

Currently, diagnostic indications for bronchoscopy include tissue sampling of pulmonary lymph nodes and nodules, evaluation of diffuse lung diseases and infectious processes, assessment of benign tracheobronchial stenosis, and management of ventilated patients in the intensive care unit. As a therapeutic modality, bronchoscopy can be used to recanalize airways with debulking instruments; place stents; remove foreign bodies; control hemoptysis; and treat early-stage bronchial cancer, emphysema, and asthma.

Some newer bronchoscopic techniques have already become part and parcel of clinical practice, whereas others are still considered to be research tools. These technological innovations, coupled with proper training and technique, will continue to shape an exciting future for IP, health care providers, and patients.

IMAGE ACQUISITION

New image-acquisition systems have revolutionized bronchoscopy. In addition to providing high-definition images and superior optical magnification, they now provide views of places that were once impossible to see with bronchoscopy: the distal tracheobronchial tree and structures outside of the bronchial walls.

Disclosures: Stefano Gasparini has no conflicts of interest to report. Ali I. Musani has served/is serving as a consultant, or has received/is receiving grants or honoraria from Olympus USA, Boston Scientific, Intuitive Surgical, CareFusion, Boehringer Laboratories, Covidien, Super Dimension, Veran, Spiration, and Allegro.
^a Division of Interventional Pulmonology, Department of Pulmonary and Critical Care Medicine, National Jewish Health, 1400 Jackson Street, J 225, Denver, CO 80206, USA; ^b SOD Pneumologia, Department of Immunoallergic and Respiratory Diseases, Azienda Ospedaliero-Universitaria "Ospedali Riuniti," Via Conca 71, Ancona 60020, Italy
* Corresponding author.
E-mail address: s.gasparini@fastnet.it

The quality of bronchoscopic images has greatly improved in recent years. We have advanced from the old fiberoptic bronchoscope with optical fibers to the video bronchoscope, which carries a video chip at its tip. New high-resolution bronchoscopes provide an outstanding level of image clarity and detail. In the near future, high-resolution scopes will be the practice standard for bronchoscopy, and the small, black spots that we used to see in bronchoscopic images (which result from breakage of flexible optical fibers) will be just a memory (**Fig. 1**).

Many bronchoscopists dream of being able to obtain an "optical biopsy," a histologic image acquired directly through the bronchoscope. This dream is about to come true with the development of optical coherence tomography (OCT) and confocal fluorescence microscopy (CFM), novel technologies that image tissues at different levels of the tracheobronchial tree with microscopic resolution. These modalities show promise for detecting preneoplastic lesions and early lung cancers[1–3] and for inspecting basement membrane integrity to differentiate carcinoma in situ from microinvasive carcinoma.[4] They may prove useful for diagnosing infiltrative, diffuse lung diseases and peripheral pulmonary lesions,[5] and for evaluating alveolar compliance and dynamics during mechanical ventilation.[6] In addition, OCT and CFM may help us to better understand the pathophysiology of lung diseases and to monitor the effects of therapy.[7] Already, these modalities have offered insights into the remodeling of airways and vascular structures in obstructive lung diseases[8–10] and the dynamics of muco-ciliary transport.[11] However, the application of these modalities has not been standardized. Robust data in the form of prospective, randomized controlled studies are lacking.[7] In the coming years, we hope to see the development of OCT and CFM technologies that will make 3-dimensional imaging of airways structures[6] possible, as well as large-scale clinical studies to validate the use of these tools in the diagnostic algorithms of different diseases.

Thanks to technological advances that have miniaturized optical fibers and video chips, ultrathin bronchoscopes are able to travel deeper into the tracheobronchial tree. These instruments have a diameter of 2.2 to 3.6 mm and allow exploration of 9th-order to 10th-order subsegmental bronchi. Ultrathin bronchoscopes have been used to diagnose peripheral pulmonary lesions, with or without the use of guidance systems (eg, virtual bronchoscopy, fluoroscopy, computed tomography [CT] fluoroscopy).[12–17] The sensitivity of ultrathin bronchoscopes for diagnosing peripheral pulmonary lesions ranges from 60% to 81%. Even though randomized trials comparing them with conventional bronchoscopes have not been done, it seems that ultrathin bronchoscopes are more sensitive for diagnosing lesions smaller than 2 cm in diameter.[18]

In addition to providing better images of the interior of the tracheobronchial tree, bronchoscopes are now able to show structures that surround the airways by incorporating endobronchial ultrasound (EBUS) (**Fig. 2**). As one of the most significant developments in IP in recent years, EBUS has revolutionized lung cancer staging. Radial EBUS probes make it possible to measure the depth of tumor invasion into the airway wall and to visualize mediastinal vascular structures and lymph nodes adjacent to the airways.[19] Thin ultrasound radial probes can be passed into peripheral airways to locate and identify peripheral lesions.[20–22] This technique has proven very useful in the diagnosis of peripheral lung nodules, where it has a sensitivity of 70% to 80%.[18] Further improvements in

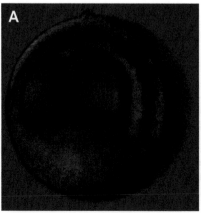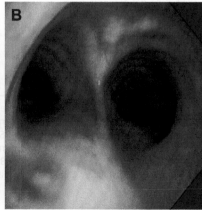

Fig. 1. Improving image quality in bronchoscopy. (*A*) Image obtained with an old fiberoptic bronchoscope. Black spots are seen where optical fibers have broken. (*B*) Image obtained with a new, high-definition bronchoscope.

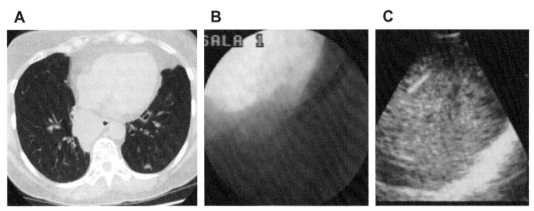

Fig. 2. (*A*) Right lower lobe consolidation adjacent to the esophagus on a CT scan. (*B*) Needle aspiration of the lesion using an EBUS scope inserted through the esophagus. (*C*) Ultrasonographic image of the lesion and the needle.

ultrasound technology have given us the linear ultrasound bronchoscope, which is equipped with a linear ultrasound transducer at its tip. This instrument facilitates transbronchial needle aspiration of lesions and lymph nodes under real-time guidance, thus reducing the risk of inadvertent blood vessel puncture. Hundreds of studies have demonstrated the safety and efficacy of EBUS-guided transbronchial needle aspiration (EBUS-TBNA), which is the new gold standard for mediastinal staging of lung cancer.[23–27]

Another fascinating technology that facilitates bronchoscopic sampling of peripheral pulmonary lesions is the electromagnetic navigation (EMN) system. An electromagnetic board placed underneath the supine patient generates a magnetic field around the patient's chest. This magnetic field pinpoints the position of a sensor probe that is inserted through the working channel of the bronchoscope while it is in the airway. The probe's position is projected on a 3-dimensional CT reconstruction that allows the operator to see the location of the probe and its spatial relationship to the target lesion. When the probe reaches the lesion, it is removed and sampling instruments can then be introduced to biopsy the lesion.

The sensitivity of transbronchial biopsy using EMN to diagnose peripheral pulmonary lesions ranges from 62% to 74%. The diagnostic yield of EMN bronchoscopy is significantly better than that of traditional fluoroscopy-guided transbronchial biopsy for nodules smaller than 2 cm in diameter.[18] Several studies have established the diagnostic utility of EMN bronchoscopy, and its use is rapidly expanding.[28–31] Emerging indications for EMN bronchoscopy are seen in the field of lung cancer treatment. Here, EMN bronchoscopy can place fiducial markers in and around pulmonary nodules for stereotactic radiosurgery.[32] It can

"tattoo" pulmonary nodules for localization before video-assisted thoracic surgery[33] and position brachytherapy probes.[34] Studies are now under way to explore how EMN bronchoscopy could be used to ablate peripheral lung cancers using modalities such as radiofrequency and microwaves.

SAMPLING INSTRUMENTS

Although innovations in image acquisition and navigation systems have revolutionized IP, improvements in sampling instruments remain disappointing. The advent of targeted chemotherapy for non–small cell lung cancer has made it increasingly important to obtain larger tumor biopsy samples for mutation analysis and molecular studies.[35] This has become a crucial issue. Several studies have shown that samples obtained by EBUS-TBNA are adequate for molecular testing for EGFR, kRas, and EML4-ALK,[36,37] but the sensitivity and specificity of this technique have yet to be clearly defined. Novel needle-forceps have been developed for both traditional TBNA and EBUS-TBNA,[38,39] but validation studies remain to be done. There is also a growing interest in the use of cryobiopsy tools, which seem to provide larger specimens from central and peripheral lesions.[40,41] However, use of cryobiopsy tools requires intubating the patient with an endotracheal tube or rigid bronchoscope. Further studies are needed to confirm the safety and diagnostic utility of these tools. Concerns about uncontrollable bleeding still loom large for cryobiopsy.

THERAPEUTIC PROCEDURES

Currently, bronchoscopic recanalization techniques, such as mechanical debulking, laser resection, electrocautery, photodynamic therapy, cryotherapy, brachytherapy, and stent placement are used routinely in the treatment of neoplastic and benign airway obstructions. New therapeutic modalities include bronchoscopic lung volume reduction (BLVR) for chronic obstructive pulmonary disease (COPD) and bronchial thermoplasty (BT) for asthma. Novel treatments for COPD that are being tested in animals and humans include unidirectional valves, coils, polymeric sealant, steam, and airway bypass. It is hoped that these new methods will be as effective as surgical lung volume reduction, but with reduced morbidity and mortality and better cost-effectiveness. Because these techniques are minimally invasive, they have the potential to help a very large population of patients suffering from severe COPD who are not candidates for surgical intervention.[42,43] For patients with severe, persistent asthma, BT has been shown in randomized controlled clinical trials to improve the quality of life and reduced need for health care use. This technique aims to reduce excessive smooth muscle in airways of patients with asthma by thermal ablation.[44,45]

TRAINING AND COMPETENCY

The future of IP will be determined not only by technological innovations, but also by how well pulmonologists, IP specialists, and surgeons are trained to use these new technologies. In fact, new modalities will benefit patients only if operators understand their proper clinical applications and are competent in all aspects of performing the new procedures. The practice of IP requires a deep understanding of chest anatomy and physiology, as well as manual dexterity, technical proficiency, and clinical judgment. In addition, IP practitioners must be knowledgeable about related fields, such as oncology, thoracic surgery, radiology, pathology, and intensive care medicine. To adapt to a rapidly changing array of IP techniques, a new emphasis on acquisition of skills and competencies is essential. The training method of "see one, do one, teach one" should be considered obsolete in the twenty-first century.

Standardized training with low-fidelity manikins and high-fidelity simulators, followed by supervised, hands-on training, will ensure that operators are properly trained in new techniques. The World Association for Bronchology and Interventional Pulmonology and regional organizations, such as the American Association of Bronchology and Interventional Pulmonology and the European Association for Bronchology and Interventional Pulmonology, should be expected to take the lead in developing and implementing rigorous IP curricula. Competency testing is also likely to become more common. In the United States, for example, in-service examination for IP fellows started in 2012 as a prelude to board certification in IP in 2013. Guidelines for competence in individual procedures performed by non-IP physicians and surgeons should also be established.

SUMMARY

The term "interventional pulmonology" supersedes the previously used term "thoracic endoscopy," a change that reflects the evolution of a specialty devoted to performing highly sophisticated and technologically advanced procedures in the lungs and chest. Continuing advances in technology promise to further expand IP's diagnostic and therapeutic frontiers. However, standardized educational programs to train and test IP physicians will be essential to maintain a high standard of practice in the field.

REFERENCES

1. Sutedja TG. New techniques for early detection of lung cancer. Eur Respir J 2003;39(Suppl):57s–66s.
2. Tsuboi M, Hayashi A, Ikeda N, et al. Optical coherence tomography in the diagnosis of bronchial lesions. Lung Cancer 2005;49:387–94.
3. McWilliams A, MacAulay C, Gazdar AF, et al. Innovative molecular and imaging approaches for the detection of lung cancer and its precursor lesions. Oncogene 2002;45:6949–59.
4. Haas AR, Vachani A, Sterman DH. Advances in diagnostic bronchoscopy. Am J Respir Crit Care Med 2010;182:589–97.
5. Thiberville L, Salaun M, Lachkar S, et al. Human in-vivo fluorescence microimaging of the alveolar ducts and sacs during bronchoscopy. Eur Respir J 2009;33:974–85.
6. Gartner M, Cimalla P, Meissner S, et al. Three-dimensional simultaneous optical coherence tomography and confocal fluorescence microscopy for investigation of lung tissue. J Biomed Opt 2012;17:071310.
7. Pare PD, Nagano T, Coxson HO. Airway imaging in diseases: gimmick or useful tool? J Appl Physiol 2012;113(4):636–46.
8. Yich CY, Von der Thusen JH, Bel EJ, et al. In vivo imaging of the airway wall in asthma: fibered confocal fluorescence microscopy in relation to histology and lung function. Respir Res 2011;12:85.
9. Thiberville L, Moreno-Swirc S, Vercauteren T, et al. In vivo imaging of the bronchial wall microstructure using fibered confocal fluorescence microscopy. Am J Respir Crit Care Med 2007;175:22–31.
10. Ohtani K, Lee AM, Lam S. Frontiers in bronchoscopic imaging. Respirology 2012;17:261–9.

11. Oldenburg AL, Chhetri RK, Hill DB, et al. Monitoring airway mucus flow and ciliary activity with optical coherence tomography. Biomed Opt Express 2012;3:1978–92.

12. Rooney CP, Wolf K, McLennan G. Ultrathin bronchoscopy as an adjunct to standard bronchoscopy in the diagnosis of peripheral lung lesions. Respiration 2002;69:63–8.

13. Fumihiro A, Yoshihiko M, Tomomichi M, et al. Transbronchial diagnosis of peripheral small lesion using an ultrathin bronchoscope with virtual bronchoscopy navigation. J Bronchol 2002;9:101–11.

14. Shinagawa N, Yamazaki K, Onodera Y, et al. CT-guided transbronchial biopsy using an ultrathin bronchoscope with a virtual bronchoscopic navigation. Chest 2004;125:1138–43.

15. Yamamoto S, Ueno K, Imamura F, et al. Usefulness of ultrathin bronchoscopy in diagnosis of lung cancer. Lung Cancer 2004;46:43–8.

16. Shinagawa N, Yamazaki K, Onodera Y, et al. Factors related to diagnostic sensitivity using an ultrathin bronchoscope under CT guidance. Chest 2007; 131:549–53.

17. Oki M, Saka H, Kitagawa S, et al. Novel thin bronchoscope with a 1.7 mm working channel for peripheral pulmonary lesions. Eur Respir J 2008; 32:465–71.

18. Gasparini S. Diagnostic management of solitary pulmonary nodules. Eur Respir Mon 2010;48:90–108.

19. Yasufuku K, Nakajima T, Chiyo M, et al. Endobronchial ultrasonography: current status and future directions. J Thorac Oncol 2007;10:970–9.

20. Herth FJ, Ernst A, Becker HD. Endobronchial ultrasound-guided transbronchial lung biopsy in solitary pulmonary nodules and peripheral lesions. Eur Respir J 2002;20:972–4.

21. Kurimoto N, Miyazawa T, Okimasa S, et al. Endobronchial ultrasonography using a guide sheath increases the ability to diagnose peripheral pulmonary lesions endoscopically. Chest 2004;126:959–65.

22. Kikuchi E, Yamazaki K, Sukoh N, et al. Endobronchial ultrasonography with guide-sheath for peripheral pulmonary lesions. Eur Respir J 2004;24:533–7.

23. Yasufuku K, Chiyo M, Sekine Y, et al. Real-time endobronchial ultrasound guided transbronchial needle aspiration of mediastinal and hilar lymph nodes. Chest 2004;11:293–6.

24. Rintoul RC, Skwarski KM, Murchison JT, et al. Endobronchial and endoscopic ultrasound guided transbronchial needle aspiration for mediastinal staging. Eur Respir J 2005;25:416–21.

25. Herth FJ, Eberhardt R, Vilmann P, et al. Real-time endobronchial ultrasound guided transbronchial needle aspiration for sampling mediastinal lymph nodes. Thorax 2006;61:795–8.

26. Herth FJ, Rabe KF, Gasparini S, et al. Transbronchial and transoesophageal (ultrasound guided) needle aspiration for the analysis of mediastinal lesions. Eur Respir J 2006;28:1264–75.

27. Annema JT, van Meerbeeck JP, Rintoul RC, et al. Mediastinoscopy vs endosonography for mediastinal nodal staging of lung cancer: a randomized trial. JAMA 2010;304:2245–52.

28. Becker HD, Herth FJ, Erns A, et al. Bronchoscopic biopsy of peripheral lung lesions under electromagnetic guidance. A pilot study. J Bronchol 2005;12: 9–13.

29. Schwarz Y, Greif J, Becker HD, et al. Real-time electromagnetic navigation bronchoscopy to peripheral lung lesions using overload CT images. Chest 2006;129:968–94.

30. Gildea TR, Mazzone PJ, Karanak D, et al. Electromagnetic navigation diagnostic bronchoscopy. A prospective study. Am J Respir Crit Care Med 2006;174:982–9.

31. Makris D, Scherpereel A, Leroy S, et al. Electromagnetic navigation diagnostic bronchoscopy for small peripheral lung lesions. Eur Respir J 2007;29: 1187–92.

32. Anantham D, Feller-Kopman D, Shanmugham LN, et al. Electromagnetic navigation bronchoscopy-guided fiducial placement of robotic stereotactic radiosurgery of lung tumors. A feasibility study. Chest 2007;132:930–5.

33. Krimsky W, Sethi S, Cicenia JC. Tattooing of pulmonary nodules for localization prior to VATS. Chest 2007;132:425a.

34. Becker HD. Electromagnetic navigation for peripheral lung lesions and mediastinal lymph nodes. Eur Respir Mon 2010;48:256–71.

35. Bulman W, Saqi A, Powell CA. Acquisition and processing of endobronchial ultrasound-guided transbronchial needle aspiration specimens in the era of targeted lung cancer chemotherapy. Am J Respir Crit Care Med 2012;185:606–11.

36. Nakajima T, Yasufuku K, Nakagawara A, et al. Multigene mutation analysis of metastatic lymph nodes in non-small cell lung cancer diagnosed by endobronchial ultrasound-guided transbronchial needle aspiration. Chest 2011;140:1319–24.

37. Sakairi Y, Nakajima T, Yasufuku K, et al. EML4-ALK fusion gene assessment using metastatic lymph node samples obtained by endobronchial ultrasound-guided transbronchial needle aspiration. Clin Cancer Res 2010;16:4938–45.

38. Gasparini S, Zuccatosta L, Sediari M, et al. Pilot feasibility study of transbronchial needle forceps: a new tool for obtaining histology samples from mediastinal subcarinal lymph nodes. J Bronchology Interv Pulmonol 2009;16:183–7.

39. Herth FJ, Schuler H, Gompelmann D, et al. Endobronchial ultrasound-guided lymph node biopsy with transbronchial needle forceps: a pilot study. Eur Respir J 2012;39:373–7.

40. Hetzel J, Eberhardt R, Herth FJ, et al. Cryobiopsy increases the diagnostic yield of endobronchial biopsy: a multicentre trial. Eur Respir J 2012;39(3): 685–90.

41. Babiak A, Hetzel J, Krishna G, et al. Transbronchial cryobiopsy: a new tool for lung biopsies. Respiration 2009;78:203–8.

42. Shah PL, Hopkinson NS. Bronchoscopic lung volume reduction for emphysema: where next? Eur Respir J 2012;39:1287–9.

43. Gasparini S, Zuccatosta L, Bonifazi M, et al. Bronchoscopic treatment of emphysema: state of the art. Respiration 2012;84(3):250–63.

44. Castro M, Rubin AS, Laviolette M, et al. Effectiveness and safety of bronchial thermoplasty in the treatment of severe asthma: a multicenter, randomized, double-blind, sham-controlled clinical trial. Am J Respir Crit Care Med 2010;181:116–24.

45. Wahidi MM, Kraft M. Bronchial thermoplasty for severe asthma. Am J Respir Crit Care Med 2012;185:709–14.

Index

Clin Chest Med 34 (2013) 611–617
http://dx.doi.org/10.1016/S0272-5231(13)00098-1
0272-5231/13/$ – see front matter © 2013 Elsevier Inc. All rights reserved.

Moving?

Make sure your subscription moves with you!

To notify us of your new address, find your **Clinics Account Number** (located on your mailing label above your name), and contact customer service at:

Email: journalscustomerservice-usa@elsevier.com

800-654-2452 (subscribers in the U.S. & Canada)
314-447-8871 (subscribers outside of the U.S. & Canada)

Fax number: 314-447-8029

Elsevier Health Sciences Division
Subscription Customer Service
3251 Riverport Lane
Maryland Heights, MO 63043

Printed and bound by CPI Group (UK) Ltd, Croydon, CR0 4YY

03/10/2024

01040378-0008